Birth Emergency Skills Training

Manual for Out-of-Hospital Midwives

Bonnie Urquhart Gruenberg

CNM, CRNP, RNC, EMT-P

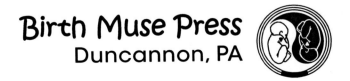

Birth Muse Press
Duncannon, PA

Library of Congress Control Number: 2008903656
ISBN 13: 978-0-9790020-0-7 ▶ ISBN 10: 0-9790020-0-1
10 9 8 7 6 5 4 3

Birth Emergency Skills Training (BEST) is also offered through Aviva Institute (http://avivainstitute.org) as an online CME course for midwives with CEUs from the Midwifery Education Accreditation Council.

Also by Bonnie U. Gruenberg
The Midwife's Journal
Essentials of Prehospital Maternity Care
Hoofprints in the Sand

What people are saying about the BEST *textbook and course*

"Bonnie Gruenberg has brought together her unique talents as an artist, an experienced Emergency Medical Technician, a Certified Nurse-Midwife and mother in a well organized, concise and creative approach to the identification, evaluation and management of care of the emergent complications of childbearing. Although the treatise is directed to midwives practicing in the out of hospital setting, it is a reference that will help all providers caring for childbearing women regardless of setting as well as all student midwives, nurses and physicians. It provides an excellent review for exams on this subject."

Kitty Ernst, President, American College of Nurse-Midwives
Mary Breckinridge Chair of Midwifery, Frontier School of Midwifery and
Family Nursing, Hyden, KY

"Birth Emergency Skills Training is written as a manual for out-of-hospital midwives but would be very useful in managing any birth emergency in a low resource setting. The book presents evidence-based, standard-of-care management of pregnancy and birth emergencies. Its systematic and clear approach to critical thinking, assessment, diagnosis and intervention when emergencies arise would provide an excellent resource for all midwifery students, as well as clinicians working in low resource settings."

Katherine Camacho Carr, PhD, ARNP, CNM, FACNM
Professor & Assistant Dean for Graduate Studies, Seattle University

"This book is phenomenal. It offers a concise discussion of obstetrical problems that will serve both out of hospital and in hospital birth practitioners as a resource in problem solving and providing safe care in the event of an obstetrical problem or emergency. The ethical responsibility of the midwife in recognizing abnormal and responding to it is importantly illustrated."

Kathleen Nishida, RN, CNM, MSN
Tokyo, Japan

"Wow, this is comprehensive!! As an NRP instructor for 20 years, I liked the section on neonatal resuscitation. . . .Great photos and resources! Loved the text and the course."

Andrea Dixon, CNM
Carmel, IN

"Love the orientation. . .how the novice vs. expert process information, communication in emergencies and acknowledging intuition as a valid skill. It really adds to a more complete picture of midwifery practice. "

Helena Wu, LM, CPM, Herbalist
Vermont

"The course was fantastic. The book is a gem! The content was thorough, easy to understand and easy to follow."

Kelly B. Brown, DC, CSCS, Colorado
Author of The Perinatal Fitness Instructor Manual

"An important book for all involved with out of hospital births."

Sally Gambill, CNM, MS, RN
Harrisburg, PA

"Amazing! The most comprehensive course ever designed. The book is full of concise, critical thinking and step-by-step cognitive actions for everyone from the beginner to the expert. The illustrations add so much to the written content."

Phyllis Block, CNM, MN
Harrisburg, PA

"The BEST Course modules were interactive and engaging, and got right to the core content very quickly. The accompanying text is a rich resource. . .before, during and after the weekend course. Bonnie Gruenberg's expertise as both a midwife with extensive out of hospital and in-hospital experience combined with her background as a paramedic gives her insight into the world of both normal and complicated births."

Kim Perry, CPM, APN, CNM, MSN
Osco, IL

"BEST will save lives. It one of the most complete and together continuing education programs I have ever seen."

Daphne Singingtree, CPM, Oregon
Academic Director, Aviva Institute
Author of Birthsong Midwifery Workbook, The Emergency Guide to Obstetric Complications, *and* Training Midwives: A Guide for Preceptors

"The information is comprehensive, thorough, and evidence-based. It gives midwives and other birth attendants a powerful guide for practice in emergency situations while continuing to emphasize that birth is normal. In addition, the manual covers conditions that are not very common but necessitate immediate recognition and treatment. Ms. Gruenberg has written an outstanding manual with clear and concise interventions while complimenting the information with relevant images, tables, and photos."

Abigail Eaves, CNM, MSN
Full Circle Midwifery Birth & Health Center

To Alex

for his loving support
through every "midwife crisis."

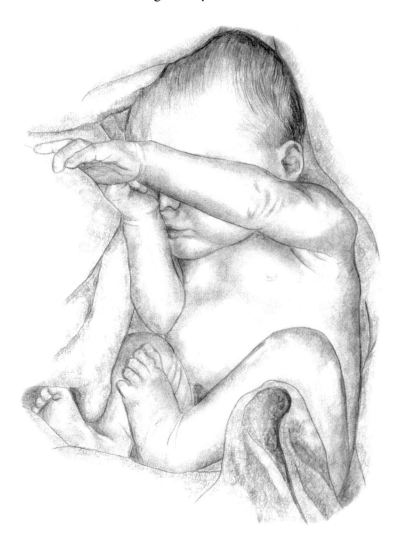

Contents

List of Tables

Reviewers

Phyllis Block, CNM, MN, holds a Master of Nursing degree from the University of Florida. She is currently in a private practice in Harrisburg, PA.

Kelly B. Brown, DC, CSCS, is a licensed Chiropractor, a Certified Strength and Conditioning Specialist, a Certified Acupuncturist, a Certified Mixed Martial Arts/Self Defense Instructor and Childbirth Educator. She is the author of *The Perinatal Fitness Instructor Manual* (Eagletree Press, 2008).

Andrea Dixon, CNM, has practiced midwifery in many settings, including home births in the California mountains; the Redding Birth Center in California, the Hospital at St. Thomas, U.S. Virgin Islands; Missouri; and most recently at both a private home-birth practice and a busy inner-city hospital practice in Indianapolis. She has served as secretary of the Missouri Midwives Association and treasurer of ACNM Chapter IV and is currently a Board Member of the Indiana Midwives Association.

Jennifer D. Hanson, LM, CPM, BA, MAT, received her undergraduate degree in psychology from Vassar College and her graduate degree in English and education from Tufts University. She taught English for 12 years and has a small home-birth practice in rural Vermont.

Kathleen Nishida, CNM, MSN, serves on the faculty of St. Luke's College of Nursing, Tokyo, Japan. She practiced clinical midwifery for eight years in a federally funded clinic in Harrisburg, PA, and is licensed to practice nursing and midwifery in the state of Pennsylvania. She is a graduate of the Yale University School of Nursing nurse-midwifery program.

Kim Perry, CPM, APN, CNM, MSN, holds a Master's degree in Nursing from the State University of New York at Stony Brook and is licensed to practice midwifery and nursing in both Illinois and Iowa. She co-founded Illinois Families for Midwifery and is a Board member of the Coalition for Illinois Midwifery. She has taught in Associate Degree Nursing programs and has precepted CPM apprentices.

Tamy Roloff LM, CPM, CD, is a graduate of Seattle Midwifery School and a Licensed Midwife with a home birth practice, as well as a La Leche League Leader, a DONA certified doula, a Certified Childbirth Educator with ICEA, and a DONA Approved Doula Trainer.

Erin Ryan, CPM, LM, has a BA in Interdisciplinary Studies from University of California-Berkeley. She attended the National Midwifery Institute and has served on its Advisory Board. She has a home birth practice in Central Vermont.

Daphne Singingtree, CPM, is the Academic Director for Aviva Institute. She is the author of the *Birthsong Midwifery Workbook*, *The Emergency Guide to Obstetric Complications*, and *Training Midwives: A Guide for Preceptors*. She has served on the Board of Directors for the Midwifery Education and Accreditation Council (MEAC) and held the post of the Education Chair for the Midwives Alliance of North America (MANA), and was the Vice President for the Oregon State Board of Direct Entry Midwifery.

Helena Wu, LM, CPM, Herbalist, is the Northeast Coordinator for Birth Arts International and a council member of the Northeast Herbal Association. She has been a La Leche League leader and childbirth educator. She studied herbal medicine at the Northeast School of Botanical Medicine. She attends home births in southwestern Vermont.

Acknowledgments

A writer's ideas emerge and evolve in response to interaction with others. I acknowledge and sincerely thank the following people, each of whom uniquely shaped this project and made it immeasurably better than it would have been otherwise.

My husband, Alex Gruenberg, has survived this latest endeavor intact, remaining understanding and helpful while I divided my waking hours between writing and midwifery. I am blessed by his unconditional love and support.

For years, my friend John Bryans, Editor-in-Chief and Publisher at Information Today/Plexus has generously helped me with manuscripts, contracts, and networking. I am always grateful for his contributions to my projects and his willingness to carve time out of his busy life to assist and advise me.

I wish to thank Daphne Singingtree and Sharon Evans of Aviva Institute, who expended tremendous time and energy to launch the BEST course, obtain CME credit, and tweak the text. I also wish to thank the faculty at Avivia that test-drove the pilot BEST course and served as reviewers for both the text and the educational program.

Special thanks to Kitty Ernst, Katherine Camacho Carr, Phyllis Block, Kathleen Nishada, Sally Gambill and Abigail Eaves, who generously agreed to read the manuscript in its early electronic form and offered valuable feedback and suggestions.

Thanks to Skip and Becky Mudge for all of their assistance. As president of Cockpit Management Resources, a company devoted to improving flight safety, Skip gave me insights into the dynamics of communication in an emergency.

The photograph of the author was taken by Tabetha Fenton, mother of Aiden and Conor. I got to know both boys as fetuses, and Aiden was born into my loving hands.

I am also grateful to the people who appear in images throughout this book, including Daelyn Gruenberg's beautiful twins Anaia and Assada, Stacie Shchouchkoff and her son Ben, Jennifer Young and her children, Amelia Lyons and her parents, Estela Difranco Field and family, Kia Fuller and her unborn twins, Peggy Boyd, Sally Gambill, Heather Mozdy, Kim Hinkson, Peter Levinson, MD, and the EMS professionals of the Plymouth, CT, Volunteer Ambulance Corps. Laura Luddy, ultrasonographer, provided many of the sonographic images used in this text. Ayodeji Bakare, MD, and Pierre Eugene, MD, generously granted me use of their surgical images.

My deepest appreciation goes to the women whom I am privileged to serve. Each day, I gain fresh insights through working with these remarkable women while following the lead of the wisdom that is within them.

Introduction

Out-of-hospital midwives have a generally low-risk clientele and may seldom encounter emergencies. Even in a low-risk practice, however, serious problems can present unexpectedly, requiring decisive intervention until the problem is solved or the client is under a physician's care. Emergencies can arise unexpectedly during an otherwise normal labor, and the outcome may depend on the midwife's expertise.

Outside the office, a midwife may face an emergency nearly anywhere at nearly any time. Some midwives greatly increase their likelihood of dealing with emergencies by helping victims of natural disasters, such as Hurricane Katrina or the 2004 Indonesian tsunami; by responding to large-scale crises of human origin, such as a sudden influx of war refugees; or simply by volunteering to attend births in developing countries or other underserved areas. Midwives working in uncontrolled environments must deal with situations that fall outside their normal scope of practice.

When emergencies occur, the lives of mothers and babies may depend on a midwife's ability to recognize and manage the situation while upholding the current standard of care. *Birth Emergency Skills Training: Manual for Out-of-Hospital Midwives* (BEST) prepares out-of-hospital midwives and other professionals to manage obstetrical emergencies with greater confidence and proficiency.

Each client, each emergency, and each provider is unique, and no book can offer exhaustive advice on every contingency. BEST therefore teaches a systematic approach to obstetrical emergencies that will serve as a framework for intervention. Like any other framework, it contains spaces to be filled in as circumstances dictate. BEST accentuates treatment modalities accepted as the standard of care in many North American settings, those interventions least likely to cause harm to mother or child, and those supported by evidence. This structure will help the out-of-hospital midwife to rapidly diagnose problems, then determine whether to treat, co-manage, or refer.

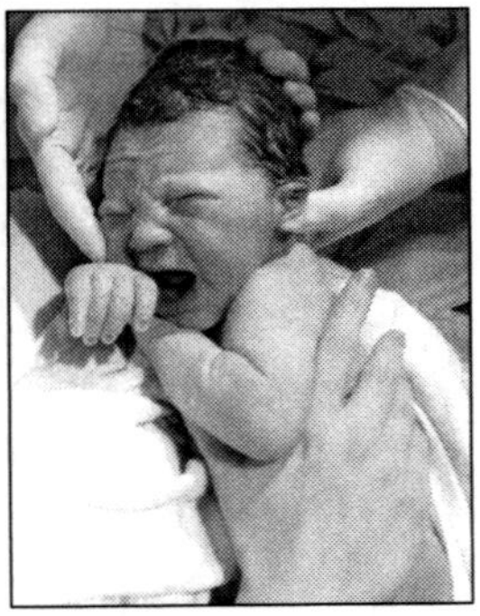

Figure 1. Midwifery is a way of life. Every midwife wants the best possible outcome for women and their babies.

Successful hands-on management of potentially life-threatening emergencies begins in the attendant's thoughts and intuition. Acquiring an expert's perceptions and habits of thinking takes time and experience, however. BEST promotes the timely acquisition of expertise by uniting "book smarts" with "street smarts" and emphasizing development of critical thinking skills.

BEST is designed primarily for the trained health care professional who attends, or may attend, out-of-hospital deliveries, but has reasonable access to emergency services and a hospital capable of surgery. Practitioners in low-resource areas can put BEST to good use by adapting its recommendations to local conditions. BEST is also offered through Aviva Institute (http://avivainstitute.org) as an online CME course for midwives and other birth professionals.

Birth Emergency Skills Training describes assessments and treatments that may not be appropriate for every practice. In many cases, an emergency-room physician or obstetrician should ideally make the initial assessment. In an actual emergency, other providers may perform many of the procedures described as performed by the midwife, such as ultrasound or laboratory tests. Procedures such as intubation and umbilical cord cannulation are described in the text because they are part of the standard of care, though many midwives do not perform them. Although electronic fetal monitoring is used infrequently outside the hospital, it is included because all midwives listen to heart tones. The provider must quickly identify abnormal fetal heart patterns, whether the heart rate is auscultated or graphed, and graphs are better suited to presentation in a book.

Where skills have been included that exceed the midwife's usual scope of practice, the purpose is to broaden knowledge. As always, midwives should function within their local standard of care, protocols, and level of training.

Because BEST course participants are midwives, and most midwives are women, the default pronouns will be feminine when referring to the provider. To avoid confusion, any references to the fetus or infant will use masculine pronouns.

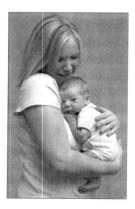

Figure 2. Every mother and baby deserves your BEST.

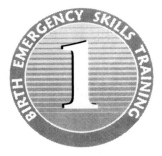

Critical Thinking in Emergencies

A Systematic Approach

OBJECTIVES

By the end of this chapter, you should be able to

▶ Explain how the beginning provider processes information differently from the expert.

▶ Describe a situation when home birth would decrease risk to mother and child, and one when it would elevate risk.

▶ List three antepartal conditions that would necessitate co-management with a physician or transfer of care.

When pregnancy and labor are normal, it is easy to be lulled into assuming that they will remain normal. This assumption is true most of the time and so comforting that it is easy to discount the early signs that a problem is evolving.

Knowledge of pathophysiology is important, but in order to recognize a problem from its earliest presentation, the provider must become a detective who pieces together a story, a pattern, or a diagnosis. Textbooks usually give the most typical presentations of disease processes along with their statistical likelihood. Statistics derived from populations, however, apply to populations, not to individuals. As often as not, when the women and babies in your care develop unexpected problems, their symptoms will not match the textbook, and signs will present with various degrees of ambiguity. Clinical judgment depends on the context of a particular situation.

Although life-threatening problems are uncommon, they carry the highest stakes. When evaluating a problem, always ask yourself, "What is the worst this could be?" and rule out life-threatening conditions first.

Clinical information is processed differently at each level of expertise. Patricia Benner (2001) observed that the novice takes a rule-based approach to a problem, moving through an internal checklist with little awareness of context. The advanced beginner is more sensitive to the nuances of the situation at hand and understands underlying principles, but needs help setting priorities. A beginner able to pass a test on clinical manifestations of disease may struggle to translate this knowledge into practical application. Beginners often feel overwhelmed and suffer incapacitating anxiety when faced with something new. Much of the beginner's discriminatory thought occurs at the conscious level. Beginners are also susceptible to tunnel vision that causes the task to become more important than the client.

The competent provider feels a sense of mastery based on experience and plans goals purposefully. She has a strong grasp of clinical know-how and understands the "why" of what she does.

The proficient provider develops a holistic perspective. She recognizes immediately when situations deviate from normal and can grasp the long-term implications of problems.

The expert provider transcends rules and trusts the intuition that arises from deep internal wellsprings of knowledge. The expert is flexible, inventing workable solutions through leaps of creativity and improvisation. Expert midwives attune to clinical data that are difficult to quantify or describe; they fit new situations into old frameworks to formulate innovative solutions. Intuition pieces the clues together into a whole that is flashed intact into the mind, not reached in an obvious linear progression. The expert does not often think consciously about her reasons for choosing actions, and she is usually unaware that she is processing knowledge at all. The salient facts just stand out. Often the flash of clinical insight may occur before quantifiable cues are identified.

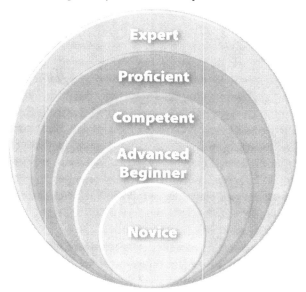

The human brain has long- and short-term memory, and these two are as different as the RAM and the hard drive in a computer. Short-term memory, like RAM, is the processing space where you manage current information. It can hold about seven separate ideas (or clusters of ideas) at once. Additional input begins to erase information already stored. Long-term memory is stored on the biological equivalent of your "hard drive," often for a lifetime. Like a file on a computer, this data is more easily retrieved if it is stored systematically. Beginning practitioners, like computers, rely on data, rules, and checklists.

Unlike computers, however, people filter information through emotions, intuition, and empathy. Reason is usually held as the standard for gathering knowledge, and emotion is often dismissed as a hindrance to reason. In truth, when providers emotionally attune to a situation, meaningful aspects stand out as important and guide their interpretations. The practicing midwife relies not just on data, but also on analyzing the situation, consulting sources, evaluating possible outcomes, taking intuitive leaps, weighing emotional responses, making tactile discriminations, considering contexts, acting on a disposition toward what is good and right, and forging empathetic connections (Benner, 2001).

DIAGNOSIS THROUGH CRITICAL THINKING

To treat appropriately, the provider must first arrive at the correct diagnosis. Accurate diagnosis involves fitting data into a coherent picture. Even seemingly incontrovertible data must be examined critically. Critical thinking generates creative ways to formulate solutions and raises questions about the strength of evidence for a given conclusion. In emergencies, this processing must be done at high speed, but not at the expense of accuracy.

Like a landscape artist, the provider must fill in the general outlines first and then refine the details. When a problem arises, the provider must consider all possible causes and develop a list of likely explanations without overcommitting to any of them. The provider must consider all relevant information before forming a working diagnosis, or she may miss data that would lead to a more accurate impression. The provider systematically analyzes and incorporates new data and notes whether it supports one hypothesis or eliminates others.

Periodically reflect on the big picture: Have all possibilities have been explored? Does the clinical impression still make sense? Are the conclusions based on evidence? Take care not to inflate the importance of clues that support your clinical impression—or ignore those that do not support it.

Remain alert to clues that contradict your working diagnosis and listen when your instincts reveal that something is not adding up. Even experienced providers can make mistakes or have blind spots. Unease about your own diagnosis often means that key elements are missing or that your original impression was inaccurate.

Do not discount intuition. Intuition is an unconscious recognition of patterns based on experience, assembled by the subconscious mind, that seems to burst into consciousness effortlessly or from an external source. Because the processing is unconscious, the experienced provider who relies on intuition often has trouble pointing to specific data that support her conviction though it tends to be highly accurate.

Intuition is a powerful tool for diagnosis and treatment, but it can be confused with training, habit, worry, preference, prejudice, or snap judgment.

Sometimes, however, intuition can be hard to distinguish from other unconscious currents. Sometimes the vague unease that a midwife feels about a variation in a client's labor, for example, is simply a focus for free-floating anxiety about her present surroundings (perhaps a remote farmhouse in a blizzard), the politics in her office, or the antics of her own teenager. Sometimes it is based on an old memory of some unpleasant event.

Midwives are geared philosophically toward nonintervention in the natural processes of pregnancy and birth. A normal labor treated as normal, for example, tends to stay normal, and every intervention in the normal process is likely to engender more interventions. Midwives often prevent obstetrical emergencies by employing gentle, natural ways of correcting a problem in the early stages.

Even while attending a normal low-risk woman in labor, the midwife should always consider the possibility of a developing problem. Through every labor, the midwife should continually ask four questions over and over in the back of her mind:

- ▶ How is the mother?
- ▶ How is the baby?
- ▶ How is the labor?
- ▶ Is everything still normal?

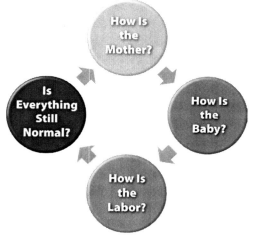

Problems can be classified using the following triage system:

- ▶ **Priority 1, "Code Red"—Critical Emergencies**
  Very uncommon, but life-threatening and requiring immediate action
- ▶ **Priority 2, "Code Orange"—Urgent Problems**
  Fairly uncommon, but potentially life-threatening, and must treated as soon as possible.
- ▶ **Priority 3, "Code Yellow"—Concerning Problems**
  Occur frequently, with the potential of developing into more significant problems, but the client is currently stable.
- ▶ **Priority 4, "Code Green"—Normal**
  Most low-risk clients will remain normal throughout labor and birth.

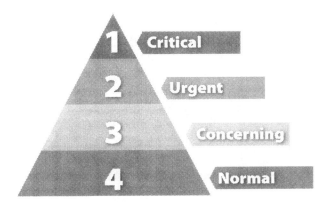

MANAGE, CO-MANAGE, OR REFER?

Only 1% of American women give birth outside a hospital (Vedam, Goff, & Nolan-Marnin, 2007). The majority of these births take place in the home or in freestanding birth centers, attended by midwives—CPMs, CNMs, CMs, or other midwives—and sometimes by physicians. With mounting evidence of the safety of out-of-hospital birth for low-risk women, it is likely that more women will choose this option. Popular birth-reality television programs and the ubiquity of Internet access in America hold the potential for disseminating the ideals of home birth and promoting its cause.

The expertise and equipment available in the hospital does not increase safety in childbirth for low-risk women. The safety advantage of a hospital birth is the availability of technological interventions if complications develop—decreasing the rate of complications for the high-risk mother and her infant. The safety advantage of home or birth-center birth is noninterventionist watchful waiting and respecting the natural process of birthing—decreasing the risk of complications for the *low-risk* mother and her infant.

High-risk mothers and babies have better outcomes in a hospital setting. Low-risk mothers and babies benefit from letting the body labor as nature intended. If complications do occur, the trained midwife can respond to the level of care available at most rural community hospitals, and stands ready to initiate transport to a tertiary-care facility. Most complications can be avoided through judicious screening of prenatal clients and transferring care for clients that are at increased risk.

Johnson and Daviss (2005) reported that low-risk North American women who had planned deliveries at home with a CPM showed a degree of safety similar to that of low-risk hospital births. A retrospective study of 49,371 deliveries in the state of Washington demonstrated that the rate of neonatal mortality was identical for licensed midwives, physicians, and nurse-midwives, and for home and hospital births (Janssen, Holt, & Myers, 1994). Columbia University researchers (Murphy & Fullerton, 1998) found home births safe for mother and infant if the birth attendant is qualified and there is provision for hospital transport in case of emergency. Schlenzka's study in California (1999) compared planned home and hospital births with similar low-risk characteristics and found the home-birth cohort to have comparable or better outcomes.

The designation of low risk is crucial to these safety statistics. The literature has demonstrated that when home births are planned with a well-screened 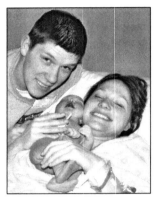 population of women and attended by professionally trained midwives carrying emergency equipment, optimum safety conditions are met and the best outcomes are achieved. "Normal" childbirth can be defined as a healthy uncomplicated term singleton pregnancy in a cephalic position with spontaneous onset and progress of labor. The inclusion of higher-risk conditions such as breech presentations, twins, and post-dates deliveries escalates mortality and morbidity well above that of women giving birth in hospitals. A study in Australia demonstrated that although home birth is safe for low-risk women, high-risk births (post-term birth, twin pregnancy, and breech presentation) and lack of response to fetal distress produced increased incidence of avoidable maternal and infant death—a finding shown previously by other research (Bastian, Keirse, & Lancaster, 1998).

Figure 3. Giving birth can be a transcendent, empowering experience.

The World Health Organization acknowledges home birth with hospital backup as a safe option for low-risk women, and contends that the best birth attendant for low-risk women is the midwife who lives in the community alongside them (Fullerton, Navarro, & Young, 2007). The position statement of the American College of Obstetricians and Gynecologists (ACOG, 2008) asserts that birth should occur in the hospital, not in the home. The American College of Nurse Midwives and the American Public Health Association support out-of-hospital maternity care services and affirm that low-risk women can safely deliver outside the hospital when attended by trained professionals.

Birth is a natural process. But when births occur in a setting inappropriate for the medical circumstances or attended by unskilled personnel, mothers and babies die. In India, where untrained attendants assist most births in the home, every 100 births bring an average of 2 maternal and 6 neonatal deaths. For each maternal death, many more women suffer from acute maternal morbidities. Of the surviving children, almost 6% will die before their fifth birthdays. Babies of deceased mothers are 3–10 times more likely to die within their first 2 years (Mathai, 2005). Clearly, home birth is a safe option only when a trained, skilled provider, and adequate supplies are available and when the risk level is appropriate for out-of-hospital delivery.

Risk can no more predict outcome than the chance of precipitation in a regional weather forecast can predict rainfall in your front yard. Risk assessment calculates whether certain outcomes are more likely or less, but in most cases cannot foretell the outcome for a particular woman.

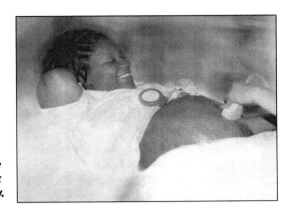

Figure 4. The hospital is the safest setting for the high-risk woman to deliver her baby.

The experience level of the midwife, the local standard of care, distance from a hospital capable of handling obstetrical complications, and the prevailing legal climate of the midwife's state of practice may factor into her decision to "risk out" a client or co-manage with another provider. The key to improving the safety to the women and babies in your care is to select clients wisely, remain vigilant for deviations from normal, establish whether the increased risk is temporary or correctable, refer judiciously, and stand ready to manage emergencies. On average, 10–20% of potential home birth clients are "risked out" for antepartum complications such as hypertension, twins, placenta previa, preterm labor, or fetal growth restriction. Of the remaining women, 5–10% require intrapartum referrals (most commonly for failure to progress), 1% postpartum referrals, and 1% neonatal referrals (Vedam, et al., 2007).

The following is a list of some situations that may require consultation, co-management, or referral.

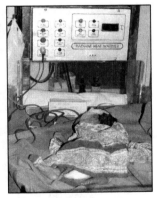

Figure 5. Infant, born at 28 weeks' gestation, in neonatal intensive care in a small community hospital in Jaipur, India. Premature infants born in small villages far from a hospital often do not survive.

Lifestyle and History

- ▶ Adverse socioeconomic conditions
- ▶ Age less than 17 years or over 40 years
- ▶ Late presentation to care
- ▶ Uncertain expected date of delivery
- ▶ Complications with prior pregnancy that are likely to recur (preeclampsia, gestational diabetes)
- ▶ Grand multipara (five or more previous births)

- ▶ Body mass index under 19 or over 35
- ▶ Poor nutrition
- ▶ Rubella during first trimester of pregnancy
- ▶ Significant use of drugs, alcohol, or other toxic substances
- ▶ History of infant over 4,500 g
- ▶ History of one late miscarriage (after 14 weeks) or preterm birth
- ▶ History of low-birth-weight infant
- ▶ Prior infant with abnormalities (cardiac anomalies, Ellis-van Creveld dwarfism, etc.)
- ▶ Less than 12 months from last delivery to present due date
- ▶ Previous hemorrhage
- ▶ History of essential or pregnancy-induced hypertension
- ▶ Repeated elective abortions
- ▶ History of long, difficult labor
- ▶ High risk for genetic disorders, hereditary disease, or anomalies
- ▶ History of cervical cerclage or incompetent cervix
- ▶ History of repeated spontaneous abortions
- ▶ History of late miscarriage or preterm birth
- ▶ History of low birth weight infant
- ▶ History of significant medical illness
- ▶ Previous myomectomy, hysterotomy, or cesarean section
- ▶ Previous neonatal mortality or stillbirth

Maternal Disease

- ▶ Blood disorders such as thrombophilias, thrombocytopenia, or certain anemias
- ▶ Cancer
- ▶ Cardiac disease
- ▶ Chronic lung disease requiring medications or treatments, such as asthma
- ▶ Deep-vein thrombosis—current or history of DVT
- ▶ Diabetes
- ▶ Hepatitis
- ▶ HIV
- ▶ Positive PPD
- ▶ Hypertension
- ▶ Cervical surgery—LEEP, cone biopsy, etc
- ▶ Lupus or other autoimmune disorder
- ▶ Marfan syndrome or other connective-tissue disease
- ▶ Renal disease or recurrent pyelonephritis
- ▶ Seizure disorder
- ▶ Syphilis
- ▶ Thyroid disorder
- ▶ Significant psychological problems

- ▶ Known uterine malformations or fibroids

Obstetrical Conditions

- ▶ Inappropriate uterine growth
- ▶ Medical conditions arising during pregnancy
- ▶ Placenta previa
- ▶ Polyhydramnios or oligohydramnios

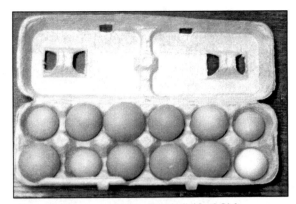

Figure 6. Every woman is a unique individual. Risk assessment calculates whether certain outcomes are more likely or less, but in most cases cannot foretell the outcome for a particular woman.

- ▶ Repeated or significant vaginal bleeding
- ▶ Persistent anemia, hemoglobinopathies, or blood dyscrasia
- ▶ Abnormal antepartum fetal assessment
- ▶ Thromboembolism or thrombophlebitis
- ▶ Hemorrhage unresponsive to therapy
- ▶ Chorioamnionitis
- ▶ Fetal anomaly
- ▶ Intrauterine fetal death
- ▶ Intrauterine growth restriction
- ▶ Incompetent cervix
- ▶ Malpresentation at term
- ▶ Maternal antibodies with potential for fetohemolytic disease
- ▶ Maternal trauma
- ▶ Multifetal gestation

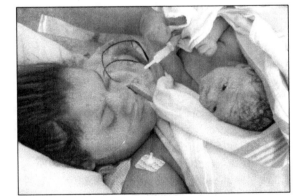

Figure 7. Social, physical, and historical risk factors can greatly increase the likelihood of complications.

- ▶ Oligohydramnios
- ▶ Preeclampsia or uncontrolled essential hypertension
- ▶ Preterm labor before 36–37 weeks
- ▶ Preterm rupture of the membranes
- ▶ Postdates by more than 2 weeks
- ▶ Suspected fetal macrosomia

- ▶ Active genital herpes
- ▶ Uterine malformations (unicornuate, bicornuate, et al.)
- ▶ Suspected or diagnosed fetal anomaly
- ▶ Acute systemic infection such as varicella, parvovirus, toxoplasmosis, cytomegalovirus, or rubella

Intrapartum Complications
- ▶ Temperature over 38°C at two or more readings
- ▶ Abnormal fetal heart-rate patterns unresponsive to therapy
- ▶ Meconium-stained fluid
- ▶ Prolapsed cord
- ▶ Bleeding more than bloody show
- ▶ Shock
- ▶ Prolonged stage of labor
- ▶ Prolonged rupture of membranes
- ▶ Retained placenta
- ▶ Primipara with unengaged fetal head in active labor

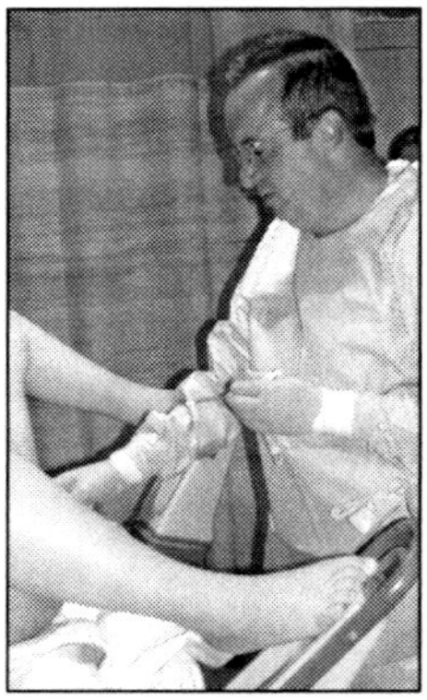

Figure 8. Intrapartum complications often require the expertise of an obstetrician and the technology of a hospital.

Postpartum Complications
- ▶ Third- or 4th-degree laceration
- ▶ Hemorrhage
- ▶ Wound infection
- ▶ Uterine infection
- ▶ Fever
- ▶ Thrombophlebitis
- ▶ Serious postpartum depression or psychosis

Newborn
- ▶ Apgar score lower than 7 at 10 min
- ▶ Seizures
- ▶ Significant congenital anomaly
- ▶ Respiratory distress
- ▶ Persistent temperature instability
- ▶ Less than 34 weeks gestational age
- ▶ Weight less than 2,500 g
- ▶ Two-vessel cord
- ▶ Cephalohematoma; other significant trauma or injury
- ▶ Congenital anomalies
- ▶ Heart rate irregular, below 100, or above 170
- ▶ Poor suck, hypotonia, abnormal cry
- ▶ Abnormal respiratory rate or pattern

- ▶ Persistent central cyanosis, pallor
- ▶ Persistent grunting and retractions
- ▶ Failure to pass urine or meconium within 24 hr of birth
- ▶ Suspected pathological jaundice
- ▶ Vomiting or diarrhea
- ▶ Infection of umbilical stump site
- ▶ Excessive weight loss, inadequate weight gain

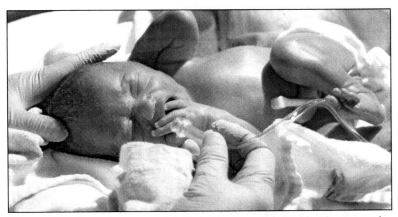

Figure 9. This 32-week premature infant requires care at a hospital with a neonatal intensive-care unit.

Risk level is not destiny; women with these indicators may enjoy an un-eventful pregnancy and birth, and low-risk women may suddenly develop problems. The midwife must remain vigilant and continually reassess as complications appear and resolve.

DECISION-MAKING CONFLICTS

Practicing midwives around the world differ in legal scope of practice and the risk level they are willing or obliged to assume. Certain higher-risk clients can become points of contention as clinicians debate whether frank breech, single previous cesarean section with prior vaginal birth, and vertex full-term twins should be considered normal variations of parturition or hazardous complications. In North America, obstetricians are increasingly unlikely to allow a vaginal birth for these clients, even in a closely monitored hospital setting.

Cesarean delivery for breech or prior cesarean decreases the risk of death or injury to the fetus in the current pregnancy. Cesarean delivery also *increases* the risk of complications for the mother in the current pregnancy *and* elevates risk in future pregnancies for both the mother and all future infants (Gabbe, 2007).

Both ACOG and SOGC recommend that the woman with one previous transverse lower uterine segment cesarean section should be offered a VBAC if there are no contraindications, but both assert that she should deliver in a hospital where immediate cesarean section is available (Martel & MacKinnon, 2005; ACOG, 2004). According to these agencies, contraindications to VBAC include previous uterine rupture, previous high vertical classical or T-shaped incision, extensive fundal uterine surgery, three or more previous cesarean deliveries, two prior uterine scars and no vaginal deliveries, medical or obstetric complications that preclude vaginal delivery, and *inability to perform emergency cesarean delivery.*

Table 1. Conditions Requiring Immediate Transport

Maternal/Fetal

Cardiac arrest

Seizures

Persistent or worsening fetal distress

Thick meconium (if birth not imminent)

Cord prolapse

Maternal fever

Foul-smelling amniotic fluid

Maternal dyspnea

Labor with malpresentation incompatible with home delivery

Bleeding in labor greater than bloody show

Postpartum hemorrhage refractory to treatment

Persistent uterine atony

Shock

Persistently abnormal vital signs

Retained placenta or placental fragments

Inability to void

Chest pain, cardiac abnormalities

Uterine inversion

Laceration requiring medical attention

Newborn

Persistent newborn pallor or central cyanosis

Seizures

Abnormal cry in newborn

Significant birth injury

Significantly abnormal feeding, voiding, or stooling

Persistently abnormal vital signs

Significant congenital anomaly

Prematurity or weight less than 2,500 g

Pathological jaundice

Even the authorities disagree about appropriate management. The World Health Organization encourages vaginal delivery if the fetus is frank breech with a flexed head, the maternal pelvis is adequate for fetal size, and the woman has not undergone prior cesarean section for cephalopelvic disproportion, but maintains that every breech delivery should ideally occur in a hospital with surgical capability. ACOG recommends cesarean delivery for breech presentations, even for a multipara with prior easy deliveries.

Second Birth Attendant

Safety for mother and infant increases significantly when two skilled providers attend the birth. In some locales, protocols mandate that two attendants trained and certified in cardiopulmonary resuscitation (CPR) and neonatal resuscitation be present at every planned out-of-hospital delivery. Ideally, this second attendant is also a midwife, responsible for auscultating the fetal heart rate, monitoring maternal vital signs, assisting at resuscitations and other emergencies, and performing other tasks.

Accountability

The midwife's actions should serve the best interests of the mothers and babies in their care, enhance the reputation of the profession, and inspire public confidence. Midwives are accountable to women and their families, their profession, regulatory bodies, state and local statutes, and local health agencies to provide proficient, ethical care. Sometimes the unrealistically optimistic client will attempt to pressure the midwife into taking on an unacceptably high level of risk.

A client can choose to give birth at home even if her risk level is dangerously high, but the midwife is under no obligation to assume or continue care in these circumstances—and may place herself in legal and ethical jeopardy if she fails to refer. Because childbirth is not an illness, and infant and maternal injuries are relatively uncommon, Americans have come to expect good outcomes and seek to hold someone accountable when complications occur, often to the tune of multimillions of dollars. Obstetrical providers are susceptible to malpractice accusations, which can raise malpractice premiums prohibitively and may restrict future practice.

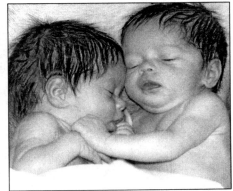

Figure 10. Mode of delivery for twins is a topic of controversy.

Documentation is crucial, and it is often the only incontrovertible evidence that a task was or was not performed. It should provide an accurate chronology of events that occurred while the client was in your care.

Communication in an Emergency

Your words and actions in a crisis situation will leave an indelible imprint. What you say and how you say it may remain with the client and her family for life. The midwife should ideally communicate sensitive information directly to the client in a private setting, without interruptions. Remember that people have different communication styles. When confronted with a crisis, some people focus on data, identifying and solving problems and forming a plan of action. Others process information emotionally and seek solutions that "feel" right. Speak at a slower speed and in a low, even tone. Sit at the client's level and make eye contact, giving nonverbal cues that communicate respect, concern, and empathy.

There is never a good time to give bad news. Critical information must be delivered immediately, regardless of the circumstances, but certain details and noncrucial decision-making can be deferred or discussed after the family has processed the initial emotional blow. Be honest and direct, but do not overwhelm the client with too much information. Provide support or helpful resources for later, as they process emotions at a deeper level. Provide hope, but not false optimism, or you will undermine your credibility and set them up for a harder fall later on. You can tailor your discussion to their knowledge gaps by asking open-ended questions, such as "What do you know about miscarriage?"

Use clear language and assess for understanding. The client in crisis quickly becomes numb and has difficulty processing information. She might not understand your explanation, and you may need to repeat the information in several different ways.

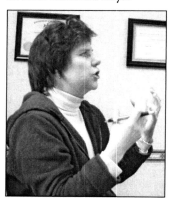

Figure 11. What you say in a crisis will impact the client for life.

Families involved in emergencies often go through all of the stages of grief. Initially they may have trouble believing that there is truly an emergency. They may feel guilty and assume they are somehow responsible or may seek to place blame. They may attempt to take control of the situation by bargaining or feel that they have somehow failed. Sometimes depression and harsh self-judgment set in. They may be angry and accusatory. They may feel cheated. Often they feel as if they were the only ones who have ever had to face this circumstance.

Sometimes the family will hold the provider responsible for the outcome or harbor unjustified resentment and hostility. Often this bitterness is redirected anger that they feel for themselves or family members, God, the universe, or Fate. It can be difficult when the angry client rejects the emotionally invested midwife who has given her best, and it can be difficult to remain kind and supportive in the face of such hostility.

Caring providers are emotionally invested in their clients, and it can be comforting for the client to know that the midwife shares her feeling of loss and frustration. Shared tears can be appropriate. In a crisis, however, emotional involvement must not obstruct rapid and decisive action.

BIBLIOGRAPHY

American College of Obstetricians and Gynecologists. (2008, February 6). *ACOG statement on home births*. Retrieved April 28, 2008, from http://www.acog.org/ from_home/publications/press_releases/nr02-06-08-2.cfm

American College of Obstetricians and Gynecologists. (2004a). *Vaginal birth after previous cesarean delivery practice guidelines* (Practice Bulletin 54). Washington, DC: Author.

Bastian, H., Keirse, M.J., & Lancaster, P.A.L. (1998). Perinatal death associated with planned home birth in Australia: Population based study. *British Medical Journal, 317* (7155), 384–388.

Benner, P. (2001). *From novice to expert: Excellence and power in clinical nursing practice.* Upper Saddle River, NJ: Prentice Hall.

Benner, P., Tanner, C, &. Chesla, C. (1998). *Expertise in nursing practice: Caring, clinical judgment and ethics.* New York: Springer Publishing Company.

Boyer, M. (2001). Root cause analysis in perinatal care: Health care professionals creating safer health care systems. *Journal of Perinatal & Neonatal Nursing, 15* (1), 40–54.

Declercq, E., & Stotland, N.E. *Home birth.* (2008). In B.D. Rose (Ed.), UpToDate. Wellesley, MA: UpToDate.

Draycott, T., Sibanda, T., Owen, L., Akande, V., Winter, C., Reading, S., et al. (2006). Does training in obstetric emergencies improve neonatal outcome? *Obstetrical & Gynecological Survey, 61* (6), 365–366.

Fullerton, J., Navarro, A., & Young, S. (2007). Outcomes of planned home births: An integrative review. *Journal of Midwifery and Women's Health 52* (4) 323–333.

Ganatra, B.R., & Hirve, S.S. (1995). Unsafe motherhood: The determinants of maternal mortality. *Journal of the Indian Medical Association, 93* (2): 34–35.

Janssen, P.A., Holt, V.L., & Myers, S.J. (1994). Licensed midwife-attended, out-of-hospital births in Washington State: Are they safe? *Birth, 21* (3):141–148.

Johnson, K.C., & Daviss, B-A. (2005). Outcomes of planned home births with certified professional midwives: Large prospective study in North America. *British Medical Journal, 330* (7505), 1416.

Mann, S., Marcus, R., & Sachs, B. (2006, January 1). Grand rounds: Lessons from the cockpit: How team training can reduce errors on L&D. *Contemporary OB/GYN.* Retrieved March 23, 2008, from http://www.modernmedicine.com/ modernmedicine/ Cover+Story/Grand-Rounds-Lessons-from-the-cockpit-How-team-tra/ArticleStandard/Article/detail/283481

Martel, M.J., & MacKinnon, C.J. (2005). Guidelines for vaginal birth after previous caesarean birth (SOGC Clinical Practice Guideline 155, electronic version). *Journal of Obstetrics and Gynaecology Canada, 27* (2), 164–174. Retrieved May 16, 2008, from http://www.sogc.org/ guidelines/public/155E-CPG-February2005.pdf

Mathai, M. (2005). Improving maternal & child survival in India. *Indian Journal of Medical Research, 121,* 624–627.

Murphy, P.A., & Fullerton, J. (1998). Outcomes of intended home births in nurse-midwifery practice: A prospective descriptive study. *Obstetrics & Gynecology, 92* (3), 461–470.

Reever, M., & Lyon, D. (2007). *Communication in crisis* (eMedicine, topic 3399). Retrieved December 22, 2007, from http://www.emedicine.com/ med/ topic 3399.htm

Rubeor, K. (2003). The role of risk management in maternal-child health. *Journal of Perinatal & Neonatal Nursing, 17* (2), 94–100.

Sackett, D.L., Straus, S.E., Richardson, W.S., Rosenberg, W., & Haynes, R.B. (2000). *Evidence-based medicine: How to practice and teach EBM* (2nd ed.). Edinburgh: Churchill Livingstone.

Schlenzka, P.F. (1999). Safety of alternative approaches to childbirth. Unpublished Dissertation, Stanford University, Palo Alto, CA.

Simpson, K. (1999). Shoulder dystocia: Nursing interventions and risk-management strategies. *American Journal of Maternal/Child Nursing, 24* (6), 305–311.

Snyder, L., & Leffler, C. (2005). Ethics manual: Fifth edition. *Annals of Internal Medicine, 142* (7), 560–582.

Stapleton, S.R. (1998). Team-building: Making collaborative practice work. *Journal of Nurse-Midwifery 43* (1), 12–18.

Vedam, S., Goff, M., & Nolan-Marnin, V. (2007). Closing the theory–practice gap: Intrapartum midwifery management of planned homebirths. *Journal of Midwifery and Women's Health, 52*(3), 291–300.

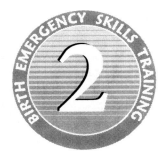

Recognizing Obstetrical Emergencies

OBJECTIVES

By the end of this chapter, you should be able to

▶ Discuss how pregnancy-related changes in cardiovascular function can be mistaken for pathology.

▶ Explain how to use OLDCART to assess pain in a pregnant woman.

▶ List three causes of airway obstruction and discuss how to manage them.

ANTEPARTUM PHYSIOLOGIC ALTERATIONS

Normal changes of pregnancy can mask or mimic pathology, and pathology can mask or mimic normal changes. Profound alterations of maternal anatomy, physiology, and psychology occur during pregnancy, especially with multifetal pregnancies. Most of the physical changes are progressive and relate to either hormonal or physical changes wrought by the developing fetus. Each organ transforms and recovers at its own rate, and some organs never return to their prepregnancy condition. With practice, the body becomes more efficient at maintaining pregnancy; firstborn children average lower birth weights than subsequent children, and even babies born after a first-trimester abortion are generally heavier than babies born to primigravidas.

Metabolism

The healthy woman who conceives with her body mass index in the optimal range will gain roughly 30 lb through the course of her pregnancy. Weight gain includes not only the fetus, but also increased uterine mass, amniotic fluid, placenta, breast glandular tissue, increased extravascular and extracellular fluid, enlarged maternal vital organs, and fat deposition.

Placental hormones affect maternal carbohydrate and lipid metabolism. The goal is to maintain a steady flow of glucose and amino acids to the fetus while supplying extra free fatty acids and glycerol as sources of maternal fuel.

Insulin-secreting pancreatic beta cells enlarge and escalate insulin production. Early in pregnancy there is an increased sensitivity to insulin, followed by progressive insulin resistance. Fasting glucose values are 10–20% lower during pregnancy because of decreased hepatic glucose production, increased storage of tissue glycogen, peripheral glucose utilization, and constant glucose consumption by the fetus (Petraglia & D'Antona, 2007). Transient maternal hyperglycemia, often noted following meals, is due to increasing insulin resistance, and transient hypoglycemia before meals and overnight is due to the unrelenting fetal requirements.

Maternal serum cholesterol increases by 50% in pregnancy, and serum triglyceride levels increase by 300%, to provide fuel to mother and fetus (Petraglia & D'Antona, 2007). Lipolysis increases, allowing the mother to burn free fatty acids, triglycerides, and ketone bodies for fuel and reserving more glucose and amino acids for fetal use.

Drug metabolism changes during pregnancy. The increase in body water may dilute medications in the bloodstream, and the decrease in plasma proteins reduces drug binding and may increase serum concentration. Some medications require higher doses to achieve therapeutic serum levels during pregnancy, creating the potential for toxicity after delivery. The gastrointestinal tract moves more slowly during pregnancy, potentially altering drug absorption. Renal filtration rates increase and accelerate excretion of some medications. The second-trimester drop in maternal blood pressure may increase the orthostatic hypotension associated with certain medications such as antipsychotics, tricyclic antidepressants, and antihypertensives.

Thermoregulatory Control

The fetus and placenta generate large amounts of heat through the process of metabolism. The maternal basal metabolic rate, and therefore heat production, also escalate during pregnancy. The pregnant woman disperses this heat through increased respiration and circulation, increased plasma volume, and by dilating blood vessels and moving heated blood to the skin. If heat is produced faster than it can be lost, for example during exercise in hot, humid conditions, the core temperature will increase. Minor temperature fluctuations bring no risk to the fetus, but sustained overheating can be damaging.

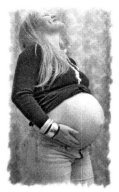

Figure 12. Uterine enlargement is one of the most obvious changes in pregnancy.

Reproductive System

Uterine enlargement is one of the most obvious changes in pregnancy. The nonpregnant uterus weighs about 100 g, but by the end of pregnancy it weighs about 1,200 g and occupies much of the abdominal cavity. Uterine enlargement is not due solely to the growing fetus and surrounding fluid; it also reflects a hormonally influenced increase in maternal muscle mass. Uterine walls thicken in early pregnancy, but thin to about 1.5 cm or less at term. By the end of pregnancy, the vascular system of the uterus contains one sixth of the mother's total blood volume.

From the second trimester on, the uterus begins contracting, presumably to tone the muscles for labor. Research suggests that pregnant women are aware of only 10–17% of these contractions. Runs of painful Braxton Hicks contractions can become false labor in the third trimester, but the contractions of progressing premature labor can be painless. It can be difficult to differentiate among Braxton Hicks contractions, false labor, and labor.

The uterus outgrows the confines of the pelvis at about 12 weeks' gestation and pushes the intestines out of place as it enlarges. It rotates to the right as it grows, displaced by the sigmoid colon on the left side of the abdomen. At term the uterus nearly reaches the liver and may displace the appendix as far as the right flank. The rising diaphragm, in turn, pushes the heart up and to the left, changing the cardiac silhouette seen in radiographs. As pregnancy advances, the uterus compresses the ureters at the pelvic brim, a situation that may allow urine to back up and distend the kidneys (hydronephrosis).

The abdominal wall supports the uterus and helps to keep its long axis upright in relation to the pelvic inlet. Repeated childbearing can slacken the abdominal wall, however, allowing the pregnant uterus to fall forward.

Throughout pregnancy, uterine blood flow increases to perfuse the growing placenta. The cervix and vagina may become so vascular and blood-engorged that they turn purplish or bluish. The cervix and uterus soften. A plug of thick mucus forms in the cervical opening to seal it against infection. The vagina produces greater amounts of thick, white, acidic discharge to discourage bacterial growth. Hormones are secreted by the corpus luteum and placenta that loosen pelvic connective tissue.

Breasts

Breasts tingle and become tender during the first 2 months of pregnancy. They enlarge and become nodular and vascular as ductal networks begin to prepare for lactation. Colostrum, the yellowish, high-protein, antibody-rich fluid that sustains the infant for the first days of breastfeeding, may leak from the breasts by the end of the first trimester.

Integumentary System

Mucous membranes become very vascular, swollen, and prone to capillary rupture. Slight bleeding may occur with tooth brushing, nose blowing, and sexual intercourse. The pregnant woman may develop a dark line on the midline of her abdomen (linea nigra), deeply pigmented nipples, and facial blotching (chloasma). Stretch marks may occur on abdomen and breast, and spider veins may appear because of the increased estrogen levels (Keltz-Pomeranz, 2007).

Cardiovascular System

The pregnant woman undergoes many hemodynamic changes to help the fetus grow optimally and as a buffer against hemorrhage at delivery. These changes are evident early in gestation, peak at the end of the second trimester, and then plateau until delivery. By the 28th week of pregnancy, the average increase in total body water is 8.5 liters. At term the placenta and uterus receive blood flow of about 600–800 ml/min. Uterine arteries dilate capaciously, while uterine arterioles increase their capacity threefold and spiral arteries supplying the placenta increase to 30 times their usual diameter (Foley, 2007). Heart rate and stroke volume increase, while systemic vascular resistance and mean arterial pressure decrease.

Extra blood is needed to perfuse the placenta and the increased vascularity of the reproductive organs, protect against orthostatic and supine hypotension, carry nutrients to the fetus, excrete waste products, dissipate excess body heat, and serve as a hemodynamic safeguard in preparation for blood loss during delivery. Blood volume increases by 45–50% over pre-pregnant levels, beginning as early as the fourth week of gestation, peaking at 28–34 weeks' gestation, then stabilizing until delivery (Gabbe, 2007).

The quantity of red blood cells begins to increase by the middle of the first trimester in response to the higher metabolic requirement for oxygen. By the end of gestation, the pregnant woman will have 20–30% more red blood cells (Gabbe, 2007). Women with inadequate iron intake may show a red blood cell increase of only 15–20%, highlighting the importance of dietary iron or supplementation (Foley, 2007).

Plasma volume increase outpaces the production of new red blood cells, creating a dilutional anemia that peaks at 24–28 weeks' gestation. This decrease in the proportion of red blood cells in the blood decreases blood viscosity that facilitates tissue perfusion and reduces cardiac workload. Mild physiological anemia is an indicator of good health in pregnancy, suggesting an expanding vascular volume. The lack of this hemodilution is associated with increased risk of stillbirth and growth restriction and may be an early warning sign of preeclampsia.

Volume expansion also has a dilutional effect on plasma proteins such as serum albumin, fibrinogen, and globulins. With a lower concentration of these proteins, body fluid has an increased tendency to "third space" from the intravascular compartment to the interstitial space, causing edema. About 50% of pregnant women will show evidence of edema (Foley, 2007). Trace edema is generally a good sign in otherwise normal pregnancies and is associated with optimal birth weights and improved neonatal survival, probably because it is an indicator of adequate volume expansion.

Cardiac output escalates throughout pregnancy as a result of lower systemic vascular resistance, increased blood volume, elevated heart rate, and an increase in stroke volume at the beginning of pregnancy. As gestation advances, cardiac output increases 30–50% over nonpregnant levels (Gabbe,

2007). Half of this increase occurs by the 8th week of pregnancy, and peak cardiac output is between 20–32 weeks' gestation.

Actual cardiac output is related to posture; it is maximal when the woman reclines on her left side, and in late pregnancy it can be decreased as much as 30% by compression of the inferior vena cava by the gravid uterus when the woman is supine (Foley, 2007). Postural hypotension, evidenced by dizziness and fainting when standing, can become pronounced during pregnancy as a result of low peripheral vascular resistance and pooling of blood in the legs.

During labor, cardiac output becomes even more robust—increasing by an additional 15% in early labor, 25% in active labor, and about 50% while pushing—as further protection against excessive blood loss (Bridges, Womble, Wallace, & McCartney, 2003). Immediately postpartum, the uterus contracts, returning as much as 500 ml of blood from the uterine vasculature to the maternal circulation and relieving pressure on the vena cava. Cardiac output increases by 60–80% above pre-labor values despite the blood loss of delivery (Foley, 2007). Women who have cardiac problems are more likely to develop pulmonary edema at the end of labor or immediately thereafter. Oxytocin, which can encourage fluid retention, may increase this risk. By 3 months after delivery, cardiac output and systemic vascular resistance return to pre-pregnancy levels.

Pregnancy increases the resting pulse by about 15–20 beats per minute (bpm). Blood pressure drops slightly during the first 2 trimesters, but returns to pre-pregnant levels by term. Because of the greater blood volume, a pregnant woman can acutely lose 30–35% of her blood without a change in vital signs (Foley, 2007). The diastolic value typically drops 16–20 mmHg, but changes in the systolic pressure are less dramatic.

Low readings such as 86/60 may be found in young women and women who exercise regularly. Recent research has indicated that persistently low blood pressure carries an increased risk of stillbirth (Warland, McCutcheon, & Baghurst, 2008). Mildly high blood-pressure readings are a much greater cause for concern in pregnant women than in nonpregnant women of childbearing age. A reading of 140/90 can indicate the onset of a life-threatening hypertensive disorder, especially if accompanied by generalized edema and symptoms such as malaise, headache, or epigastric pain. Some previously normotensive women will become transiently hypertensive after delivery as the peripheral vasculature resumes its prepregnancy tone.

Blood clots more easily in pregnancy. Increased levels of clotting factors and fibrinogen and reduced anticoagulation factors decrease the mother's risk of hemorrhage, but amplify her risk of venous thrombosis. Pregnant women are also prone to varicose veins in the legs, rectum, vulva, and pelvis because of vascular dilation and venous compression from the heavy uterus. This combination of dilated veins, sluggish venous return, and an increased tendency to clot predisposes a pregnant and newly postpartum woman to developing blood clots. These clots can migrate to the lungs to become pulmonary emboli—a leading cause of maternal death.

Normal maternal cardiovascular adaptations to pregnancy often mimic pathological processes. The pregnant woman may feel short of breath and become easily fatigued, especially with exercise. Rib flaring, costochondritis, and indigestion may cause chest pain. Syncope becomes more likely in pregnancy. On chest radiographs, the heart of a pregnant woman often appears enlarged, and the left ventricle looks hypertrophied. Pitting edema is common, especially in warm weather.

The simple act of lying flat on the back for 3–10 min may induce supine hypotensive syndrome. When supine posture causes the inferior vena cava to become compressed between the spine and the gravid uterus, the maternal heart rate escalates, blood pressure declines, and the pulse pressure (the difference between systolic and diastolic blood pressure) decreases. The woman may remain asymptomatic or become lightheaded, short of breath, panicky, nauseated, and syncopal.

The heart sounds louder to auscultation from the first trimester, and most pregnant women develop a subtle third heart sound. The provider may hear exaggerated splitting of S-1 and a systolic ejection murmur up to grade 2/4 over the pulmonary and tricuspid areas. Although systolic murmurs are almost universal in pregnancy, diastolic murmurs are an unusual finding and may suggest a pathological process.

The growing uterus causes the diaphragm to lift; the ribs to flare, and the heart to rotate to the left, anterior, and transverse, resulting in a 15°–20° left axis deviation on a 12-lead EKG. Transient ST segment and T wave changes, the presence of a Q wave, and inverted T waves may be normal in pregnancy, but should prompt a cardiology consult (Foley, 2007). Arrhythmias such as supraventricular tachycardia and ventricular extrasystoles are frequently noted in normal pregnant women, but should prompt a referral to a specialist if she reports persistent symptomatic palpitations.

Gastrointestinal System

Pregnant women often experience an alteration in taste, which leads to cravings and food aversions. Gingivitis is likely to occur in pregnancy, probably related to hormonally induced vascular and immune changes. Epulis, a benign granuloma of the oral mucosa, sometimes develops. Ptyalism, overproduction of saliva, may be vexing.

Gastric emptying and intestinal transit times are delayed in pregnancy by hormonal and mechanical factors. Rising hormone levels and blood-sugar fluctuations make nausea and vomiting common during the first trimester. The lower esophageal sphincter pressure decreases as the gravid uterus pushes the stomach up under the diaphragm, causing almost half of pregnant women to experience heartburn. Hormonal changes may cause abdominal bloating and constipation, which may be exacerbated by iron supplementation.

Stomach sphincter relaxation and the pressure of the gravid uterus result in frequent heartburn. Although the stomach does not take longer to empty, small bowel and colonic transit times are prolonged in late pregnancy, probably because of increased levels of progesterone and compression by the fetus. Increased intra-abdominal pressure and relaxation of the lower esophageal sphincter predisposes pregnant women to gastric aspiration during surgery or sedation.

About 30–40% of pregnant and postpartum women develop hemorrhoids (Sinclair, 2004). The pressure of the gravid uterus restricting blood return from the rectal veins causes these varicosities of the anal canal. Many women develop prominent varicosities in the labia and vagina by the same mechanism.

Serum alkaline phosphatase values in hepatic-function panels may increase markedly because of placental metabolism. Gallbladder function is altered during pregnancy. Progesterone seems to retard gallbladder emptying, leading to stasis of bile and increased formation of gallstones. Slow movement of bile can cause generalized skin itchiness from bile salts.

Musculoskeletal System

Progressive lordosis or "swayback" normally occurs in pregnancy as the woman compensates for the heavy uterus weighing down the front of the body, while the neck flexes forward and shoulders move down. The pelvis tilts anteriorly, causing increased use of hip extensor, abductor, and ankle flexor muscles. Abdominal muscles stretch, weaken, and separate, altering posture and straining paraspinal muscles. Lordosis contributes to the low-back pain commonly experienced by pregnant women. Balance is affected by changes in posture and center of gravity, increasing the likelihood of falls. The sacroiliac joints and pubic symphysis become wider and more mobile. Hormones loosen joints to maximize pelvic expansion during delivery, when an extra centimeter may be crucial, but they also loosen joints throughout the body. The weight gain of pregnancy increases the stress on the hips and knees by as much as 100% during weight-bearing exercise such as running (Bermas, 2007). Healthy joints may become painful, and unstable or arthritic joints may suffer further damage. One third to two thirds of all pregnant women develop back pain, and 41% report first-time back pain during pregnancy (Bermas, 2007).

Endocrine System

A comprehensive discussion of reproductive endocrinology is beyond the scope of this book, but a few key concepts will prove useful.

The thyroid enlarges by about 30% in pregnancy. In early pregnancy, thyroid stimulating hormone may be low because circulating HCG (which is a structurally similar molecule) confuses the feedback system. The levels of T3 and free T4 are in balance, and the woman usually remains euthyroid. Hyperemesis gravidarum is sometimes linked to hyperthyroidism.

In the pancreas, the cells of the islets of Langerhans increase in size while the beta cells and insulin receptors increase in size and number. Fasting glucose tends to run lower in pregnancy, but postprandial glucose levels tend to elevate. The hormones of pregnancy increase insulin resistance progressively as pregnancy advances, and insulin production is doubled (Petraglia & D'Antona, 2007). The renal threshold for glucose decreases and may cause glucose to spill into the urine.

The hypothalamus regulates and coordinates much of maternal endocrine function and sends releasing hormones to the pituitary.

The anterior lobe of the pituitary gland enlarges up to threefold during pregnancy as the hormonal milieu changes: growth hormone production declines, adrenocorticotropic hormone (ACTH) increases, and prolactin increases throughout pregnancy and is further elevated during lactation. Thyroid stimulating hormone (TSH) levels may be somewhat decreased through the first trimester and may be slightly elevated at term.

The intermediate lobe of the pituitary also grows larger during pregnancy. It increases production of melanocyte-stimulating hormone (MSH), the hormone responsible for the hyperpigmentation (linea nigra, chloasma) common to pregnancy.

The posterior lobe of the pituitary gland stores oxytocin and antidiuretic hormone, both of which are important to pregnancy. Antidiuretic hormone influences plasma osmolality and sodium concentration. Oxytocin causes uterine contractions and the "let down" of milk during lactation. Maternal plasma concentrations rise continuously across gestation, and the uterus becomes more sensitive to its effects around the time of labor. Nipple stimulation stimulates oxytocin release, which in turn causes contraction of myoepithelial cells in ductal smooth muscle and milk ejection.

Progesterone is produced by the corpus luteum until the placenta takes over production at 8–12 weeks' gestation. Progesterone and testosterone levels rise through pregnancy, peaking at term.

Renal and Urinary System

The mucosa of the bladder, like mucosa elsewhere in the body, becomes increasingly vascular and edematous during pregnancy. Progesterone relaxes the bladder muscle and increases its capacity until the enlarging uterus squeezes it flat.

Urinary frequency, nocturia, dysuria, urgency, and stress incontinence are commonplace during pregnancy. Urinary output increases as a result of higher fluid intake, plasma volume expansion, and increased renal filtration rate. Urinary incontinence occurs in response to uterine pressure on the bladder as well as hormonally influenced changes to the suspensory ligaments of the urethra.

Progesterone relaxes the tone and decreases peristalsis of the ureters, and pressure from the gravid uterus may cause them to become displaced, elongated, and winding. The uterus, displaced to the right by the colon, compresses the right ureter and sometimes the left against the pelvis, blocking drainage (hydroureter). This dilated collecting system may contain 200–300 ml of retained urine, which may encourage bacterial growth and lead to pyelonephritis. Almost all women will show some degree of hydroureter and hydronephrosis during pregnancy. It may progress to the point of pain or even renal failure and may necessitate stent placement. Renal calculi (kidney stones) are more common in pregnancy, and they can obstruct flow and cause or worsen ureteral dilatation.

Increased cardiac output results in increased renal perfusion and filtration. Kidneys enlarge during pregnancy, and glomerular filtration rates increase more than 50% by the end of the first trimester (Varney, 2004). The pregnant woman may have altered drug metabolism because the kidneys excrete drugs faster.

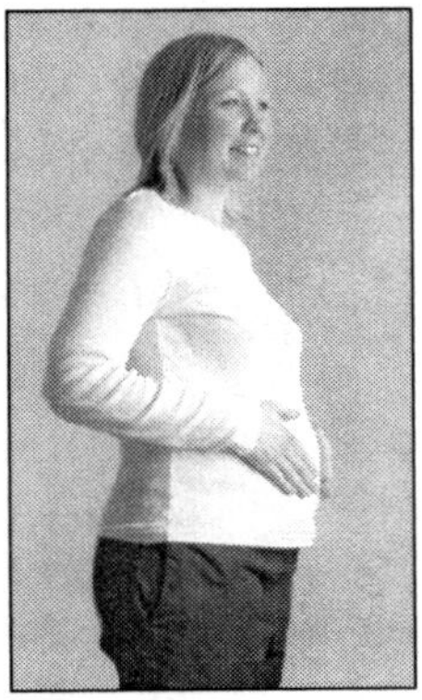

Pregnant women excrete more glucose, amino acids, and beta microglobulin in the urine and may develop glycosuria in the absence of hyperglycemia. Urinary protein excretion may be double the values for nonpregnant women, often reaching 80–200 mg per 24 hr in the third trimester.

Respiratory System

Increased estrogen levels cause the mucous membranes of the upper respiratory system to engorge with blood. They also cause glandular hyperactivity, increased phagocytic activity, and increased mucopolysaccharide content. The result: complaints of nasal stuffiness and epistaxis.

Figure 13. The diaphragm rises and the chest diameter expands, growing wider front to back.

The ribs flare early in pregnancy, long before the gravid uterus rises into the abdomen. The diaphragm rises and the chest diameter expands, growing wider front to back. Pregnancy is a state of relative hyperventilation, for increased levels of progesterone stimulate the respiratory drive. Minute ventilation increases by almost 50% at term because of a 40% increase in tidal volume (Weinberger, 2007). The rate of breathing remains unchanged, however. The pregnant woman moves more air and extracts more oxygen with each breath. These changes in respiratory physiology may make the woman feel short of breath even when her breathing is not compromised.

Pregnant women use 20% more oxygen to meet the demands of the placenta, fetus, and maternal organs, but this increase is more than satisfied by the increase in minute volume (Weinberger, 2007). Blood levels of oxygen rise while carbon dioxide levels decrease, creating mild compensated respiratory alkalosis. The kidneys compensate by excreting bicarbonate, maintaining the arterial blood pH about 7.40–7.45.

Nervous System

Laxity of joint articulations and shifts in posture may put pressure on nerves, causing shooting pains such as sciatica. Carpal tunnel syndrome may develop, causing the woman pain and numbness, especially upon waking, and difficulty grasping. Carpal tunnel syndrome in pregnancy is partially attributable to lordosis, which puts pressure on nerves in the neck and shoulders.

RESPONDING TO EMERGENCIES

The home-birth provider can avoid many emergencies through careful management, close observation, referral of high-risk clients, and adhering to clinical guidelines. Some crises, however, will arise unexpectedly despite optimal care and monitoring. Every midwife should maintain current certification in CPR, the Heimlich maneuver, and neonatal resuscitation and should stay current with the management of complications that may be encountered in practice.

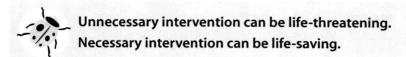

Unnecessary intervention can be life-threatening.
Necessary intervention can be life-saving.

When an emergency arises, it is essential to identify the problem at its earliest presentation. Early detection generally yields better outcomes. Calmly take charge; a single leader helps avoid confusion. If extra hands are needed or transport is required, get help early on, as indicated. Avoid leaving the woman unattended. Gather information quickly, process it logically, and then act decisively and boldly.

Initial Assessment

Sometimes the unexpected happens. The midwife may hear a crash and find the client twitching on the bathroom floor or arrive at her home to find her unresponsive. The provider may encounter an unconscious pregnant woman in a public place and know nothing about her circumstances. When the situation at hand deviates from normal, the provider must conduct a rapid problem-oriented evaluation of the client and establish priorities of care based on existing and potential problems.

The goal of the initial assessment is to identify and correct potentially life-threatening conditions such as airway compromise, hemorrhage, and inadequate breathing. For the provider, it is a gathering and rapid processing of information gleaned from the history, physical assessment, environment, mechanism of injury, and instinct.

Use the mnemonic AVPU to categorize whether the client is alert, responds to verbal or painful stimuli, or is unresponsive.

AVPU
ALERT—Awake; eyes open; may be oriented to time, place, and person or disoriented.
VERBAL—Appears asleep, but rouses when spoken to. Take note of any confusion or disorientation.
PAINFUL STIMULI—Not responsive to verbal stimulation, but responds to painful stimuli. Pinch her fingernails or drag your knuckles over her sternum and observe her reaction. Purposeful responses include awakening, moaning, pushing you away, or withdrawing. Nonpurposeful responses to painful stimuli include decorticate posturing (arms flexed, legs extended) and decerebrate posturing (arms and legs extended), both of which can indicate grave neurological damage.
UNRESPONSIVE—Comatose, no response to any stimulus.

Sometimes the nature of the illness is not readily apparent. On first assessment, the client herself is often the best source of information. If she is unable to answer, gather information from bystanders, family members, or the surroundings.

When assessing emergencies, think **AACT and ReACT:**

AACT and ReACT
ALERT—Be alert ▶ Exercise hypervigilant attention
ANALYZE—Think about possible causes
CONSIDER—Use OLDCART ▶ Gather data
TREAT—Make first response ▶ Proceed to definitive care
**ReACT	ReAssess ▶ ReConsider ▶ Re-Treat**

Know Your ABCs

In any emergency, rapidly assess the basic vital signs.

AIRWAY—Oxygen is the most vital need of the body because minutes without it will cause death. Ensuring a clear airway is the first step in treating any emergency. If your client is talking to you, she has an open airway.

The most common airway obstruction in the unconscious person is the tongue blocking the flow of air. If trauma is not a concern, open the airway by using the head-tilt chin-lift maneuver and repositioning the head. Place your hand on the forehead of the client and lift the chin with the fingers of your other hand. For the trauma victim, stabilize the cervical spine and perform the jaw-thrust maneuver by placing your hands on the client's cheeks and lifting up on the angle of the jaw with your fingers. With babies and children, gently extend the head and neck, taking care not to hyperextend or hyperflex the airway, either of which can cause obstruction.

Look for chest rise and listen to the flow of air. Snoring occurs when the tongue partially blocks the airway. Gurgling indicates secretions or foreign material. High-pitched stridor indicates an upper-airway obstruction that can become lethal if not rapidly resolved. A foreign body lodged in the airway, swelling, anaphylaxis, or respiratory burns can cause stridor. Crowing is a high-pitched upper airway sound resulting from a partial airway obstruction, most commonly heard in children with croup or epiglottitis.

If the woman cannot move air, she is in respiratory arrest. If a foreign body obstructs the airway and the client is moving minimal air or is losing consciousness, employ the Heimlich maneuver.

The unresponsive woman may be unable to protect her airway, so the provider must ensure that it remains patent with suctioning, positioning, and airway adjuncts if available.

BREATHING—After opening the airway, look, listen, and feel for breathing. Assess for ineffective breathing such as labored respirations, speaking in broken sentences, retractions, use of accessory muscles of the neck and abdomen, audibly noisy breaths, and nasal flaring. The hypoxic client will often be confused, restless, or agitated. Respiratory rates less than 10 or greater than 30 may indicate inadequate air exchange.

Observe the respiratory pattern. Rapid, deep respirations (tachypnea with hyperpnea) suggest acidosis and indicate that the body is trying to correct a dangerously low pH by expelling acids through the respiratory tract. Diabetic ketoacidosis presents with deep, rapid, respirations and a fruity odor to the breath. Cheyne-Stokes respirations—a sequence of decreasing rate and depth alternating with apnea and Biot's respirations (irregular, short, and gasping)—indicate serious brain injury. Agonal respirations are the last slow gasps before total apnea.

If breathing is compromised but the client is moving adequate air, supply high-flow oxygen and be prepared to assist ventilation. If the client is unresponsive but is breathing adequately, monitor the airway for continued patency and supply high-flow oxygen. If the woman is unresponsive and has apnea or agonal breathing, give two rescue breaths with any delivery method available—mouth-to-mouth, mouth-to-mask, bag-mask device (with or without oxygen), or an advanced airway. Watch for chest rise. If the chest does not rise, readjust the airway and reattempt ventilation.

CIRCULATION—Initially assess for adequate circulation by feeling for a strong pulse. If the client is breathing, she has a pulse; but if her blood pressure is low, that pulse may not be palpable. The presence of a carotid pulse in an adult suggests a systolic blood pressure above 60, a femoral pulse suggests systolic pressure greater than 70, and a radial pulse suggests systolic pressure greater than 80. Infants have short, inaccessible necks, so pulse is palpated in the brachial artery of the arm or auscultated apically.

Severe bradycardia (less than 50 bpm) presents with cardiac problems, medication overdose, head injury, or vasovagal syncope. Some causes of tachycardia (greater than 110 bpm) include shock, exposure to chemicals like caffeine or medications, dehydration, hypothermia, lung problems, thyroid disorders, hypoglycemia, cardiovascular problem like arrhythmia or pulmonary embolism, panic disorder, pain, or fear. An irregular pulse may indicate a cardiac arrhythmia (Bledsoe, Porter, & Cherry, 2003).

If the client is unresponsive and not breathing, check for a carotid pulse (adult) or brachial pulse (infant). If the pulse is absent, begin chest compressions as per American Heart Association guidelines. If the pulse is present, but adequate respirations are absent, continue rescue breathing. If a pulse is present, check for skin color—pallor indicates poor perfusion, and cyanosis indicates hypoxia. Flushed red skin indicates hyperthermia, and rarely indicates advanced carbon monoxide poisoning. Clammy, pale skin indicates that circulating blood is being shunted away from the skin to the vital organs.

ABCs with POP
AIRWAY—Taking care with the spine
BREATHING
CIRCULATION—With attention to bleeding
Placenta **O**ptimally **P**erfused

As you move thorough the initial survey, correct critical problems as you find them. Open the airway, apply oxygen, and stop bleeding. Ask yourself
- What is going on here?
- Is this a trauma? Do I need to stabilize the c-spine?
- What is the level of consciousness?
- Are ABCs stable or unstable?
- What are my priorities?

EVALUATING THE PRESENT COMPLAINT

The provider can evaluate most complaints and pains using the OLDCART mnemonic.

Taking a History Using OLDCART—Ask the Client:
ONSET—When did the problem start? What were you doing? Was the onset gradual or rapid? In what order did the symptoms occur?
LOCATION—Where does it hurt? Did the pain start there or has it moved? Is it localized, or does it radiate?
DURATION—How long have you had the symptoms? Do they come and go? Have you experienced them before?
CHARACTERISTICS—Quality and quantity of the pain—sharp? Dull? Frequency? On a scale of 0–10, with 10 being the worst pain you ever had and 0 being no pain at all, what number would you give this pain?
ASSOCIATED symptoms—What other symptoms are you experiencing?
RELIEVING/aggravating factors—What makes your symptoms better? What makes them worse?
TREATMENT—Have you treated the symptoms (with medications, herbs, remedies, hot soaks, etc.)? Did the treatment help or make things worse?

From Essentials of Prehospital Maternity Care, *by Bonnie U. Gruenberg, 2005, Upper Saddle River, NJ: Prentice Hall. Copyright 2005 by Prentice Hall. Reprinted with permission.*

OLDCART is a systematic method of gaining data that will help you to understand the nature of the problem. Often several possible conditions fit the clinical presentation, and the correct diagnosis emerges only as the provider solicits further clues, processes information, and reformulates treatment.

When seeking the cause of an obstetrical emergency, organize your initial impressions by asking yourself, "What is the most likely cause?" and "What is the worst it could be?" By considering these two questions first, you will focus your attention on the essentials. Identify the problem that is most likely to explain the symptoms while considering, "Could this problem be life-threatening?" Using this technique, you will give your initial attention to the most important aspects—identifying the most likely and most dangerous diagnoses—while keeping your mind open to other explanations as you gather data.

First Thought, Worst Thought

**Organize your initial impressions using
FIRST THOUGHT, WORST THOUGHT
"What is the most likely cause?"
"What is the worst it could be?"**

Determine the sequence of events: did she faint and then fall, or fall, then lose consciousness? Even if the problem is obvious, such as cord prolapse, continue to consider the possibilities. Are fetal heart tones present? If so, what rate? Is there more than one baby? Is there malpresentation? Is the baby term?

Because the mother is the life-support system for the fetus, the best way to care for the fetus is usually to stabilize the mother. The provider must consider potentially life-threatening conditions in the mother before turning attention to the fetus.

When seeking the cause of an obstetrical emergency, if two or more hypotheses explain the observed facts, use the simplest until contradictory evidence emerges.

Transport Plan

Transport unstable clients immediately. EMS is often the best option for transport, especially if advanced life support is available, because the ambulance is better suited for resuscitation should the client require CPR or other procedures. Many EMS providers carry a variety of medications and are able to intubate or start intravenous lines.

In some circumstances, the mother and fetus or newborn should be transported to a facility that offers comprehensive services for high-risk pregnant women and neonates. A neonatal intensive-care unit can make a lifelong difference to a baby with anomalies or extreme prematurity. The practicing midwife and her backup physician can determine together which local and regional hospitals offer the services required by an individual client.

A hospital with level-I neonatal intensive-care facilities cares primarily for normal mothers and babies as well as most emergencies. A level-II facility can handle the majority of maternal and neonatal complications. A level-III facility offers the full range of maternal and neonatal services and can provide care for critically ill infants. Regional tertiary hospitals provide the highest acuity services, including managing clients with rare diseases.

Table 2. Danger Signs in Pregnancy and Possible Causes

Sudden gush of fluid

Premature rupture of membranes, urinary incontinence, vaginal infection.

Vaginal bleeding

Placenta previa, placental abruption, bloody show, polyps, lesions of cervix or vagina. Sometimes a woman will spot after a recent vaginal examination or sexual intercourse.

Abdominal pain

Preterm labor, placental abruption, appendicitis, round-ligament pain, gallbladder, urinary-tract infection, renal calculi, hydronephrosis, pancreatitis.

Dizziness

Many causes, some of them benign. May relate to hypertension, medications, low blood sugar, or orthostatic hypotension.

Visual disturbances

Preeclampsia.

Severe vomiting

Hyperemesis gravidarum, gastroenteritis, or other gastro-intestinal disorder. May occur with appendicitis, head injury, or other condition. Client requires hospital evaluation if intake and output are poor.

Edema of hands, feet, or face

Preeclampsia. Pedal edema is often normal in pregnancy.

Severe headache

May be related to preeclampsia or may result from tension, migraine, or head injury.

Severe leg pain

Thrombophlebitis—or may be leg cramps.

Seizure

Preeclampsia—or may result from preexisting seizure disorder or head injury.

Epigastric pain

Preeclampsia, gallbladder inflammation, heartburn.

Reduced urine output

Preeclampsia, poor fluid intake, renal dysfunction.

Painful urination

Urinary-tract infection, vaginal or vulvar infection.

Absence of or decrease in fetal movement

Fetal compromise or death, maternal distraction, medication, maternal obesity.

Preterm contractions

Premature labor; may also be triggered by urinary-tract infection, dehydration, or uterine irritability.

Elevated temperature, chills

Infection.

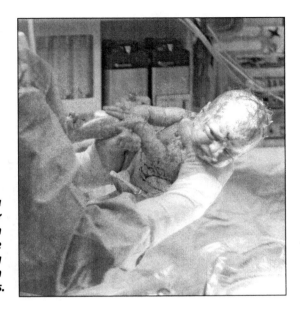

Figure 14. Rapid transport to a hospital with the capacity for immediate cesarean section and a neonatal intensive-care unit can make a lifelong difference to a baby in an obstetrical crisis.

BIBLIOGRAPHY

American College of Obstetricians and Gynecologists. (2004a). *Vaginal birth after previous cesarean delivery practice guidelines* (Practice Bulletin 54). Washington, DC: Author.

Bermas, B.L. (2007). Pain related to the musculoskeletal system during pregnancy. In B.D. Rose (Ed.), *UpToDate*. Wellesley, MA: UpToDate.

Bledsoe, B., Porter, R., & Cherry, R. (2003). *Essentials of paramedic care.* Upper Saddle River, NJ: Prentice Hall Health.

Bridges, E.J., Womble, S., Wallace, M., & McCartney, J. (2003). Hemodynamic monitoring in high-risk obstetrics patients I: Expected hemodynamic changes in pregnancy (Electronic version). *Critical Care Nurse, 23* (4), 53–62. Retrieved March 24, 2008, from http://ccn.aacnjournals.org/ cgi/content/full/23/4/53

College of Midwives of British Columbia. (2005). *Home birth handbook for midwifery clients.* Retrieved July 28, 2007, from http://www.cmbc.bc.ca/ docs/model_of_care/HomeBirthHandbook.pdf

Draycott, T., Sibanda, T,. Owen, L., Akande, V., Winter, C., Reading, S., et al. (2006). Does training in obstetric emergencies improve neonatal outcome? *Obstetrical & Gynecological Survey, 61* (6), 365–366.

Dunphy, L., Winland-Brown, J.E., Porter, B., & Thomas, D. (2007). *Primary care: The art and science of advanced practice nursing* (2nd ed.). Philadelphia:, F.A. Davis.

Foley, M.R. (2007). Maternal cardiovascular and hemodynamic adaptation to pregnancy. In B.D. Rose (Ed.), *UpToDate*. Wellesley, MA: UpToDate.

Keltz-Pomeranz, M.K. (2007). Physiologic changes of the skin, hair, nails, and mucous membranes during pregnancy. In B.D. Rose (Ed.), *UpToDate*. Wellesley, MA: UpToDate.

Petraglia, F., & D'Antona, D. (2007). Maternal endocrine and metabolic adaptation to pregnancy. In B.D. Rose (Ed.), *UpToDate*. Wellesley, MA: UpToDate.

Sinclair, C. (2004). *A midwife's handbook.* St. Louis: Saunders.

Varney, H. (2004). *Varney's midwifery* (4th ed.). Sudbury, MA: Jones & Bartlett.

Warland, J., McCutcheon, H., & Baghurst, P. (2008). Maternal blood pressure in pregnancy and stillbirth: A case-control study of third-trimester stillbirth. *American Journal of Perinatology, 25* (5), 311–317.

Weinberger, S.E. (2007). Dyspnea during pregnancy. In B.D. Rose (Ed.), *UpToDate*. Wellesley, MA: UpToDate.

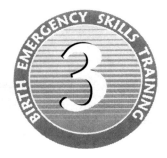

Bleeding in Pregnancy

OBJECTIVES

- ▶ Contrast and compare etiologies of vaginal bleeding, including
  - ▶ Spontaneous abortion
  - ▶ Hydatidiform mole
  - ▶ Ectopic pregnancy
  - ▶ Cervical/mucosal bleeding
- ▶ Briefly discuss the pathophysiology of disseminated intravascular coagulation.
- ▶ Compare and contrast the presentation of placental abruption versus placenta previa, including
  - ▶ Etiologic/predisposing factors
  - ▶ Signs and symptoms
  - ▶ Pathophysiology
  - ▶ Indicated diagnostic workup
  - ▶ Maternal and fetal complications

ANTEPARTAL BLEEDING— FIRST HALF OF PREGNANCY

AACT and ReACT
ALERT—Be alert ▶ Exercise hypervigilant attention
ANALYZE—Think about possible causes
CONSIDER—Use OLDCART ▶ Gather data
TREAT—Make first response ▶ Proceed to definitive care
ReACT | ReAssess ▶ ReConsider ▶ Re-Treat

✎ AACT—Alert

First-trimester vaginal bleeding occurs commonly in both viable and non-viable pregnancies. Twenty to 40% of women experience bleeding during the first trimester, and many of these deliver healthy babies at term (Tulandi & Al-Fozan, 2006). Most bleeding in early pregnancy results from one of five causes. These causes are contained in the mnemonic TEMPT:

TEMPT
THREATENED abortion
ECTOPIC pregnancy
MATERNAL pathology of uterus, vagina, or cervix
PHYSIOLOGICAL bleeding
TRAUMA

Taking a History Using OLDCART—Ask the Client:
ONSET—When did the problem start? What were you doing? Was the onset gradual or rapid? In what order did the symptoms occur?
LOCATION—Where does it hurt? Did the pain start there or has it moved? Is it localized, or does it radiate?
DURATION—How long have you had the symptoms? Do they come and go? Have you experienced them before?
CHARACTERISTICS—Quality and quantity of the pain—sharp? Dull? Frequency? On a scale of 0–10, with 10 being the worst pain you ever had and 0 being no pain at all, what number would you give this pain?
ASSOCIATED symptoms—What other symptoms are you experiencing?
RELIEVING/aggravating factors—What makes your symptoms better? What makes them worse?
TREATMENT—Have you treated the symptoms (with medications, herbs, remedies, hot soaks, etc.)? Did the treatment help or make things worse?

*From **Essentials of Prehospital Maternity Care**, by Bonnie U. Gruenberg, 2005, Upper Saddle River, NJ: Prentice Hall. Copyright 2005 by Prentice Hall. Reprinted with permission.*

AACT—Analyze

- ▶ Why is she bleeding?
- ▶ Differential diagnoses

Table 3. Possible Causes of Early-Pregnancy Bleeding

Threatened abortion

Loss of one fetus in multiple pregnancy

Hydatidiform mole

Ectopic pregnancy

Maternal pathology of uterus vagina, or cervix

Polyp, cervicitis, cervical carcinoma

Cervical hemangioma

Condyloma, neoplasm, foreign body, laceration, ulceration

Infection——bacterial vaginosis, trichomonas, chlamydia, gonorrhea

Physiological

Implantation bleeding

Cervical ectropion (columnar epithelium exposed by eversion of the endocervix)

Trauma

Vaginal, cervical, vulvar laceration

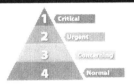

Early pregnancy bleeding can be priority 1, 2, 3, or 4. Determining acuity is an important aspect of management.

Ectopic Pregnancy

Priority 1 or 2

The incidence of ectopic pregnancy in the United States has tripled since 1970 to 1 in every 44 pregnancies. It is the leading cause of first-trimester maternal death. *Always consider ectopic pregnancy a possibility unless the conceptus has been sonographically confirmed in the uterus.* Because the consequences of a ruptured extrauterine pregnancy can be so devastating, suspect ectopic pregnancy in any woman of reproductive age with lower abdominal pain, vaginal bleeding, and amenorrhea. Normally, conception occurs in the fallopian tubes, and the conceptus reaches the uterus within about a week. There it encounters the thick, hormonally-primed endometrium and taps into the mother's bloodstream for life support.

Ectopic ("out of place") pregnancy occurs when the embryo embeds somewhere outside the uterus. The most common site is the fallopian tube (95%), but occasionally the embryo will implant on the ovary (4%), cervix (1%), or even in the abdominal cavity (<1%) (Tulandi, 2007a).

None of these structures is suitable for supporting a growing embryo, and the fragile, vascular fallopian tube is vulnerable to rupture. Ectopic pregnancy begins as clinically indistinguishable from intrauterine pregnancy (IUP), but in time it begins to distend the tube and invade blood vessels. Placental and corpus luteal function falter, and hormone levels begin to drop. The decidua, no longer maintained by a healthy corpus luteum, begins to shed, causing bleeding. If the ectopic pregnancy ruptures the tube or erodes through the tube wall, the woman will hemorrhage into her abdominal cavity, potentially creating the hemodynamic equivalent of a shotgun blast to the abdomen.

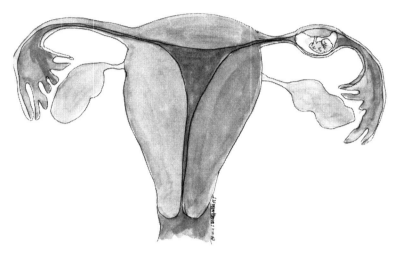

Figure 15. The most common site for an ectopic pregnancy is the fallopian tube.

In other cases, the ectopic pregnancy will die and spontaneously resolve, form a chronic hematoma, or abort out the end of the tube, sometimes reimplanting as an abdominal pregnancy. Rupture can initially present as a small defect in the tube with minimal pain and bleeding that grows gradually worse or as massive hemorrhage. Fortunately, using modern diagnostic techniques, most ectopic pregnancies may be diagnosed before they rupture.

The woman with an ectopic pregnancy may not realize that she is pregnant. Pain and bleeding usually appear by 6–8 weeks' gestation, but symptoms can occur as early as 5 weeks' gestation or (rarely) as late as 14–16 weeks (Tulandi, 2007a). Half of women with extrauterine pregnancy have no symptoms prior to tubal rupture and have no known risk factors (Tulandi, 2007a).

The classic presentation of ectopic pregnancy is the woman with amenorrhea and diffuse abdominal pain, progressing to severe unilateral lower abdominal pain. In most cases, pain onset is abrupt and severe; but in some cases, the woman may have chronic discomfort with irregular spotting for days before becoming acutely symptomatic. Rupture of the fallopian tube rapidly progresses to hypovolemic shock with rapid, weak pulse; confusion and restlessness; pale, clammy skin; collapsed neck veins; hypotension; and syncope. Three of four clients will have abdominal pain with rebound tenderness, rigidity, and distention. (Rebound tenderness is sudden severe pain when the hand is rapidly released following abdominal palpation.) Free blood in the abdomen may cause nausea, vomiting, and diarrhea and irritate the phrenic nerve (which runs under the diaphragm), causing referred pain to the right shoulder.

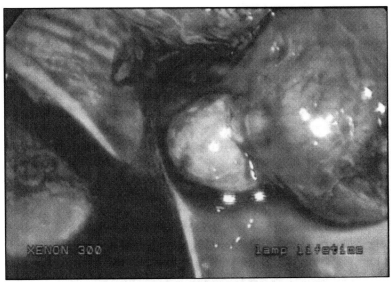

Figure 16. Laparoscopic photograph of ectopic pregnancy with free blood in the abdomen. Courtesy of Dr. Pierre Eugene.

Vaginal bleeding occurs in 40–50% of women with extrauterine pregnancy, but the degree of shock exceeds that accounted for by visible blood loss (Tulandi, 2007a). Blood pooling in the cul de sac may cause a sensation of rectal pressure. A rare finding is Cullen's sign, a blue tint beneath the umbilicus indicating free blood in the abdomen.

In other cases of intrauterine pregnancy, symptoms can be vague and variable. In the absence of unambiguous symptoms, the process of diagnosis is imprecise. On the client's first visit to the emergency department, physicians fail to correctly diagnose ectopic pregnancy more than 40% of the time; consequently, ruptured ectopic pregnancy remains the major cause of pregnancy-related maternal mortality in the first trimester (Tenore, 2000).

The chief complaint may be vague pain low in the pelvis. Vital signs may be normal if rupture has not yet occurred. Some women present with only syncope or profound shock (20%) (Tulandi, 2007a). Differential diagnoses include spontaneous abortion, ruptured ovarian cyst, appendicitis, salpingitis (infection of the fallopian tube), torsion (twisting) of the ovary, round-ligament pain, torsion or degeneration of a uterine fibroid, kidney stone, abscess, and urinary-tract infection.

Rarely, extrauterine gestation establishes itself someplace other than the fallopian tube. A cervical pregnancy presents with profuse, almost painless bleeding. A pregnancy implanted in a hysterotomy scar causes bleeding, abdominal pain, and eventual rupture of the scar if untreated. Ovarian pregnancies can be difficult to differentiate from hemorrhagic ovarian cysts or pregnancy in the distal tube, and they are usually treated surgically. An interstitial or cornual pregnancy can be difficult to distinguish from an IUP, but is likely to rupture before 12 weeks if untreated. Heterotopic pregnancy consists of one embryo in the uterus, one ectopic, and is rare except among women undergoing in vitro fertilization.

Abdominal pregnancy carries a high mortality rate for both mother (20%) and fetus (40–90%), and congenital deformities from compression are common (Tulandi, 2007a). The placenta attaches to the outer uterus, bowel, mesentery, liver, spleen, bladder, or ligaments and may separate anytime during pregnancy, causing uncontrollable hemorrhage. Oligo-hydramnios, poor placental definition, abnormal fetal lie, and an empty uterus low in the pelvis are visible on ultrasound, although late in gestation the thickened gestational sac may be misidentified as an IUP by an unsuspecting sonographer.

Risk factors for ectopic pregnancy include previous pelvic or tubal surgery, history of infertility, smoking, maternal age over 35, use of an intrauterine device (IUD) for contraception, altered hormone levels, and congenital anomalies of the fallopian tubes. Prior ectopic pregnancy correlates with an 8–14% recurrence rate (Tulandi, 2007a). Chlamydia or gonorrhea infection can damage the intrafallopian cilia, encouraging ectopic implantation.

About 7 women per 1,000 will conceive an ectopic pregnancy within 10 years of tubal ligation (Tulandi, 2007a). Women who have undergone tubal reanastomosis (reversal of tubal ligation to achieve pregnancy) are also at greater risk.

Implantation Bleeding
Priority 4

Implantation bleeding occurs about 10–14 days after fertilization and is thought to be caused when the implanting embryo disrupts the blood vessels of the uterine lining. Implantation bleeding results from vascular disruption as the embryo burrows into the endometrial tissue. Implantation bleeding can be scanty or profuse; it usually occurs 5–6 weeks after the last menstrual period and lasts a day or two.

 About 30% of early pregnancy losses occur before a pregnancy has been clinically recognized.

Threatened Abortion

Priority 1, 2, or 3

Spontaneous abortion is the clinical term for what is commonly termed a miscarriage. Pregnancy loss is the most common complication of human gestation. About one third to one half of women who experience vaginal bleeding in the first trimester will lose the pregnancy. In many cases, the cause of spontaneous abortion is not clear. One quarter to one half of conceived embryos never implant. About 11% of women with a positive pregnancy test will miscarry, 80% of these during the first trimester (Tulandi & Al-Fozan, 2006). Risk increases with each consecutive miscarriage. After 15 weeks, the risk of miscarriage for normal fetuses decreases to 6 per 1,000 (Tulandi & Al-Fozan, 2006).

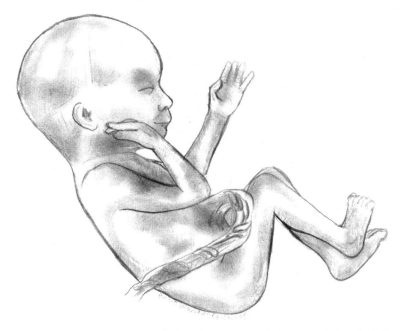

Figure 17. Midtrimester pregnancy loss may result from infection, antiphospholipid syndrome, diabetes, substance abuse, genetic disorders, uterine or placental abnormalities, cervical trauma, or cervical incompetence, but many losses remain unexplained.

Bleeding or abdominal pain with an IUP and closed cervix is termed a threatened abortion. Ultrasound may show a visible fetal heartbeat, empty gestational sac, or an empty uterus if gestational age is very early. Most women with bleeding beyond 7 weeks' gestation with documented fetal heart activity will not miscarry; but the presence of first-trimester bleeding increases the likelihood of adverse pregnancy outcome, including growth restriction, preterm delivery, and stillbirth, especially when the bleeding is heavy or extends into the second trimester.

In most cases, the bleeding results from a small abruption or subchorionic hematoma. Often this separation of the placenta from the decidua cannot be visualized on ultrasound; but if the hematoma is visible and symptomatic, pregnancy loss is more likely. (Incidental findings of small, asymptomatic subchorionic hematomas do not increase risk.)

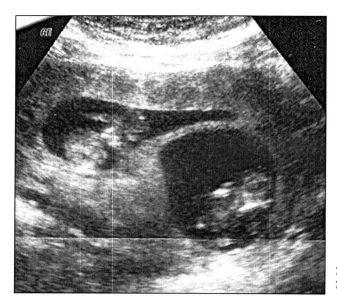

18. Twin gestation, 11 weeks.

The most common cause of pregnancy loss is chromosomal abnormality: too many or too few chromosomes, defective or missing genes, or missing chromosomal segments. The majority of early miscarriages are autosomal trisomies (three copies of a chromosome), including trisomy 21 (Down syndrome), trisomy 18, and trisomy 13. Parents may carry a rearrangement of chromosomes (usually a translocation or inversion) or each parent may carry a harmless single copy of problematic gene that is lethal as a homozygous pair. Advanced maternal age increases the risk of pregnancy loss due to poor egg quality, a less receptive endometrium, and endocrine dysfunction. Embryos fathered by men with a high percentage of abnormal sperm are also less likely to survive.

Pregnancy loss may be caused by toxins such as anesthetic gases, agricultural chemicals, cocaine, moderate to high alcohol consumption, and tobacco use, and by infections such as *Listeria monocytogenes*, *Toxoplasma gondii*, cytomegalovirus, and primary genital herpes. Urinary-tract infections are a risk factor for spontaneous abortion.

More than 10% of women with repeated pregnancy loss have congenital uterine anomalies that interfere with implantation or uterine distention, such as bicornuate or unicornuate uterus (Tulandi & Al-Fozan, 2007). Women with an untreated septate uterus have greater than 60% risk of pregnancy loss, probably because inadequate blood supply to the septum causes implantation failure (Tulandi & Al-Fozan). Submucous leiomyomas can also interfere with implantation, as can intrauterine adhesions and endometrial abnormalities that develop after pregnancy-related dilation and curettage (D&C) procedures.

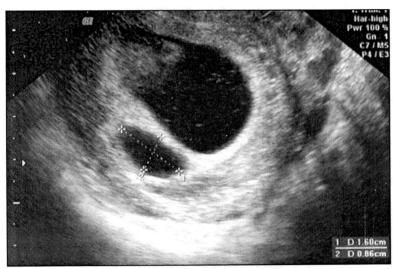

Figure 19. Vanishing twin (bottom) with surviving twin (top) 7.4 weeks.

Endocrine factors such as decreased thyroid function, inadequate progesterone production, and abnormal prolactin levels play a significant role in recurrent pregnancy loss. Poorly controlled diabetes with hA1C above 8% can cause congenital anomalies and both early and late pregnancy loss (Tulandi & Al-Fozan, 2007). The maternal immune system can cause pregnancy loss by attacking and killing the conceptus. Thrombophilias can cause clotting within spiral arteries and the intervillous space on the maternal side of the placenta, causing abnormalities of the uteroplacental circulation that can lead to pregnancy loss, intrauterine growth restriction (IUGR), abruption, or preeclampsia.

About one third of the spontaneous abortions occurring before 9 weeks' gestation are "blighted" or anembryonic (Tulandi & Al-Fozan, 2006). The gestational sac and placenta develop, but no yolk sac or embryo. On ultrasound examination, the gestational sac will be 20 mm or more, but no embryo will be visible. Severe bleeding, abdominal or back pain, passage of tissue, and cervical dilation indicate inevitable pregnancy loss. This condition progresses to either complete abortion or incomplete abortion. In early pregnancy, the woman may be given the option to complete the miscarriage naturally, or a D&C may be performed to hasten the process and limit blood loss and pain.

Incomplete Abortion

Priority 1 or 2

In incomplete abortion, some of the products of conception are expelled while other parts—usually placental fragments—are retained in the uterus. When a pregnancy loss occurs early in the first trimester, the body can usually expel the products of conception without surgical intervention. With advancing gestation, placental tissue is often left in the uterus, causing bleeding that can result in hypovolemic shock. The woman may be in intense pain, her cervix is usually dilated, and tissue may be lodged in the cervical os. Beta-HCG levels are plateaued or slowly falling. Ultrasound indicates retained products in the uterus or thickened, irregular endometrium (greater than 5 mm double stripe). The woman must have a (D&C) operation to complete the process and stop the bleeding.

Missed Abortion

Typically priority 2 or 3

In a missed abortion, the products of conception are retained in utero after the fetus has died. Expulsion occurs days or weeks later. The nausea, breast tenderness, and urinary frequency of pregnancy may subside, and vaginal spotting may occur, though the cervix usually stays closed. Ultrasound detects no fetal heartbeat. In early pregnancy, management can be expectant; but with advancing gestational age or prolonged retention of pregnancy, intervention is recommended.

Vanishing Twin

First trimester priority 3.5

A vanishing twin is a singleton pregnancy that involves loss of a multiple gestation in the early weeks of pregnancy. It occurs in about 36% of multifetal pregnancies (Chasen & Chervenak, 2007a). The lost twin may be reabsorbed or "mummified" (compressed into a *fetus papyraceus*), or it may regress to a subtle lesion on the placenta such as a cyst or fibrin deposit. If a twin is lost after the 20th week, the risk of morbidity increases for both the mother and surviving fetus.

Septic Abortion

Priority 1 or 2

In septic abortion, infection invades the uterine cavity during the abortion process. Septic abortion may occur after conception with an intrauterine device (IUD) in place; with prolonged, undiagnosed rupture of membranes; or after attempts by unqualified individuals to end a pregnancy. Symptoms of septic abortion include fever, malaise, abdominal pain, tachycardia, vaginal bleeding, and foul-smelling bloody yellow discharge. On examination, the uterus is boggy and tender, rebound and cervical-motion tenderness are present, and the cervix may be open or closed. Ultrasound scan shows thickened endometrium or retained products of conception. The microorganisms responsible are most often *Staphylococcus aureus*, gram-negative bacilli, or gram-positive cocci, but the infection can be polymicrobial. Sepsis involving *Clostridium sordellii* has occurred after mifepristone-induced abortion.

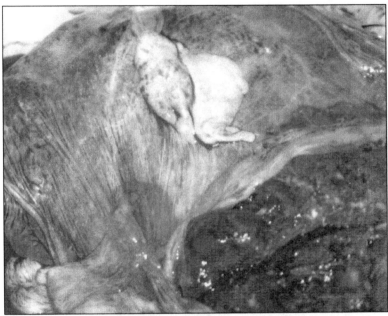

Figure 20. Fetus papyraceus. This fetus died in utero at 11 weeks, but his twin delivered full term. At birth, the barely-recognizable fetus was found attached to the placenta.

Hydatidiform Mole

Priority 2 or 3; some complications (such as related preeclampsia) are priority 1

Hydatidiform mole, also known as a molar pregnancy or gestational trophoblastic disease, occurs in about 1 per 1,000 conceptions in the United States. Some parts of Asia have a rate that is significantly greater. In a complete molar pregnancy, a sperm that duplicates its own chromosomes fertilizes a defective egg without a nucleus. Consequently, there is no maternal genetic contribution and no embryo, only a malformed placenta that proliferates as rapidly growing, grapelike fluid-filled vesicles. A partial molar pregnancy usually begins with a normal egg, which is either fertilized by two sperm or fertilized by one sperm followed by duplication of paternal chromosomes. The pregnancy can be triploid (69 XXX or 69 XXY instead of 46 XX or 46 XY) or even tetraploid, and can include fetal parts. An embryo begins to develop, but soon dies, and the abnormal placental tissue fills and distends the uterus as with a complete mole.

The pregnancy with hydatidiform mole includes a uterus is large for dates, and quantitative HCG levels are much greater than expected. Hyperemesis gravidarum, hyperthyroidism, and early-pregnancy preeclampsia commonly develop. As molar tissue separates from the decidua, the woman experiences vaginal bleeding, which is often the color of prune juice, but may be bright red. Diagnosis is made by ultrasound, and the mole is removed by surgical evacuation. Women with a history of molar pregnancy are at increased risk for choriocarcinoma, an aggressive cancer of the uterus.

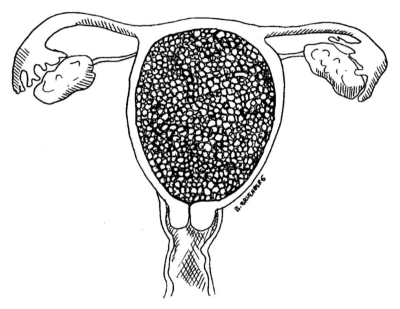

Figure 21. A hydatidiform mole involves a malformed placenta that proliferates as rapidly growing, grapelike fluid-filled vesicles.

✍ AACT—Consider

When a woman complains of lower abdominal pain and bleeding in early pregnancy, it is important to identify or exclude an ectopic pregnancy. With early diagnosis, treatment is less invasive, and the likelihood of tubal rupture is reduced. Always suspect ectopic pregnancy when a woman of childbearing age presents with lower abdominal pain or vaginal bleeding, even if she denies that she could be pregnant, has not missed a period, or has undergone tubal ligation. Assess for hemodynamic instability or significant vaginal bleeding, take orthostatic vital signs, and perform abdominal and pelvic examinations. Initiate emergency fluid resuscitation in cases of orthostatic hypotension, and move fast.

Begin your assessment by doing a primary survey, taking an OLDCART history, and forming a general impression. Is she alert and animated, or distracted and withdrawn? Assess for skin color, temperature, and moisture—pink and well perfused or pale and clammy?

Table 4. Sample OLDCART History for Bleeding in First Half of Pregnancy
ONSET—When did you first start to bleed? What were you doing? Was the onset gradual or rapid? Which came first, pain or bleeding? Did you have recent intercourse or put anything inside your vagina before the bleeding started?
LOCATION—Are you sure the blood is coming from your vagina? Could it be from your bladder or rectum? Where do you feel the pain? Is it on one side or right in the middle? Does it start in one place and radiate to somewhere else? Where?
DURATION—How many weeks pregnant are you? When was your last period? Was it normal? How long have you been bleeding? Has it been steady or does it come and go?
CHARACTERISTICS—Was the blood brown red or pink? How long does it take to soak a pad? How many pads have you soaked since the bleeding began? Large pads or small pads? Is the blood on the tissue when you wipe, soaking through your underwear, or turning the toilet water red? Are you passing clots? Did you pass any tissue? Is the pain sharp, dull, or crampy? How would you rate the pain on a scale of 0–10, with 10 being the worst pain imaginable?
ASSOCIATED symptoms—Any nausea, vomiting, fever, dizziness or fainting? Any foul-smelling vaginal discharge?
RELIEVING/aggravating factors—Do you get a fresh gush of blood or clots when you have been lying down for a while? Does your pain increase when you empty your bladder?
TREATMENT—Has a provider evaluated your bleeding previously? What did they recommend? Have you had a sonogram? How many weeks pregnant were you then? Did they see a heartbeat? Did they say the baby was in the uterus? Did they say anything about your placenta?

Evaluate vital signs by taking pulse and blood pressure supine, then standing. If blood loss has caused her to become hypovolemic, the provider may observe a drop of at least 20 mmHg of systolic pressure, or a diastolic blood pressure decrease of at least 10 mmHg with tachycardia within 3 min of standing. If the woman has symptomatic orthostatic hypotension, she will become light-headed or presyncopal upon standing, so use caution.

Polyps, infection, cervical or vaginal cancer, or capillary bleeding after intercourse usually presents with light, intermittent, and painless bleeding. The woman who reports hemorrhage, passing clots or tissue, significant pelvic pain, and lightheadedness is probably having a miscarriage or an ectopic pregnancy. Assess for risk factors; a woman with a history of two or more consecutive pregnancy losses, bicornuate uterus, or a thrombophilic disorder is at increased risk for spontaneous abortion, and a woman with a history of repeated chlamydia infections or tubal reanastomosis is at increased risk for ectopic pregnancy.

First Thought, Worst Thought

What is the most likely cause of first-trimester pain and bleeding?
Spontaneous abortion.
What is the worst it could be?
Ectopic pregnancy.

Gently percuss or palpate the woman's abdomen to check for pain, starting where she is feeling the least pain and examining the painful area last. Spontaneous abortion usually presents with midline pain, while ectopic pregnancy typically involves unilateral pain that may radiate to the right shoulder. Is her stated gestational age concordant with your physical assessment?

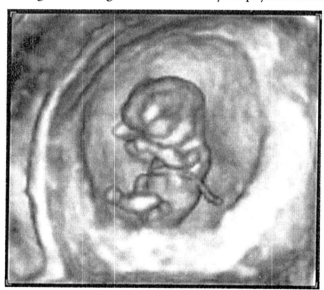

Figure 22. Three-dimensional sonogram of 10-week fetus

After examining the external abdomen, proceed to the pelvic examination to identify the source of bleeding. Examine the external genitalia and anus for any potential sites of bleeding. Gently insert a speculum and inspect the vaginal vault, sidewalls, and cervix for signs of vaginitis, trauma, vaginal or cervical neoplasia, warts, or polyps. If the woman is multiparous, the external os may appear open, but the internal os should be closed in a viable pregnancy. If the inner os is open and bleeding is heavy, suspect retained products of conception. If the woman is febrile and the uterus is tender, suspect concomitant infection.

Cervical insufficiency usually presents with vague symptoms, which can include bleeding, change in vaginal discharge, pressure, and vague uncomfortable sensations. On sonograms, a shortened cervix is evident often with funneling of the amniotic membranes. On speculum examination, the provider may view the whiteness of amniotic membranes through the dilated cervical os.

The cervix is very friable during pregnancy and prone to light bleeding after being bumped during a pelvic examination or by the penis during coitus. Cervical ectropion is common in pregnancy and may bleed on contact.

Use sponge sticks or gauze sponges on ring forceps to remove pooled blood and clots. Remove products of conception that have wedged in the os with ring forceps and send them to pathology; often this removal will control the bleeding of an incomplete abortion. Examine any tissue passed. Probe blood clots for products of conception. Women often mistake a large solid blood clot for fetal tissue. In actuality, the fetus will probably be passed whole. If the woman passes tissue, membranes appear as cellophane-like material, and placental tissue has feathery chorionic villi. The villi are more identifiable when floated in water. Usually, the products of conception are light-colored—tan or gray—and blood clots are dark red. The vesicles of a hydatidiform mole are grapelike, appearing like red currant jelly in prune juice.

If the laboratory identifies chorionic villi, the provider can assume that the products of conception have passed. If the miscarriage is complete, the cervix may be either open or closed, the uterus will feel small and tightly contracted and bleeding and cramping will become minimal. If there is not incontrovertible evidence that all products of conception have passed, follow serial HCG levels until they become undetectable.

A uterus enlarged by fibroids is irregularly shaped, while multiple pregnancy or hydatidiform mole causes uniform enlargement. If an ectopic pregnancy is present, the provider may palpate an adnexal mass or uterine enlargement or elicit pain with cervical motion or adnexal palpation; but often the examination reveals no unusual findings.

After 9–12 weeks, the fetal heart rate can often be detected with a Doppler device. The heart rate may be easier to hear if the uterus is elevated by the examining fingers during a bimanual examination while the other hand holds the Doppler suprapubically. The presence of normal heart tones by Doppler eliminates the possibility of missed abortion and makes ectopic pregnancy unlikely, but a fetal heartbeat does not guarantee a viable pregnancy. Inability to find heart tones by Doppler late in the first trimester is not always worrisome—a retroverted uterus or anterior placenta can render heart tones inaccessible by Doppler until the second trimester.

A physician sometimes performs culdocentesis during the pelvic examination by passing an 18- to 20-gauge needle through the posterior fornix and aspirating for fluid. Non-clotting frank blood in the cul-de-sac indicates ectopic pregnancy, while thin, pink fluid indicates a ruptured ovarian cyst. A physician may perform uterine curettage on the woman with low or abnormally rising beta-HCG levels, or those with levels above the discriminatory zone with no IUP visible on ultrasound. This procedure is performed to avoid unnecessary methotrexate treatment for women without ectopic pregnancy, but it carries the risk of disrupting a viable pregnancy. If HCG levels do not fall by 15% within 12 hr of D&C, ectopic pregnancy is likely (Tulandi, 2007a).

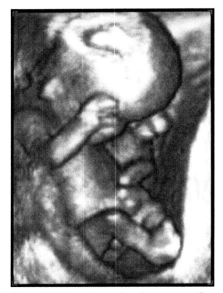 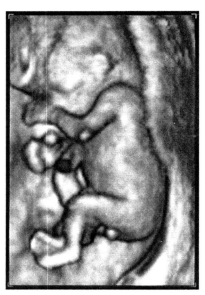

Figure 23. Three-dimensional sonogram of 11-week fetus.

Figure 24. Three-dimensional sonogram of 11-week fetus.

Laboratory and imaging tests can refute or confirm the clinical impression, but are not always absolute. Often, the actual cause of bleeding is never discovered. In the absence of an unequivocal diagnosis, the provider must focus on whether the bleeding is dangerous to the well being of the mother or child, or is a symptom of serious underlying pathology.

Human Chorionic Gonadotropin

Human chorionic gonadotropin (HCG) is primarily produced by placental tissue, and on occasion by malignant tumors, although men and nonpregnant women may produce minute amounts. This hormone is detectable in serum and urine as soon as 8 days after ovulation if pregnancy has occurred.

In early pregnancy, HCG levels can be measured over time to help clinical diagnosis in pregnancies too early for ultrasound diagnosis. Every pregnancy takes a unique interval to establish itself in the uterus. Ovulation does not always occur midcycle, and sperm can live up to 5 days after intercourse, lingering in the fallopian tubes awaiting the ovum. After fertilization, the conceptus may take as many as twelve more days to implant in the uterus, causing even sensitive pregnancy tests to delay recognizing a viable pregnancy. The normal HCG concentration varies widely from pregnancy to pregnancy, and there is variability among laboratories as well. Serial results are more accurate when performed by the same laboratory.

Table 5. HCG Levels during Pregnancy		
After Conception— Week of Pregnancy		**Normal HCG Levels mIU/ml**
1		5–50 (avg. 14)
2		5–50 (avg. 21)
3		5–50 (avg. 42)
4		10–425
5		19–7,340
6		1,080–56,500
7–8		7,650–229,000
9–12		25,700–288,000
13–16		13,300–254,000
17–24		4,060–165,400
25–40		3,640–117,000
The HCG level doubles approximately every 2.2 days during the first trimester of pregnancy. Values vary widely from laboratory to laboratory and from woman to woman.		

Serum HCG rises rapidly until about 41 days of gestation. It is first detectable 7–10 days after ovulation, doubles every 1.6 days during the 5th week, every 48 hr during the 6th week, and every 2.7 days during the 7th week (Sinclair, 2004). HCG then slows its rate of increase until it reaches a peak of approximately 100,000 mIU/ml at 10 weeks and declines to a plateau of approximately 10,000–20,000 mIU/ml in the second and third trimesters.

Quantitative serum blood tests can detect beta-HCG levels as low as 1 mIU/ml. The most sensitive urine tests have a minimum detection threshold of about 20–25 mIU/ml, and become positive about 8–9 days after ovulation. A blood serum level of less than 5 mIU/ml (5 IU/l) can be considered negative and anything above 25 mIU/ml (25 IU/l) positive for pregnancy. Values that fall between these thresholds are equivocal and necessitate further testing.

A single HCG measurement is of little clinical benefit, but serial measurements taken 2 or 3 days apart are helpful in distinguishing a healthy pregnancy from an abnormal one. Monitor the woman at high risk for ectopic pregnancy with serial HCG levels soon after conception to identify an extrauterine pregnancy before symptoms appear. With a viable intra-uterine pregnancy, beta-HCG levels rise an average of 66% every 48 hr in the first 40 days of pregnancy. Only 15% of viable pregnancies will have a rate of increase lower than this, and all viable pregnancies will show at least a 55% increase (Tulandi, 2007a). Levels of HCG that remain steady or rise slowly over 48 hr can also indicate an ectopic pregnancy. Although more than half of all ectopic pregnancies show normal doubling early in gestation, as gestation advances the doubling falls to or below the minimum-doubling threshold of a viable pregnancy.

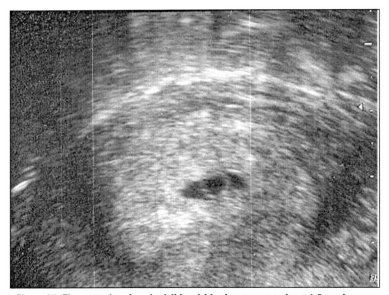

Figure 25. The gestational sac is visible within the uterus at about 4.5 weeks, or when beta-HCG levels reach about 1,800.

Progesterone levels remain constant through the first 10 weeks of pregnancy. Pregnancies associated with a progesterone level under 5 ng/ml are usually nonviable IUPs or ectopic pregnancies, while progesterone levels above 25 ng/ml usually indicate a thriving gestation. Values that fall between these levels are not as useful to diagnosis. Some clinicians supplement with progesterone vaginal suppositories if levels are low, but even administering progesterone to women with luteal-phase defects does not reduce the risk of abortion—and may increase the risk of congenital anomalies (Sinclair, 2004).

 Estimated HCG levels can be remembered by the "rule of 10s": 100 mIU/ml at missed menses, 100,000 mIU/ml at 10 weeks, and 10,000 mIU/ml at term.

The clinician should repeat the HCG level in 72 hr, which will help to correctly classify viable pregnancies that are slow to double. If the HCG levels rise without doubling over 72 hr, the pregnancy is either ectopic or will eventually abort. Once the pregnancy has advanced enough to be visible on sonogram, HCG monitoring is no longer useful.

Dropping levels of beta-HCG can indicate either a nonviable IUP or a spontaneously resolving ectopic pregnancy. Weekly serum HCG levels should be obtained until the result is negative.

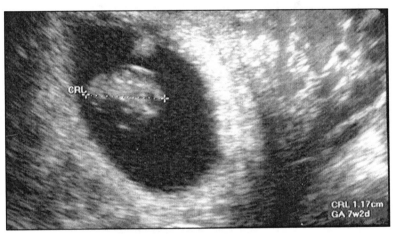

Figure 26. Intrauterine pregnancy at 7 weeks, 2 days.

Ultrasound Examination

Transvaginal ultrasound is the most important tool for confirming the presence or absence of an early IUP, identifying structures at an earlier stage of gestation with greater accuracy than transabdominal scanning. When transvaginal ultrasound and beta-HCG levels are used together, ectopic pregnancy is diagnosed with great accuracy. The discriminatory zone is the HCG level above which a gestational sac should be visible on ultrasound scan. The absence of an intrauterine gestational sac at HCG concentrations greater than 1,800 IU/l (greater than 1,800–3,500 IU/l transabdominally) strongly suggests an ectopic or nonviable IUP. Ectopic pregnancies with a high level of beta-HCG (>10,000 IU/l) are at critical risk for catastrophic tubal rupture.

If at this time transvaginal ultrasound shows a complex adnexal mass and an empty uterus, ectopic pregnancy is almost certain. However, early gestation with multiple embryos can cause high HCG levels without visualization of a pregnancy, and an adnexal mass is not always identified. Less common causes of bleeding, such as hydatidiform mole or partial loss of a multifetal gestation can also be identified on ultrasound. The accuracy of the ultrasound scan vary with the skill of the ultrasonographer, the quality of the equipment, the presence of uterine anomalies, fibroids, or multiple gestation, and the laboratory characteristics of the HCG assay used.

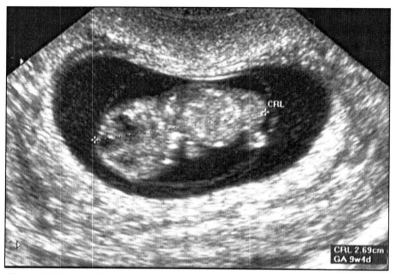

Figure 27. Intrauterine pregnancy at 9 weeks, 4 days.

With ectopic pregnancy, a pseudosac of accumulated fluid in the uterus can be mistaken for a gestational sac, as can endometrial cysts. On Doppler ultrasound, a tubal pregnancy has 20–45% greater blood flow than in the opposite tube, with low impedance and sometimes circular flow (Tulandi, 2007a). Other signs of ectopic pregnancy include visualization of a fluid-filled adnexal mass surrounded by an echogenic ring (bagel sign) and free fluid in the peritoneal cavity or pouch of Douglas. This fluid could indicate bleeding from an ectopic pregnancy or ruptured ovarian cyst. This fluid can also be identified through culdocentesis, but ultrasound is less invasive and yields about the same amount of useful information.

A negative sonogram with HCG levels below the discriminatory zone could indicate an early IUP that may or may not be viable, or an ectopic pregnancy.

Visualization of an IUP excludes the diagnosis of ectopic pregnancy except in rare cases when the embryo has an ectopic twin or is implanted in the uterine cornua. The first sonographic evidence of an IUP is a round gestational sac, visible on transvaginal ultrasound at 4.5–5 weeks' gestation, positioned eccentrically within the uterine fundus beneath the endometrial surface and surrounded by two echogenic rings of chorionic villi. It is visible around the time HCG levels reach 1,800 (Ailsworth, Anderson, Atwood, Bailey, & Canavan, 2006). From 5–6 weeks until about 10 weeks, the yolk sac is visible as a round, echogenic structure within the gestational sac. The embryo first appears as a thickening along the edge of the yolk sac and grows swiftly at the rate of 1 mm/day. By the time the sac is 2 cm in size, an embryo should be seen. When the embryo measures about 5 mm, a heartbeat should be identified on ultrasound, about 3.5–4 weeks post-conception or 5.5–6 weeks after the last menstrual period.

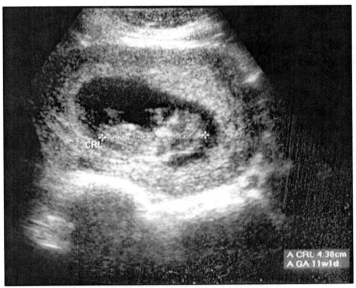

Figure 28. Intrauterine pregnancy at 11 weeks, 1 day.

Table 6. Sonographic Crown-Rump Length and Menstrual Age			
5.7 weeks	0.2 cm	10.4 weeks	3.5 cm
6.1 Weeks	0.4 cm	10.9 Weeks	4.0 cm
7.2 Weeks	1.0 cm	11.7 Weeks	5.0 cm
8.0 Weeks	1.6 cm	12.1 Weeks	5.5 cm
8.6 Weeks	2.0 cm	13.2 Weeks	7.0 cm
9.2 Weeks	2.5 cm	14.0 Weeks	8.0 cm
9.9 Weeks	3.0 cm	Menstrual age (weeks) = Crown-Rump Length (cm) + 6.5	

A misshapen, enlarged, free-floating, or calcified yolk sac is associated with a poor prognosis, as is small sac size or fetal bradycardia below 100 bpm at 5–7 weeks' gestation. A subchorionic hematoma greater than 25% of the gestational sac volume doubles the rate of pregnancy loss, but small or moderate hematomas do not appear to affect outcome (Tulandi & Al-Fozan, 2006). Serial examinations with beta-HCG levels 4–7 days apart can establish viability if findings are unclear or other signs of poor prognosis are present.

A normal yolk sac and fetal heartbeat are reassuring, but not a guarantee of a viable pregnancy, especially for women over 35 and women with repeated pregnancy losses. A separating placenta is difficult to identify on ultrasound examination unless a sizable blood clot has formed behind it. If the ultrasound scan identifies an embryo greater than 5 mm crown to rump without a heartbeat or a gestational sac greater than 18 mm with no fetal pole, the pregnancy is not viable.

✍ AACT—Treat

First Response

> ▶ Early pregnancy bleeding—vital signs stable

Medical treatment is not usually indicated for initial onset of minor spotting.

Bed rest has not been shown to improve outcomes, but the woman should avoid strenuous activity and sexual intercourse.

If bleeding stops, follow up in routine office visit.

For heavy, recurrent or persistent bleeding, or significant pain, refer to physician, assess for viability and for ectopic pregnancy.

> ▶ Vital signs unstable (or likely to become unstable)

The out-of-hospital obstetrical provider's role with the unstable woman with bleeding or lower abdominal pain task is to stabilize her as well as possible, then transfer her care to an appropriate facility as quickly as possible.

Table 7. Ultrasound Dates in Early Pregnancy

When beta-HCG levels reach 1,800–2,000, the gestational sac should be visible on transvaginal ultrasound

If the gestational sac is >10 mm, a yolk sac should be visible

If the gestational sac is 18–25 mm, an embryo should be visible

If the embryo is greater than 5 mm, cardiac motion should be visible

---

Definitive Care

Upon arrival at the hospital, the physician will evaluate laboratory results and perform an ultrasound. If the client's vital signs are not stabilized with infusion of crystalloid solutions, type-specific cross-matched blood transfusion is indicated.

After confirmation of ectopic pregnancy, the physician will determine whether expectant management, laparoscopic or open surgery, or medical management is indicated. Expectant management may be an option when the HCG levels are below 1,000 mIU/ml and dropping, ectopic mass of less than 3 cm, no embryonic heartbeat, and the woman is hemodynamically stable. Women with low, rapidly declining HCG levels can safely choose this option, but it is essential to select clients who are reliable, live near the hospital, and will present for serial blood work until their HCG results are negative.

Table 8. Differential Diagnoses of Vaginal Bleeding in Early Pregnancy

Condition	Usual Symptoms	Symptoms Sometimes Present
Threatened abortion	Bleeding—light or heavy Closed cervix Uterine size equals dates	Cramping and pain in lower abdomen
Ectopic pregnancy	Light bleeding Abdominal pain Closed cervix Empty uterus on ultrasound Complex adnexal mass Beta-HCG slow to rise, plateaued, or slowly dropping Free blood in cul de sac	Fainting Tender adnexal mass Amenorrhea Cervical motion tenderness Peritoneal irritation
Inevitable abortion	Heavy bleeding, clots Dilated cervix Cramping and pain in lower abdomen, may be severe Beta-HCG dropping	No expulsion of products of conception
Incomplete abortion	Heavy bleeding Dilated cervix Partial expulsion of products of conception Cramping and pain in lower abdomen	Fever and foul discharge if infection present Uterine tenderness
Molar pregnancy	Heavy bleeding—often the color of prune juice Dilated cervix Uterus larger than dates and unusually soft Passage of grape-like vesicles Beta-HCG elevated and rising faster than normal Molar tissue visualized on ultrasound	Nausea/vomiting Spontaneous abortion if partial molar pregnancy Cramping and pain in lower abdomen Large cystic ovaries Early-onset preeclampsia No evidence of a fetus

Ectopic Pregnancy

Immediate surgical excision is the definitive treatment if the woman is hemodynamically unstable, the tube has ruptured, an adnexal mass greater than 4 cm is visible on ultrasound, HCG levels are above 5,000 mIU/ml, a fetal heartbeat is detected, or if the woman is unable or unwilling to comply with a medical treatment regimen. In the past, ectopic pregnancy was usually treated with salpingectomy, but today treatment of unruptured ectopic pregnancy usually involves laparoscopically incising the tube and milking the pregnancy out of the distal ampulla. This approach is minimally invasive and preserves tubal function. Alternatively, the section of the tube that contains the embryo is removed, with or without reanastomosis. Laparoscopic surgery decreases blood loss and formation of postoperative adhesions, while reducing cost, hospitalization, and convalescence period. Sometimes laparoscopy is necessary to confirm the diagnosis of ectopic pregnancy when IUP has not been confirmed

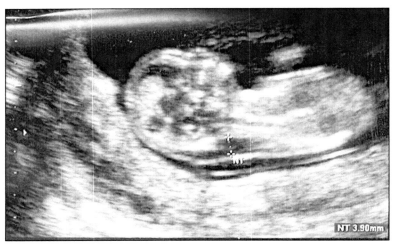

Figure 29. This 12-week fetus has an abnormally wide nuchal translucency measurement, indicating a greater risk of abnormalities.

Women who are hemodynamically unstable or who have cornual pregnancies are treated through laparotomy. Laparotomy is also used in cases of obesity, multiple dense adhesions, and when the surgeon is not experienced in the laparoscopic surgery.

If the ectopic pregnancy is identified early and the woman is compliant with follow-up, medical management with methotrexate injection may be appropriate. Medical therapy is less invasive and easier to recover from than surgery. It may cause less damage to the tube, it is cost effective, and it avoids the need for hospitalization and anesthesia.

Methotrexate is a folic acid antagonist also used to treat leukemia, lymphoma, and carcinomas, for immunosuppression, and in the treatment of severe psoriasis and rheumatoid arthritis. It works by blocking DNA synthesis and cell division, and therefore is lethal to embryos. Methotrexate is especially useful for treating pregnancy implanted on the cervix, ovary, or in the interstitial or the cornual portion of the tube, because in these situations surgical treatment carries a high risk of hemorrhage and may necessitate hysterectomy or oophorectomy. Candidates for methotrexate therapy are hemodynamically stable, reliable for follow-up, and at less than 6 weeks' gestation; their HCG levels are less than 5,000 mIU/ml, their tubal mass is less than 4 cm in diameter on ultrasound, and no embryonic heartbeat is present. About 90–95% of women treated with methotrexate will successfully resolve ectopic pregnancy. The remainder require repeated methotrexate therapy or surgery (Tulandi, 2007a). Serial beta-HCG levels are followed until the results are under 5mIU/ml. If a client receiving methotrexate experiences increased pain, increasing vaginal bleeding, dizziness, tachycardia, palpitations, or syncope, suspect ruptured ectopic pregnancy. Women who are Rh-negative should have an IM injection of anti-D immunoglobulin 300 mcg IM to guard against Rh isoimmunization.

Table 9. OOH Management of Early-Pregnancy Bleeding

(Order of steps may vary)

Airway, breathing, circulation, vital signs

Explain concerns to the woman and her family

Call for EMS and implement emergency transport plan

If the client is hypotensive or tachycardic, start two large-bore intravenous lines of normal saline or lactated Ringer's, run wide

Place in Trendelenberg position

Administer high-flow oxygen

Conduct pelvic examination to localize source of bleeding and check uterine size and tenderness

Remove any tissue from the cervical os and take cultures as indicated

If gestation is beyond first trimester, massage uterus to control bleeding

Consider oxytocin for severe bleeding in incomplete abortion (10–20 units in 1 L of normal saline or lactated Ringer's, wide open)

Transport rapidly to a facility with the capacity for immediate surgery

Chart essential data and history for the receiving facility

Obtain CBC, type, and screen. Consider Anti-D immune globulin

Obtain urinalysis with culture and sensitivities

Less than 8 weeks—obtain quantitative beta-HCG levels every 2–3 days and a single serum progesterone

8–10 weeks—transvaginal ultrasound

10 weeks or greater—fetal heart rate with a Doppler device. If heart tones are not heard or bleeding is significant, proceed to ultrasound.

Spontaneous Abortion

Most early miscarriages complete spontaneously without medical involvement. Medical and surgical interventions are beneficial in the case of incomplete abortion, excessive bleeding or pain, prolonged symptoms, or infection. For the woman with an early fetal demise or blighted ovum, expectant management may be an option for an interval, but curettage or aspiration procedures or misoprostol are of greater benefit. Some women will opt for a surgical evacuation of the uterus at the earliest opportunity

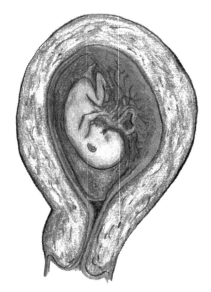

Figure 30. If the pregnancy survives beyond 12 weeks' gestation, odds are good that it will continue to term.

to circumvent the risk of pain and heavy bleeding and because of psychological resistance to carrying a dead fetus. Intravaginal misoprostol is a safe and effective alternative to surgery in these circumstances, increasing blood loss, but causing less pain, trauma, and infection than surgical intervention. Obstetric indications remain an "off-label" use for misoprostol.

After the uterus is empty, methylergonovine (Methergine) 0.2 mg PO may be given to decrease bleeding every 4 hr for 6 doses. Ibuprofen 800 mg PO q6–8 hr prn is effective for pain, If risk factors for infection are present, doxycycline 100 mg PO may be prescribed bid for 4–7 days.

Considerations for Limited-Resource Settings

Misoprostol treatment is valuable in limited-resource settings, including developing countries, because it is inexpensive, easy to store, and is appropriate for use in locations without surgical capabilities. The dose is 400mcg by mouth or 600–800 mcg intravaginally.

ANTEPARTAL BLEEDING— SECOND HALF OF PREGNANCY

AACT and ReACT
ALERT—Be alert ▶ Exercise hypervigilant attention
ANALYZE—Think about possible causes
CONSIDER—Use OLDCART ▶ Gather data
TREAT—Make first response ▶ Proceed to definitive care
ReACT | ReAssess ▶ ReConsider ▶ Re-Treat

✍ AACT—Alert

Antepartum and intrapartum hemorrhage are defined as significant bleeding after 20 weeks' gestation. Major causes include placenta previa (20%) and placental abruption (30%) (Norwitz & Park, 2007). Other common causes include trauma secondary to a pelvic examination or sexual intercourse; infection; or bloody show—capillary disruption associated with term or preterm labor. Less often, late-second and third-trimester bleeding may indicate uterine rupture, vasa previa, cervical hemangioma, or cervicovaginal neoplasm. Many causes of third-trimester bleeding—placental abruption, uterine rupture, vasa previa, and placenta previa—are obstetrical emergencies that may result in hypovolemic shock and fetal death.

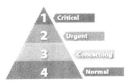

Late-pregnancy bleeding can be priority 1, 2, 3, or 4. Determining acuity is an important aspect of management.

Table 10. Possible Causes of Late-Pregnancy Bleeding	
Placenta previa	Uterine rupture
Abruptio placentae	Vasa previa
Trauma	Cervical hemangioma
Infection	Cervico-vaginal neoplasm
Labor	

✍ AACT—Analyze

▶ Why is she bleeding?

Placenta Previa

Significant bleeding from placenta previa—priority 1 or 2

Placenta previa refers to placental implantation in the lower uterine segment, partially or completely covering the cervical os. In the third trimester, when the lower uterine segment gradually thins in preparation for the onset of labor, this placental attachment begins to shear, and painless bleeding results. Thrombin release from the bleeding sites stimulates uterine contractions, which in turn cause more separation and bleeding.

Bleeding occurs before 36 weeks' gestation in almost two thirds of women with placenta previa, and half of this number present with bleeding before 30 weeks' gestation. Typically, the first bleeding episode is minimal, and each subsequent hemorrhage is more copious. The initial bleeding usually resolves, and then recurs with labor. As the cervix dilates, the placental implantation site is disrupted, and free flowing hemorrhage may result. Placenta previa carries a perinatal mortality rate up to 10% (Gilbert, 2007).

Placenta previa and low-lying placenta can be found in 5% of all second-trimester pregnancies, often identified as an incidental finding on ultrasound at 20–24 weeks' gestation. Ninety percent of these will resolve by 30 weeks' gestation (Ailsworth, et al., 2006). The lower uterine segment develops as pregnancy

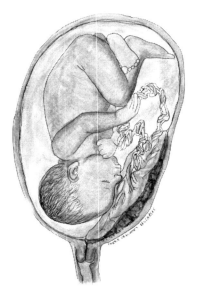

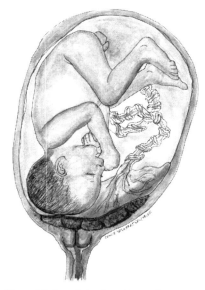

Figure 31. Marginal placenta previa occurs when the placental edge is near or partially overlaps the cervical os.

Figure 32. Complete placenta previa occurs when the placenta completely covers the cervical os.

progresses, and by term placenta previa affects only 3–5 pregnancies per 1,000. The condition is more likely to persist if the placenta completely covers the os or overlaps the os by more than 2.5 cm, or if there is a history of prior cesarean delivery. Multiple cesarean sections increase the risk of previa to as much as 10% (Ailsworth, et al.).

Endometrial or myometrial damage and conditions that prevent placental migration increase risk of placenta previa (Gilbert, 2007). Other risk factors include age over 35, multiparity, assisted reproduction, multiple gestation, erythroblastosis, Müllerian anomalies such as bicornuate uterus, closely spaced pregnancies, tobacco or cocaine use, and short interpregnancy interval. The recurrence rate in future pregnancies is 4–8% (Gilbert).

Placenta previa is classified in relation to how much placenta encroaches across or near the os.

▶ **Marginal placenta previa** (25–50%)—placenta encroaches on the edge of the cervical os.

▶ **Partial placenta previa** (30%,)—placenta partially covers the cervical os

▶ **Complete or total placenta previa** (20–45%)—placenta occludes the cervical os.

▶ **Low-lying placenta**—placenta implants in the lower part of the uterus, within 2–3 cm from the os. A low-lying placenta may resolve as the pregnancy progresses.

Half of women with placenta previa deliver prematurely, increasing perinatal mortality. Some obstetricians place a cerclage in hope of decreasing the risk of preterm birth, but as of this writing the practice has yet to become standard of care. Placenta previa is also associated with fetal malformations and intrauterine growth restriction.

Women with bright red, painless vaginal bleeding in the second half of pregnancy are suspected to have placenta previa until proven otherwise. Abruption or labor may also be present, causing the woman to experience pain unrelated to the previa itself. Do not perform a digital examination until the diagnosis of placenta previa is excluded; if the placenta is over the os, the examiner's finger could disrupt the placenta and create an uncontrollable hemorrhage.

First Thought, Worst Thought

What is the most likely cause of late-pregnancy bleeding?

Postcoital spotting or other capillary disruption

What is the worst it could be?

Placental abruption, placenta previa, uterine rupture, preterm labor, vasa previa.

Placental Abruption
Usually priority 1 or 2

Placental abruption (*abruptio placentae*) refers to partial or complete separation of the placenta from the uterine wall prior to delivery of the fetus. Most abruptions result from an ongoing pathologic vascular process, but some follow acute events, such as trauma. The complications of severe abruption can be devastating, including severe blood loss, fetal anoxia, disseminated intravascular coagulation (DIC), the need for hysterectomy, and even death. Even a small abruption can cause prematurity, intrauterine growth restriction, and fetal anemia. The amount of vaginal bleeding does indicate the extent of abruption, but fetal demise suggests that more than half the placenta has detached. If abruption is severe enough to cause fetal death, the woman is likely to develop DIC within an hour or two after abrupting.

Placental abruption is a major cause of perinatal mortality and morbidity. Risk increases with trauma, prior abruption, placental abnormalities, inherited thrombophilias such as factor V Leiden, oligohydramnios, male fetus, and prior cesarean delivery, trauma, uterine anomaly or fibroids, preterm premature rupture of the membranes, unexplained elevated   levels, bleeding disorders, and rapid decompression of a uterus overstretched by multiple pregnancy or polyhydramnios. The placenta that implants over a uterine abnormality or myoma is poorly anchored and unstable and thus prone to abruption. Grand multiparas are at increased risk, probably due to the placental sites of prior pregnancies causing endometrial scarring, or aberrant uterine vasculature. Older pregnant women are more likely to have vascular disease and therefore are more likely to have faulty placentation and subsequent abruption. One in 10 women who use cocaine in the third trimester will experience an abruption.

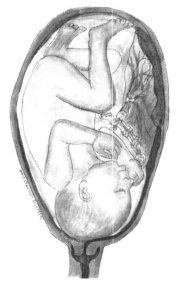 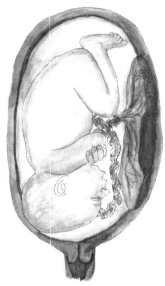

Figure 33. Marginal abruption occurs when the edge of the placenta separates from the uterine wall, causing bleeding.

Figure 34. Concealed abruption involves bleeding behind the placenta while the margins remain intact, forming a painful hematoma that blocks perfusion without frank bleeding.

Women who smoke before and during pregnancy are at much greater risk of abruption than non-smokers; for every 10 cigarettes smoked daily, the risk increases by 20%. The woman with chronic hypertension or preeclampsia is more likely to suffer abruption severe enough to cause stillbirth, probably due to abnormal trophoblastic invasion of uteroplacental arteries in the first and second trimesters. Antihypertensive medications do not reduce this risk. Smoking not only contributes to hypertension, it also synergistically increases the likelihood of abruption if hypertension occurs because nicotine constricts vessels already compromised by hypertension.

When abruption occurs, bleeding develops behind the placenta as defective maternal vessels in the decidua basalis rupture at the interface with the placental villi. The collecting blood separates the placenta from the uterus and creates a barrier between the villi and the maternal blood supply. A hematoma forms. In the case of a severe abruption, the hematoma may dissect through the placental-decidual interface until most of the placenta has detached and is unable to unable to exchange gases and nutrients.

Prostaglandin release and irritating free blood causes uterine spasm, which also interferes with perfusion. The fetus becomes hypoxic from the impaired

3: BLEEDING IN PREGNANCY

gas exchange of the separating placenta and the uterine contraction squeezing off the blood supply.

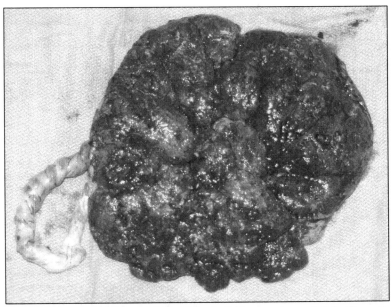

Figure 35. Placenta of heavy smoker at 37 weeks. Tobacco use is associated with small, calcified placentas and high risk of abruption, stillbirth, and preterm delivery.

The same placental/decidual inflammation that can cause abruption can also cause preterm rupture of the membranes. Neutrophils are attracted to fibrin deposits formed by thrombin at the site of decidual hemorrhage, and release material that breaks down membranes. Thrombin may also cause uterine contractions. Conversely, a long latency between rupture of membranes and delivery increases the risk of abruption, most likely secondary to progressive inflammatory processes.

Trauma such as a fall or motor vehicle accident commonly causes abruption through rapid deceleration, even without direct injury to the abdomen. Because the uterine myometrium is more elastic than the comparatively rigid placenta, the uterus stretches, but the placenta does not. Instead, it shears from the uterine wall. Abruptions related to trauma are often catastrophic, and are most likely to present within 24 hr of the incident.

Diagnosis can be difficult. Because there is no definitive test to diagnose abruption with any accuracy, the provider must rely on signs and symptoms confirmed by evaluation of the placenta after delivery. Most typically, the woman will have a small to moderate amount of bleeding with or without abdominal or back pain, an inconclusive sonogram report, and a reassuring fetal heart rate.

Placental abruption may present with vaginal bleeding (>80%), abdominal pain (>50%), uterine hyper stimulation (contractions may be tetanic or frequent with no break between), uterine rigidity, backache, and uterine tenderness (Gillen-Goldstein, 2008). Fetal heart-rate abnormalities or fetal demise can result from maternal hypotension or from a significant decrease in the functional placental surface area perfused.

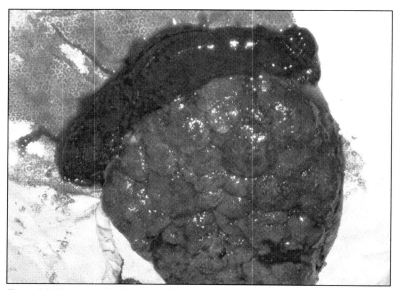

Figure 36. Placenta with abruption. This placenta's small size, congested appearance, and abundant calcification indicate that the woman was at high risk for abruption. The large adherent clot and smaller clots in other locations indicate that the abruption was severe and involved a large portion of the placental surface area. Fortunately, emergency cesarean section was performed, and mother and baby were stabilized.

Bleeding may occur behind the placenta while the margins remain intact, forming a painful hematoma which blocks perfusion without frank bleeding. In other cases, bleeding is torrential, and can even include passage of placental fragments through the vagina. Sometimes blood moves through the membranes to dye the amniotic fluid a distinctive "port wine" color or extravasates into the uterine muscle (Couvelaire uterus). Disseminated intravascular coagulation (DIC) may occur, especially when abruption is severe enough to cause fetal death.

Treatment involves consideration of gestational age and the stability of mother and fetus. Abruption at term or cases of maternal or fetal compromise should be delivered. Vaginal delivery in a tertiary care hospital may be an option if mother and infant are stable. Labor complicated by abruption is usually turbulent and quick. If mother or viable fetus is unstable or labor fails to progress, cesarean delivery is indicated. Cesarean is sometimes necessary for maternal indications alone.

If mother and a fetus are relatively stable, the provider can manage the client expectantly, and consider tocolysis and betamethasone as clinically indicated.

Tocolytics delay delivery by an average of 7 days, which buys enough time to derive maximal benefit from corticosteroid therapy.

The severity of placental abruption can be categorized by grade:

▶ Grade 0—Retrospective diagnosis of placental abruption, no obvious symptoms

▶ Grade 1—vaginal bleeding only

▶ Grade 2—vaginal bleeding, concealed hemorrhage, uterine tenderness, nonreassuring fetal heart rate

▶ Grade 3—vaginal bleeding, shock, extensive concealed hemorrhage, uterine tenderness, and fetal death. One third of grade-3 clients will have coagulopathy.

Vasa Previa and Velamentous Umbilical Cord
Priority 1 if bleeding

A velamentous cord has vessels that run through the fetal membranes instead of being insulated in a layer of Wharton's jelly. This usually involves the section of the umbilical cord nearest the placental insertion, or it involves vessels running between lobes of a placenta. Velamentous insertion occurs in about 1 singleton pregnancy out of 100, but occurs more often with monochorionic twins and placenta previa. A two-vessel umbilical cord has a velamentous insertion about 12% of the time (Russo-Stieglitz & Lockwood, 2007).

Although velamentous cord insertion is sometimes identified on ultrasound, diagnosis is usually not made during pregnancy, and failure to recognize the condition antenatally is not a breach of the standard of care. Velamentous umbilical cord is sometimes associated with intrauterine growth restriction, premature delivery, congenital anomalies, low Apgar scores, retained placenta, and bleeding. Velamentous vessels can also rupture, causing fetal hemorrhage and often death.

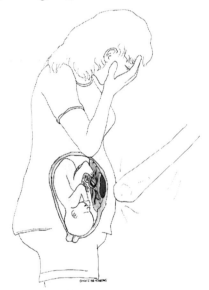

Figure 37. Blunt abdominal trauma can cause placental abruption.

Vasa previa is a rare condition in which the velamentous vessels cross the membranes of the lower uterine segment in front of the fetal presenting part. If these vessels rupture, the fetus can exsanguinate. Rupture of the vessels can occur with or without rupture of the membranes, resulting in a vaginal hemorrhage consisting of fetal blood. These vessels are also vulnerable to compression from the fetal presenting part.

Vasa previa is more common in pregnancies with a second-trimester low-lying placenta or placenta previa even if it has resolved, pregnancies resulting from assisted reproductive technologies, and women with bi-lobed and succenturiate lobe placentas in the lower uterine segment. On ultrasound examination, vasa previa can be differentiated from a funic presentation (cord is presenting part) by repositioning the mother into Trendelenberg; a cord will shift position, a vasa previa will not.

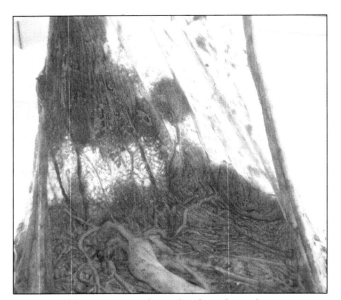

Figure 38. Velamentous vessels running through membranes to a succenturiate lobe.

Rarely, vessels are palpable on vaginal examination across the presenting membranes. Consider vasa previa when vaginal bleeding occurs with rupture of membranes, along with a nonreassuring fetal heart pattern such as sinusoidal. In the case of vasa previa, only an emergent cesarean section can save the fetus. The hemorrhage consists of fetal blood, and a term fetus only contains about 250 ml of blood. Suggested management for an antenatally diagnosed vasa previa is twice weekly nonstress testing at 28–30 weeks' gestation, and possible hospital admission with continuous monitoring after 32 weeks, prepared for emergency delivery if fetal distress or hemorrhage occur. The goal is delivery by cesarean once fetal lung maturity has been established.

Uterine Rupture
Priority 1

Uterine rupture is defined as the full-thickness separation of the uterine wall and the overlying serosa. This is an infrequent complication, even for the woman with a previously scarred uterus, but carries serious consequences for both mother and fetus, including hemorrhage, fetal distress, and expulsion of the fetus into the abdominal cavity. Uterine rupture requires rapid delivery by cesarean section and may necessitate hysterectomy, and it carries a 5% mortality rate for the mother and 50% for the fetus. Thirteen percent of uterine ruptures happen outside the hospital (Ailsworth, et al., 2006).

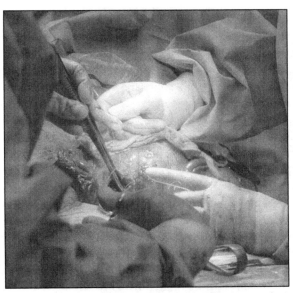

Figure 39. Uterine repair. A uterus scarred by prior cesarean is at higher risk for uterine rupture, but most cases involve uterine-scar dehiscence rather than frank rupture.

Uterine scar dehiscence is the separation of a prior uterine scar without disrupting the visceral peritoneum, often involving minimal bleeding and no fetal distress (Cunningham, et al., 2005). The fetus, placenta, and umbilical cord remain within the uterus. While uterine rupture during pregnancy is rare and catastrophic, uterine scar dehiscence is more commonplace and seldom results in poor maternal or fetal outcome. Uterine scarring from a prior cesarean is a significant risk factor for uterine rupture, but in most cases it involves uterine-scar dehiscence rather than frank uterine rupture.

Risk for uterine rupture for a woman with a normal, unscarred uterus is about 1 in 7440 pregnancies (Nahum & Pham, 2008). The risk of uterine rupture is increased by fetal macrosomia; short interpregnancy interval; malformed uterus; obstructed labor; multiparity (four or more prior deliveries); malpresentations; labor induction; blunt trauma; cocaine use; and uterine surgeries such as cesarean section, uterine myomectomy, or repair of a Müllerian defect. Pasupathy and Dobbie (2004) found that while uterine rupture is not more common in smaller hospitals, it is three times more likely to result in death of the infant at these facilities. A meta-analysis in the *British Medical Journal* found that compared with elective repeat cesarean delivery, trial of labor increased the risk of uterine rupture by 2.7 per 1000 cases and did not increase maternal mortality (Guise, et al., 2004). The additional risk of perinatal death from rupture of a uterine scar was 1.4 per 10,000 and the additional risk of hysterectomy was 3.4 per 10,000. They concluded that obstetricians would need to perform 370 elective cesarean deliveries to prevent one symptomatic uterine rupture.

Any uterine scarring increases the risk for uterine rupture. The woman with a "classical" vertical uterine incision is especially vulnerable, with one third of these ruptures occurring before labor begins. It is important to obtain the operative report: a woman may have a horizontal scar across her abdomen and a vertical one on the uterus. One study showed that women who deliver vaginally after two previous cesarean deliveries had a rupture risk 5 times greater than the woman who had a single previous cesarean. History of a prior successful vaginal birth reduces the risk, and the 2004 ACOG guidelines suggest that the woman with a prior vaginal delivery and two previous cesareans can be a candidate for vaginal birth after cesarean (VBAC). Risk increases when a woman with prior cesarean has a lower uterine segment thickness of less than 3.5 mm on transabdominal ultrasonography at 36–38 weeks' gestation.

Major fetal morbidity develops within 10–37 min of uterine rupture and includes acidosis, hypoxic-ischemic encephalopathies with impaired motor development, and death (Nahum & Pham, 2008). Maternal morbidity includes significant bladder injuries such as ruptured bladder or accidental cystotomy, severe blood loss often resulting in hypovolemic shock, or the need for hysterectomy. Maternal death is rare in developed nations, but in developing countries 5–10% of women suffering uterine rupture will die (Nahum & Pham).

Uterine rupture is a true emergency requiring rapid and decisive intervention. Classic signs and symptoms include fetal heart-rate abnormalities, decreased baseline uterine tone, loss of uterine contractility, abdominal pain, recession of the presenting fetal part, hemorrhage, and shock. In actual practice, the signs and symptoms are ambiguous.

Prolonged, late, or recurrent variable decelerations or fetal bradycardias are often the only signs of uterine rupture. Maternal abdominal pain is an unreliable sign, and occurs in only about 22% of uterine ruptures (Nahum & Pham, 2008). Uterine tetany (contraction > 90 seconds) and hyperstimulation (more than 5 contractions in 10 minutes) are not often associated with uterine rupture. Decreased uterine tone and diminished uterine activity are also uncommon signs. Vaginal bleeding is present in 11–67% of uterine ruptures, and maternal hypovolemic shock occurs in 29–46% (Nahum & Pham).

The longer fetal bradycardia or decelerations persist before delivery, the greater the risk of asphyxia. Sudden uterine rupture is least likely to result in poor outcomes for the baby if he has good reserves at the time of rupture and is delivered immediately via cesarean. Rapid intervention decreases mortality, but does not necessarily prevent severe metabolic acidosis or serious neonatal disease. Long-term outcomes are good for the vast majority of babies delivered 18–37 min after onset of bradycardia or decelerations (Nahum & Pham, 2008).

A 2004 study of women attempting to VBAC in out-of-hospital birth centers showed a 0.2% incidence of uterine rupture for women with a single prior cesarean and gestational age <42 weeks. Half of uterine ruptures and 57% of perinatal deaths involved women with more than one previous cesarean delivery or who were ≥42 weeks' gestation (Lieberman, Ernst, Rooks, Stapleton & Flamm, 2004). Researchers included CNMs who hoped to demonstrate the safety of VBAC in birth centers. Instead, they concluded that birth centers should refer women with prior cesarean births to hospitals for delivery because of the high rate of complications associated with VBAC.

AACT—Consider
Evaluating Bleeding
Heavy bleeding in the second half of pregnancy is almost always serious. A careful speculum examination can help to localize the source of bleeding. If the cervix has begun to open, you may observe the white bulge of membranes in the cervical os. A large balloon of membranes can mean complete dilation or a partially dilated cervix with membranes protruding hourglass-fashion through the cervix. Take care not to jostle the cervix with the speculum, as this can disrupt a placenta previa and cause torrential hemorrhage. Observing blood coming through the cervix differentiates a uterine etiology from a vaginal cause.

While a digital examination is an important part of the evaluation of a woman with early pregnancy bleeding, this procedure can trigger uncontrollable hemorrhage in the client with placenta previa. Defer the digital examination until after placenta previa has been excluded. Ultrasound is necessary to localize the placental location, but it is unlikely to show abruption. Transvaginal ultrasound can determine whether the placenta is across the cervical os and identify a shortened or funneling cervix indicating preterm labor.

In a classical presentation of placenta previa, vaginal bleeding is bright red and painless, and it tends to recur. The uterus is soft and not tender. The fetus is easy to palpate, out of the pelvis and is likely to be a breech or transverse presentation. Heart tones are usually reassuring.

In contrast, placental abruption classically presents with abdominal pain; rigid, tender uterus; fetal parts difficult to palpate; and sometimes shock with symptoms beyond vaginal blood loss. In other cases, abruption with a Couvelaire uterus may cause uterine atony, which can lead to postpartum hemorrhage severe enough to require hysterectomy. Mark the fundal height and time directly on the abdomen with an ink pen—concealed abruption may show a progressive rise in fundal height over time.

Uterine rupture can present subtly or dramatically, typically with nonspecific signs and symptoms. Often, by the time the diagnosis is evident, mother and fetus are already compromised. Symptoms include bleeding, nonreassuring fetal heart rate, increasing abdominal girth, maternal tachycardia, sudden change in the character of labor pain at the peak of a contraction, increased abdominal tenderness (or unusual patterns of pain radiation), or severe shock. The woman may feel the sensation of "something tearing inside" or may experience very little discomfort.

Contractions often continue after uterine rupture. Free blood in the peritoneal cavity can cause chest or shoulder pain, mimicking pulmonary embolism. The fetus may suddenly become easy to palpate if it has been expelled from the uterus into the abdomen. The fetus may kick violently upon rupture, then fall still.

✎ AACT—Treat

First Response

When a woman is bleeding significantly in the second trimester, act quickly and decisively, considering the worst case scenario first. The priority is rapid transport and stabilization. Emergency treatment of antepartal hemorrhage begins with ABCs and treatment of shock. Signs of shock include a rapid and thready pulse; pale, clammy skin; restlessness and anxiety; and nausea. Blood pressure usually remains stable until about 30% of blood volume is lost, then plummets when the woman is no longer able to compensate (Gilbert, 2007).

If you can begin to stabilize the woman without delaying transport she will benefit, but rapid transport to a hospital with the capacity for immediate surgery is vital. Give high flow oxygen, position the woman on her left side with her head at or below heart level and feet elevated on a thick pillow. Start two large-bore (16- or 18-gauge) IV lines and replenish the intravascular volume with crystalloid solution like lactated Ringer's or normal saline until blood products are available. Monitor the fetal heart tones closely. If blood loss has caused severe hypovolemia, EMS may utilize pneumatic anti-shock garments. Bloodwork includes hematocrit, platelet count, fibrinogen, prothrombin time, activated partial thromboplastin time, blood type and Rh, and Betke (KB) test. Providers at the hospital will probably crossmatch 2–4 units of packed red blood cells.

If no laboratory is available, test fibrinogen levels by drawing 5 ml of blood into a red-top tube and putting it aside. If fibrinogen levels are normal, a clot should form within 10 min. If the fibrinogen level is abnormally low, the blood will not clot.

Definitive Care

In the hospitalized nonpregnant client, blood products are usually transfused when the estimated blood loss from hemorrhage exceeds 30% of blood volume or when the hemoglobin is less than 10 g/dl. These values, however, may reflect the pregnant woman's baseline, so the provider must closely monitor bleeding, blood pressure, maternal and fetal heart rates, peripheral perfusion, and urine output to determine when transfusion is indicated. If 2 L of crystalloid fails to correct hypotension, a transfusion may be beneficial.

Rh (D)-negative women should receive Rh (D)-immune globulin when bleeding occurs. It may be necessary to redose the Rh-negative mother if bleeding occurs after 3 weeks or in the case of a large fetomaternal hemorrhage. A Kleihauer-Betke test quantifies the amount of fetal cells in the maternal circulation and determines the amount of Rh (D)-immune globulin necessary to prevent isoimmunization.

If the fetus is viable, the fetal heart rate is continuously monitored for non-reassuring patterns such as loss of reactivity, minimal variability, tachycardia, late decelerations, or a sinusoidal heart rate. Some hospitals monitor the maternal heart rhythm on a cardiac monitor. Maternal vital signs and urine output are closely followed. Vaginal blood loss can be accurately measured by weighing perineal pads.

The obstetrician will move to immediate delivery for uncontrolled maternal hemorrhage, major vaginal bleeding after 34 weeks' gestation, or fetal distress not improved by maternal oxygen therapy, left-sided positioning, and intravascular volume replacement.

Placental Abruption

The provider must consider the gestational age of the fetus, wellbeing of mother and fetus, and the Bishop score of the cervix when considering delivery options. Placental abruption accounts for about 15% of all neonatal deaths, and 30% of deaths from abruption occur within 2 hr of arrival at the hospital (Simpson & Creehan, 2007). Conservative management is an option for minor abruption if the woman is remote from term. The client is managed in the hospital until her bleeding has stopped and her lab work and fetal status are reassuring. The risk of a second abruption is high. The provider should consider corticosteroid administration between 24 and 34 weeks' gestation to accelerate lung maturation in the event of preterm delivery. In some cases of stable abruption with preterm labor, tocolytics are employed to prolong the pregnancy until corticosteroids take effect.

At or near term, immediate delivery is usually the safest option. If the woman is parous and hemodynamically stable, if labor is progressing normally, and if fetal status is reassuring, vaginal birth might be attempted. The provider must exercise caution; abruption is often associated with rapid, intense labor that can decrease placental perfusion and can cause fetal hypoxia.

Cesarean delivery may be indicated in the case of severe hemorrhage or DIC, uterine rigidity, previous uterine surgery, or nonreassuring fetal heart-rate tracing. In abruption, blood loss may be greater with vaginal delivery than with surgical birth. When abruption occurs at the threshold of viability, maternal risks of cesarean section may outweigh the potential benefit to the fetus.

Placenta Previa

Women with placenta previa should be informed of the risk of severe intra-partum and postpartum bleeding, including the possible need for transfusion and hysterectomy. Hemorrhage secondary to placenta previa is an obstetrical emergency and immediate delivery is necessary. Placenta previa almost always necessitates cesarean delivery. While the stable woman with a reassuring fetal heart tracing may have regional anesthesia, emergent cesarean performed for heavy bleeding usually requires general anesthesia.

Occasionally vaginal delivery can be accomplished with an anterior marginal previa, because the descending fetal head may compress the placental bed and decrease bleeding. Because the lower uterine segment is less able to contract following delivery, potential for postpartum hemorrhage is great. Vaginal delivery of a complete previa is infrequently considered in the case of fetal demise or pre-viable fetus, if blood loss is not excessive. If placenta is low-lying, women can often deliver vaginally without hemorrhage if the placenta is greater than 2.0 centimeters from the internal os.

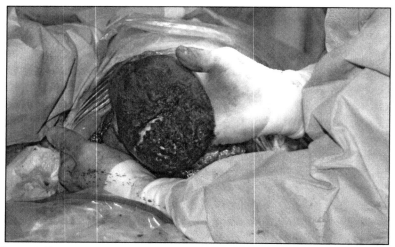

Figure 40. The woman with bleeding episodes of increasing severity or frequency or with a shortened cervix or persistent contractions is delivered expeditiously by cesarean.

Most women with symptomatic placenta previa (i.e., any amount of bleeding) are admitted to the antepartum unit and managed expectantly. Recurrent bleeding episodes can occur unexpectedly and may be copious. Some providers will discharge women with placenta previa 48 hr after bleeding stops if they can get to the hospital quickly if bleeding recurs, are compliant with bed rest, and are willing to accept the risks of outpatient management.

About half of these women are still pregnant a month after the first episode of bleeding. Even women with blood loss greater than 500 cc can often maintain pregnancy for an additional 2 weeks or more. Tocolysis may be indicated if bleeding has stopped and contractions persist and the fetus is less than 34 weeks. The provider should initiate corticosteroid therapy if bleeding from placenta previa occurs at 24–34 weeks' gestation.

If the woman is stable, amniocentesis is typically performed at 36 weeks' gestation to determine fetal lung maturity. Preemptive cesarean is performed when the fetal lungs are developed to minimize the risk of emergent delivery and hemorrhage. If lungs are immature at 36 weeks, amniocentesis is repeated at 37 weeks. If the fetal lungs are still immature, the baby will be delivered at 38 weeks without repeat testing.

Blood transfusion is often required during surgery if hemorrhage is excessive. Five to 10% of previas are also placenta accreta, making cesarean hysterectomy sometimes necessary.

Uterine Rupture

Successful outcome for uterine rupture is directly related to early recognition of signs and symptoms and short interval between onset and surgical treatment. Hysterectomy is the definitive treatment for intractable uterine bleeding, multiple rupture sites, or longitudinal laceration. The surgeon may elect to repair the uterus for a low transverse laceration without extension to the broad ligament or cervix, if hemorrhage is controlled, there is no evidence of coagulopathy, and the woman wants to have more children.

BIBLIOGRAPHY

Ailsworth, K., Anderson, J., Atwood, L.A., Bailey, R.E., & Canavan, T. (2006). *ALSO: Advanced life support in obstetrics* (4th ed.). Leawood, KS: American Academy of Family Practice Physicians.

Chasen, S.T., & Chervenak, F.A. (2007a). Antepartum assessment of twin gestations. In B.D. Rose (Ed.), *UpToDate*. Wellesley, MA: UpToDate.

Cunningham, F., Grant, N., Leveno, K., Gilstrap, L., Hauth, J., & Wenstrom, K. (2005). *Williams obstetrics* (22nd ed.). New York: McGraw-Hill.

Gabbe, S.G., Niebyl, J.R., & Simpson, J.L., Eds. (2007). *Obstetrics: Normal and problem pregnancies* (5th ed.). New York: Churchill Livingstone.

Gilbert, E.S. (2007). *Manual of high risk pregnancy and delivery* (4th ed.). St Louis: Mosby.

Gillen-Goldstein, J. (2008). Clinical features and diagnosis of abruptio placentae. In B.D. Rose (Ed.), *UpToDate*. Wellesley, MA: UpToDate.

Gruenberg, Bonnie U. (2005). *Essentials of prehospital maternity care.* Upper Saddle River, NJ: Prentice Hall.

Guise, J.-M., McDonagh, M.S., Osterweil, P., Nygren, P., Chan, B.K.S., & Helfand, M. (2004). Systematic review of the incidence and consequences of uterine rupture in women with previous caesarean section [Electronic version]. *British Medical Journal, 329* (7456), 19–25. Retrieved May 10, 2008, from http://www.bmj.com/ cgi/content/full/329/7456/19

Hamman, A.K., Wang, N.E., & Chona, S. (2006). The pregnant adolescent with vaginal bleeding: Etiology, diagnosis, and management. *Pediatric Emergency Care, 22*(10), 761–767.

Heppard, M., & Garite, T. (2002). *Acute obstetrics: A practical guide* (3rd ed.). St. Louis: Mosby.

Hladky, K., & Yankowitz, J. (2002). Placental abruption. *Obstetrical and Gynecological Survey, 57* (5), 299–305.

Ladewig, P., London, M., Moberly, S., & Olds, S. (2002). *Contemporary maternal-newborn nursing care.* Upper Saddle River, NJ: Prentice Hall.

Leung, L.L.K. (2007). Clinical features, diagnosis, and treatment of disseminated intravascular coagulation in adults. In B.D. Rose (Ed.), *UpToDate*. Wellesley, MA: UpToDate.

Lieberman, E., Ernst, E.K., Rooks, J.P., Stapleton, S., & Flamm, B. (2004). Results of the national study of vaginal birth after cesarean in birth centers. *Obstetrics & Gynecology, 104* (5), 933–942.

Lockwood, C.J., & Russo-Stieglitz, K. (2008a). Management of placenta previa. In B.D. Rose (Ed.), *UpToDate*. Wellesley, MA: UpToDate.

Nahum, G.G., & Pham, K.Q. (2008). *Uterine rupture in pregnancy* (eMedicine, topic 3399). Retrieved May 10, 2008, from http://www.emedicine.com/ med/ topic 3746.htm

Newberry, L. (Ed.). (2003). *Sheehy's emergency nursing: Principles and practice* (5th ed.). St. Louis: Mosby.

Norwitz, E.R., & Park, J.S. (2007). Overview of the etiology and evaluation of vaginal bleeding in pregnant women. In B.D. Rose (Ed.), *UpToDate*. Wellesley, MA: UpToDate.

Pearlman, M., Tintinalli, J., & Dyne, P. (2004). *Obstetric and gynecologic emergencies: Diagnosis and management*. New York: McGraw-Hill.

Queenan, J., Hobbins, J., & Spong, C. (Eds.). (2005). *Protocols for high-risk pregnancies* (4th ed). Hoboken, NJ: Wiley-Blackwell.

Ratcliffe, S.D., Baxley, E.G., Cline, M.K., & Sakornbut, E.L. (2008). *Family medicine obstetrics* (3rd ed.). Philadelphia: Mosby Elsevier.

Russo-Stieglitz, K., & Lockwood, C.J. (2007). Placenta previa and vasa previa. In B.D. Rose (Ed.), *UpToDate*. Wellesley, MA: UpToDate.

Simpson, K.R., & Creehan, P.A. (2007). *AWHONN's perinatal nursing* (3rd ed.). Hagerstown, MD: Lippincott Williams & Wilkins.

Sinclair, C. (2004). *A midwife's handbook*. St. Louis: Saunders.

Smith, G.C.S., Pell, J.P., Pasupathy, D., & Dobbie, R. (2004). Factors predisposing to perinatal death related to uterine rupture during attempted vaginal birth after caesarean section: Retrospective cohort study. *British Medical Journal, 329* (7462), 375–377.

Tenore, J.L. (2000). Ectopic pregnancy [Electronic version]. *American Family Physician, 61* (4), 1080–1088. Retrieved May 10, 2008, from http://www.aafp.org/ afp/20000215/1080.html

Tulandi, T. (2007a). Cervical pregnancy. In B.D. Rose (Ed.), *UpToDate*. Wellesley, MA: UpToDate.

Tulandi, T. (2007b). Clinical manifestations, diagnosis, and management of ectopic pregnancy. In B.D. Rose (Ed.), *UpToDate*. Wellesley, MA: UpToDate.

Tulandi, T., & Al-Fozan, H.M. (2006). Spontaneous abortion: Risk factors, etiology, clinical manifestations, and diagnostic evaluation. In B.D. Rose (Ed.), *UpToDate*. Wellesley, MA: UpToDate.

Tulandi, T., & Al-Fozan, H.M. (2007). Definition and etiology of recurrent pregnancy loss. In B.D. Rose (Ed.), *UpToDate*. Wellesley, MA: UpToDate.

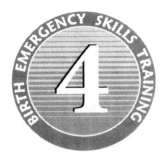

Postpartum Hemorrhage

OBJECTIVES

▶ Compare and contrast expectant management and active management of the third stage of labor.

▶ List three definitions of postpartum hemorrhage.

▶ Formulate a plan of management for third-stage hemorrhage, including pharmacological therapy.

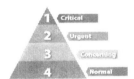

PPH is priority 2, Urgent. If it is uncontrolled or involves coagulopathy or blood loss greater than 1,500–2,000 cc, it is priority 1.

⚠ AACT—Alert

Postpartum hemorrhage (PPH) is responsible for the majority of maternal mortality worldwide. It causes about 8% of maternal deaths in the United States and 25% in developing countries (Smith & Brennan, 2006). PPH can lead to shock, renal failure, acute respiratory distress syndrome, coagulopathy, and Sheehan's syndrome (ischemia of the posterior pituitary causing lactation dysfunction or failure). Even moderately heavy blood loss can interfere with new motherhood by causing orthostatic hypotension, anemia, and exhaustion.

Primary or early PPH develops within 24 hr of delivery, while secondary or late PPH occurs 24 hr to as much as 12 weeks after delivery. Risk factors include obesity; high parity; Asian or Hispanic race; precipitous labor; preeclampsia; uterine overdistention related to multiple gestation, polyhydramnios, or macrosomia; long, difficult labor; rapid, intense labor; preterm delivery; prior postpartum hemorrhage; and previous cesarean delivery. The risk of hemorrhage is also increased if the time between the birth of the baby and the birth of the placenta exceeds

30 min. Often PPH occurs in the absence of risk factors—any woman who gives birth is potentially vulnerable.

How much bleeding is too much, and how is this blood loss measured? Authorities disagree, variously defining PPH as

- ▶ Symptomatic bleeding (lightheadedness, vertigo, syncope, hypotension, tachycardia, or oliguria), or
- ▶ Estimated blood loss ≥500 ml after vaginal birth or 1,000 ml after cesarean delivery, or
- ▶ 10% decline in postpartum hemoglobin concentration from antepartum levels.

All of these definitions are problematical. The classic definition of hemorrhage as blood loss greater than 500 cc was based nonscientific estimations. Recent studies with accurate measurement mechanisms reveal that *average* blood loss at a vaginal delivery is actually 600–650 cc. More than half of vaginal deliveries would meet this definition of PPH.

First Thought, Worst Thought

What is the most likely cause of postpartum hemorrhage?
Atony.
What is the worst it could be?
Uncontrollable hemorrhage, DIC, shock.

Hemoglobin measurement is a retrospective diagnosis; usually the hemorrhage has been controlled by the time the lab values are assessed. Further, preeclampsia, dehydration, overhydration, and timing of the test may alter hemoglobin values irrespective of blood loss.

Symptomatic hypovolemia is a better indication of excessive blood loss, but a healthy pregnant woman usually does not show signs until blood loss tops 1,500 cc, or 25% of her circulating volume. The loss of a given amount of blood may be compensated for in one woman, but may lead to ischemic injury in another. Conversely, the preeclamptic woman does not undergo the usual blood volume expansion of pregnancy, and will show signs of shock with blood loss that a healthy woman would tolerate asymptomatically. PPH, then, is best defined by the provider who deems blood loss significant enough to warrant intervention.

Blood flow to the pregnant uterus at term is 800–1,000 ml/min. Maternal vessels that pass through a latticework of interwoven uterine muscle fibers abundantly supply the placenta. Uterine myometrium has the unique ability to retract, that is, to remain shortened after each successive contraction. After the baby vacates the uterus, the uterus contracts, and the site of placental attachment shrinks, causing the placenta to buckle and separate from the suddenly uneven interface. A hematoma forms behind the placenta, accelerating the process of separation. After delivery of the placenta, the body achieves hemostasis through uterine contraction, which compresses the vasculature supplying the placental bed. The muscle bundles act as "living ligatures" and squeeze the vessels closed, staunching the flow of blood. Local decidual hemostatic factors and systemic coagulation components such as platelets also play a role by creating a fibrin "mesh" over the placental site.

Hemorrhage? Get on TRAC:
TRAUMA (20%)
RETAINED products (10%)
ATONY (>70%)
COAGULATION defects (1%)

Postpartum hemorrhage usually consists of heavy vaginal bleeding that can rapidly progress to shock, or blood may accumulate less obviously in an atonic uterus or collect behind an undelivered placenta. Slow trickle bleeding may add up to excessive blood loss and result in shock.

AACT—Analyze

Postpartum hemorrhage occurs for four major reasons. No individual case is limited to a single etiology.

Atony

Uterine atony is the insufficient contraction and retraction of the uterine myometrial fibers. At least 80% of cases of PPH result from ineffective uterine contraction during the first 4 hr following delivery (Jacobs, 2007). About 5% of women will experience this uterine atony. In some cases, the fundus will feel firm, but bleeding continues because a focal area of the uterus is atonic, or the uterus not sufficiently or uniformly contracted.

Trauma

When bleeding continues despite a well-contracted uterus, consider perineal, vaginal, or cervical lacerations or uterine rupture. Lacerations of the upper reproductive tract are unusual in the out-of-hospital-delivery, but may occur, especially if the woman has friable tissue secondary to condyloma or other lesions. Cervical lacerations may occur spontaneously, particularly if the woman forcefully pushes before fully dilated. Vaginal sidewall lacerations may occur in association with compound presentation. Manipulations to resolve shoulder dystocia can also cause lacerations.

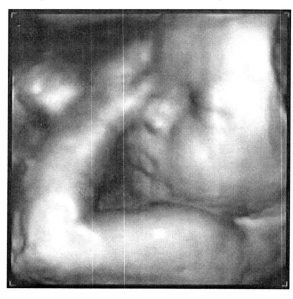

Figure 41. Polyhydramnios increases the risk of postpartum hemorrhage by overdistending the uterus. This 34-week fetus is easily visualized on three-dimensional ultrasound because of the increased amniotic fluid volume.

Retained Products

If products of conception or blood clots remain in the uterus after delivery, uterine contraction is thwarted and bleeding ensues. Often the culprit is a succenturiate or accessory lobe left behind after the primary placenta delivers. Carefully examine the placenta for torn vessels, a rough edge, or fetal vessels reaching the placental edge and ending at a tear in the membranes. Deliveries involving pre-viable or early preterm fetuses are more likely to involve retained placentas. If the placenta remains attached, manual or surgical removal may be necessary upon arrival at the hospital.

Coagulation Defects

Bleeding is initially controlled by uterine contraction, but within hours or days, clotting and fibrin deposits over the placental site begin to influence hemostasis. Coagulopathy associated with HELLP syndrome, abruption, DIC, sepsis, fetal demise, amniotic fluid embolism or functional abnormalities of platelets may promote bleeding. Dilutional coagulopathy can also follow aggressive resuscitation with crystalloids.

MANAGEMENT OF THIRD-STAGE LABOR
✍ AACT—Consider

The two primary options for the management of third-stage labor are physiological (or expectant) management and active management. These two approaches represent the opposite ends of a continuum. Many providers practice somewhere in the middle, using techniques from each method.

Strict physiological management involves allowing the mother's body to complete the third stage naturally. The cord is not clamped until pulsations cease, and the uterus is left to deliver the placenta on its own timetable, within an hour after birth. Oxytocics are used only if the woman begins to hemorrhage.

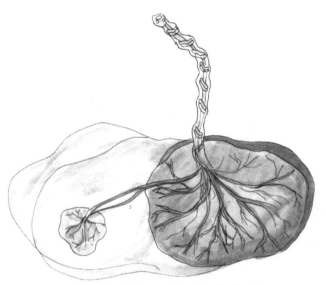

Figure 42. A succenturiate lobe may be retained in the uterus.

To actively manage third-stage labor, the provider administers oxytocin with the birth of the anterior shoulder or soon thereafter and delivers the placenta with controlled cord traction.

 Early cord clamping can reduce the amount of blood the newborn receives at birth by more than 50%. As long as the cord pulses, oxygen exchange continues between infant and mother as it did in utero, helping the newborn make the transition to extrauterine life. Once the cord is cut, the baby loses this maternal assistance. Most of the placental blood volume is transfused within 3 min after delivery.

Early cord clamping was once part of this regimen, but research showed that keeping the cord intact for about a minute after delivery does not affect the rate of hemorrhage. The American Academy of Pediatrics and the

World Health Organization endorse delayed cord clamping to reduce neo-natal anemia and improve circulation to the infant's brain, lungs, extremi-ties, and intestines, and to protect against persistent pulmonary hyperten-sion of the newborn.

In 2003, the International Confederation of Midwives and the Inter-national Federation of Gynecologists and Obstetrics published a joint statement recommending active management of the third-stage of la-bor and administering oxytocin within 1 min of the birth of the baby (or ergometrine or misoprostol if oxytocin is not available). The cord is clamped after pulsations cease, and controlled cord traction is used with uterine counterpressure. After the placenta is out, fundal massage should be performed.

Table 11. Performing Controlled Cord Traction

After cord pulsations stop, place a clamp on the cord near the introitus.

Watch for signs of detachment.

Grasp the lower segment of the uterus just above the symphysis pubis. With a uterine contraction, exert steady pressure upward and backwards.

Your other hand holds the clamp on the cord at the level of the introitus and puts steady traction on the cord *downward* and backwards.

Encourage the mother to push.

Start with light traction at first and carefully increase tension. Aggressive cord traction can cause uterine inversion or cord avulsion.

If the placenta does not deliver after 30–40 seconds, wait for the next contraction and repeat.

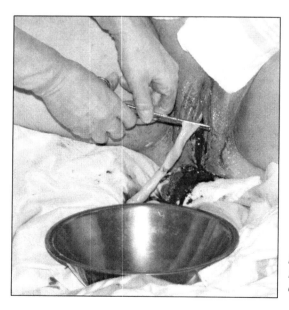

Figure 43. Active third-stage management. Place a clamp on the cord near the introitus.

The evidence is strong (at least in hospital settings) that active management of the third stage of labor reduces blood loss. Randomized controlled trials and a Cochrane meta-analysis involving more than 6,000 women show a 60% reduction in PPH when active management is employed rather than physiological management, assisted only by gravity or nipple stimulation (Smith & Brennan, 2006). Researchers propose that 1 parturient woman out of every 12 could be spared PPH if active management were instituted with every delivery. Medical organizations worldwide advocate this technique, and it is taught in the Advanced Life Support Obstetrics course designed by the American Academy of Family Practice Physicians (Ailsworth, et al., 2006).

Researchers disagree about whether the same benefit can be achieved if oxytocin is given after placenta delivery. While some studies showed that PPH was best prevented by starting oxytocin with the birth of the baby, most studies conclude that oxytocin was equally effective when given after delivery of the anterior shoulder, delivery of the placenta, or cord clamping (Ailsworth, et al., 2006).

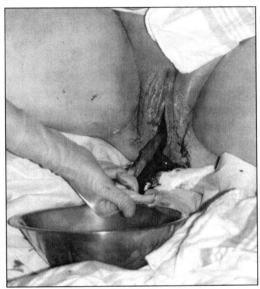

Figure 44. Active third-stage management. Wait for the uterus to contract. Then, with one hand bracing the uterus above the pubic bone, begin careful, controlled cord traction

While research unequivocally demonstrates that the parturient woman will lose less blood with active management of third stage labor, opponents argue that for the average healthy woman, this reduction in blood loss is not clinically relevant. Hemorrhage with a vaginal birth is classically defined as blood loss greater than 500 cc, an unrealistic definition because more than half of women will lose more than this. A nonpregnant woman can donate 500 cc to a blood bank without suffering hemodynamic consequences. A woman undergoing a cesarean section can lose twice this amount before it is considered excessive.

Blood volume increases 45–50% during pregnancy, serving in part as a safeguard against excessive blood loss during delivery. Healthy women with adequate antepartum hemoglobin and hematocrit levels generally tolerate 1,000–1,500 cc of blood loss without hemodynamic consequence.

Women delivering out of the hospital are usually at lower risk for PPH than those in a hospital setting, due to lower risk status, minimal interventions, and often better overall health. Many procedures that are performed exclusively in hospital births are associated with a higher rate of PPH, such as instrumental vaginal delivery, episiotomy, and oxytocin induction or augmentation. Women who deliver in the hospital setting are more likely to have risk factors for hemorrhage, such as preeclampsia or chorioamnionitis. Although active management may be the routine management of choice in the hospital setting, more research is needed to determine whether healthy women delivering outside a hospital derive the same benefit.

✍ AACT—Treat

The diagnosis of PPH is established by assessing the quantity of blood loss and the client's clinical condition, including level of consciousness and vital signs. Treatment of PPH includes identifying the cause, appropriate therapy, and fluid resuscitation.

A Stepwise Approach to Management of PPH

Postpartum hemorrhage usually begins abruptly and, with proper treatment, ends quickly. The provider should learn the steps of controlling PPH in sequence and institute them swiftly if hemorrhage occurs. The provider should decisively move from one intervention to the next while considering modifications that might apply to the individual woman.

Consider:

▶ Is the bladder empty?
▶ Is the placenta out?
▶ Is an intravenous line in place?
▶ Are appropriate medications readily available?
▶ Is the woman accessible for procedures? (Move her from the tub, etc.)

Removing the Placenta

If the woman is hemorrhaging and the placenta is undelivered, deliver it with controlled cord traction. Care must be taken because the risk of uterine inversion is greater if the uterus remains poorly contracted. The Cochrane group (Carroli & Bergel, 2004) demonstrated that umbilical-vein injection of saline solution plus 30–50 IU of oxytocin decreases the incidence of retained placenta.

Perform manual removal if the placenta is not easily delivered or the cord is avulsed. Stop massaging and allow the uterus to relax. Insert your entire hand by holding your thumb and fingers together. Control the uterine fundus with your other hand. Remove the placenta if it is in the lower segment. If it is not there, look for the placental edge. Use your hand as a spatula and insert your fingers into the cleavage plane between the placenta and the uterine wall. Work your fingers beneath the entire placenta, gather the entire placenta in your palm, and remove it as one piece if possible. When the placenta is out, perform bimanual massage while an assistant examines the placenta for missing pieces.

Postpartum Hemorrhage—Remember DAMIT To Dam the Flow of Blood
DELIVER placenta
AGGRESSIVELY massage uterus **A**SSESS for retained products, coagulopathy, and trauma
MEDS—oxytocin, methylergonovine, or prostaglandins
IV, shock positioning, oxygen, bimanual compression
TRANSPORT rapidly

If you cannot identify the cleavage plane, transport for surgical removal of the placenta. Consider the possibility of invasive placenta. Sometimes the physician must relax the uterus with terbutaline, IV nitroglycerin, or general anesthesia to accomplish removal, and this relaxation can trigger torrential hemorrhage. Rarely, emergency hysterectomy is necessary to control the bleeding. Manual removal of the placenta often results in infection and late postpartum hemorrhage.

Uterine Atony

Most PPH is due to uterine atony, so your initial action is to find the fundus through the abdominal wall and assess tone while massaging the uterus. Massage stimulates uniform contraction of the myometrium and expresses clots that have accumulated in the uterine interior. If the uterus is boggy, massage briskly and give oxytocin as an infusion of 20–40 units in 1 liter of NS at 10–15 ml/min rapidly. If there is no IV access, give 10 units IM.

Oxytocin is the first-line agent for preventing and treating PPH because it is effective and has few side effects. Conventional wisdom holds that a 10-unit direct IV bolus of oxytocin carries a risk of hypotension, but a randomized controlled trial found no adverse affects associated with this route.

Administration of oxytocin before delivery of the placenta does not increase the likelihood of retained placenta.

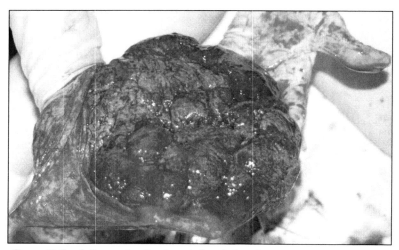

Figure 45. Carefully examine the placenta for missing pieces.

Empty the bladder with a catheter if there is any chance of distention. If she is still bleeding, proceed to bimanual massage. Place one hand on the fundus, and insert the other entire hand in the vagina, anterior to the cervix. Avoid worsening any lacerations that may be present. Remove any blood clots from the vagina, cervix, and lower uterine segment that might be interfering with uterine contraction.

Place the vaginal hand in the anterior fornix and make a fist. Grasp the posterior aspect of the fundus with your other hand and bend it onto the fist that is inside the vagina. Compress the uterus between your two hands to remove clots and stimulate contraction. Bimanual compression compresses the blood vessels, staunching blood flow and encouraging it to clot. About 10 minutes of bimanual compression tends to decrease bleeding even in the absence of adequate contraction and can control the bleeding from a ruptured uterus. Sometimes a similar hemostasis can be achieved externally by grasping the uterus through the abdominal wall and holding firm compression for 10 minutes.

If bleeding is significant and there is a delay in definitive treatment, aortic compression can be performed to temporarily control bleeding and encourage clotting of the attachment site. Make a fist with your left hand and place it on her abdomen with your index finger at the umbilicus and your knuckles in line with her spine. Press straight down to compress the aorta against her spine. You will feel a strong pulse under your hand. Palpate for a femoral pulse with your right hand. Compress until the femoral pulse disappears. This procedure can be very painful, but can prevent exsanguination while the woman is transported to the hospital. If her legs become numb and tingly, release pressure somewhat to allow her some circulation, then resume.

If oxytocin and uterine massage fail to achieve hemostasis, consider ergot alkaloids. These are derived from a fungus that infects rye grain. Methylergonovine (Methergine), ergometrine, and ergonovine cause tetanic contraction of the upper and lower uterine segments, effectively controlling hemorrhage. The usual dose is 0.2 mg IM, which may be repeated every 2–4 hr, sometimes followed by a short course of oral Methergine. Ergot alkaloids can also cause nausea and vomiting, and hypertension is a contraindication because ergots can elevate blood pressure. Recent research failed to show ergotamines more beneficial than oxytocin alone.

Prostaglandins vasoconstrict and stimulate uterine contraction. IM carboprost (Hemabate) 250 mcg is also an option for the second-line agent, repeated every 15 min to a maximum of 2 mg (8 doses). Use with caution with asthma and hypertension. Carboprost is 80–90% effective in resolving hemorrhage refractory to oxytocin and Methergine, but side effects can be problematic (Smith & Brennan, 2006). Vomiting, diarrhea, and general malaise are associated with carboprost. Carboprost is not as useful for the woman who is in shock, because poor tissue perfusion results in poor absorption of the IM medication.

Misoprostol is a prostaglandin E1 analog first developed for the treatment of stomach ulcers. It is used "off-label" to stimulate uterine contraction. Recent studies have demonstrated that misoprostol is a safe and effective agent, ideal for low-resource settings because it is safe, effective, and inexpensive ($1.00 per 600-mcg dose) and does not require refrigeration. Semi-skilled birth attendants in developing countries can give misoprostol orally, rectally, sublingually, or vaginally. PPH is treated with doses ranging from 200–1,000 mcg. It may be used in the woman with asthma. Side effects include fever, nausea, and diarrhea.

Retained Tissue

After delivery, inspect the placenta to identify missing fragments or lobes. If bimanual compression, massage, and uterotonics fail to control the hemorrhage, perform manual exploration of the uterus to remove clots, membrane, and placental fragments. You may consider wrapping gauze around one hand, then carefully inserting it into the uterus to remove retained placenta tissue by gently sweeping the inner wall of the uterus. Removal of retained tissue can be difficult and painful. Persistently adherent placental fragments may require curettage by a physician in the operating room. After exploration and evacuation of the uterus, continue massage and uterotonics. Often bleeding will be controlled by removal of clots and placental fragments, but in some cases surgical management is necessary. After manual uterine exploration, broad-spectrum antibiotics are commonly administered to reduce the risk of endometritis.

Trauma

If bleeding persists despite a well-contracted uterus, consider trauma. Start with the external genitalia and work your way in. Inspect the genital tract from perineum to cervix and palpate the uterine cavity for defects indicating uterine rupture. Clitoral and periurethral lacerations can bleed persistently. If you identify a bleeding laceration, apply pressure, and suture the wound if direct pressure does not stop the bleeding.

Insert a speculum and grasp the anterior cervix with a ring forceps. Place a second ring forceps at the 2-o'clock position, and systematically inspect the entire cervix by placing one forceps ahead of the next, proceeding around the circumference. Suture cervical lacerations only if they are actively bleeding. A cervical laceration larger than 2 cm is repaired by grasping each edge of the laceration with ring forceps starting a continuous, interlocking stitch above the apex of the tear. If you cannot find the apex, place the stitch as high as possible and sew proximally, using gentle traction on the suture line to pull the apex into view. A retractor may be necessary to expose the area in need of suturing. Sutures placed superior to the fornix have been known to accidentally ligate the ureters (Jacobs, 2007).

Check for evidence of uterine rupture. Dehiscence of a lower-segment scar does not usually cause PPH. Severe lacerations may involve the uterus or lead to broad ligament or retroperitoneal hematomas, although trauma of this severity is rare outside the hospital.

Hematomas are uncommon and may occur whether or not the woman has had a laceration. Clients with lower-genital-tract hematomas usually present with intense pain and localized, tender swelling with tachycardia and hypotension greater than what is explained by visible blood loss. Broad-ligament hematomas may be palpated as masses adjacent to the uterus. Occasionally, the woman with severe pain, pallor, diaphoresis, and a palpable mass will have not a hematoma, but a severely distended bladder.

Lower-genital-tract hematomas can be managed expectantly; but if they are expanding, they require incision and drainage. Ultrasound, CT scanning, and MRI all may be used to assess broad ligament and retroperitoneal hematomas, and if the lesion continues to evolve, arterial embolization may be performed.

Coagulopathy

If the uterus is well contracted and there are no placental fragments, consider coagulopathy. In developed countries, coagulopathies are rare causes of out-of-hospital hemorrhage because most clotting disorders (such as idiopathic thrombocytopenic purpura, thrombotic thrombocytopenic purpura, von Willebrand disease, and hemophilia) are identified antepartum, and hospital birth would be planned. DIC can uncommonly develop in the client with severe preeclampsia, amniotic fluid embolism, sepsis, placental abruption, or prolonged retention of fetal demise.

The woman with coagulopathy-related hemorrhage will bleed without clots and ooze blood from puncture sites. Lab work includes platelet count, prothrombin time (PT or INR), partial thromboplastin time (PTT), fibrinogen, and fibrin split products (D-dimer). Blood-product replacement is necessary to achieve hemostasis, and rapid transport is crucial.

Surgical Management

When hemorrhage is persistent, the physician may insert a device into the uterus to tamponade the bleeding. A Sengstaken-Blakemore tube, Bakri tamponade balloon, or #24 Foley catheter with a 30-ml balloon controls PPH through internal compression of the placental bed. Sometimes the surgeon will pack the uterus with gauze that has been saturated with 5,000 units of thrombin in 5 ml sterile saline to enhance clotting. Even condoms and surgical gloves have been used successfully to control bleeding in low-resource settings.

Arterial embolization by an interventional radiologist is an option at some facilities for the hemodynamically stable woman. A catheter is inserted into a femoral artery and internal iliac arteriography is performed. An occlusive thrombotic agent is administered through the catheter to occlude the arteries responsible for the hemorrhage.

Rarely, surgical intervention is needed to stop PPH. The surgeon will enter the abdomen with either a subumbilical vertical incision or Pfannenstiel incision, remove any free blood, and examine the pelvic organs for laceration, rupture, or hematoma. In the case of uterine rupture, the surgeon must quickly decide whether to repair the defect or perform a hysterectomy. If atony is the cause of the hemorrhage, the surgeon will compress and massage the uterus and may inject oxytocin, carboprost, or methylergonovine directly into the uterine muscle.

Uterine-artery ligation is the highly effective technique of tying off the vessels that supply approximately 90% of uterine blood flow. After the uterine arteries are ligated, atony may persist, but the uterus will grow pale and blood loss will slow or cease. The ovarian artery and internal iliac (hypogastric) artery are also sometimes closed off to control bleeding within the genital tract, usually if uterine artery ligation fails.

The B-Lynch technique entails compressing the uterine walls with single large suture by opening the lower uterine segment, suturing through the posterior wall and over the fundus, and then tying the suture anteriorly. A comparable procedure can be accomplished without opening the uterus. Menstrual flow and fertility are not impaired by these procedures.

Arterial embolization may be useful in situations when preservation of fertility is desired, surgical options have been exhausted, and when managing hematomas. Pelvic arterial embolization is performed by placing an angiographic catheter in the abdominal aorta and injecting contrast material while imaging the pelvis. If the images show the source of the hemorrhage, a catheter is passed into the bleeding vessel and gelatin sponge pledgets are introduced to occlude the vessel. If the source cannot be identified, the internal iliac artery is targeted bilaterally. Hysterectomy is sometimes required when bleeding fails to respond to any other therapy, and it should be performed without delay if control of hemorrhage is necessary to prevent death.

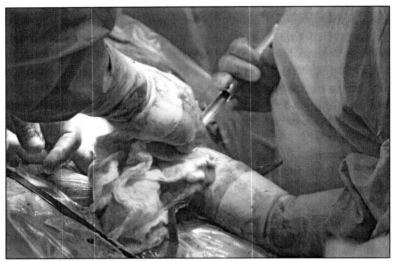

Figure 46. Staunching the flow. Surgical management is sometimes necessary to control postpartum hemorrhage.

Fluid Resuscitation

When a woman is hemorrhaging, start two large-bore IV lines and infuse isotonic crystalloid solution such as normal saline (NS) or lactated Ringer's with the goal of expanding intravascular volume. Low-osmolality solutions such as 5% dextrose in water or diluted NS in 5% dextrose are not useful for hemorrhage because they move rapidly into the interstitial space rather than remaining in the vessels. Even isotonic fluids extravasate much faster than would blood—every liter of blood loss requires replacement with 3 L of crystalloid to offset the shift into the interstitial space. The healthy woman is not likely to develop a dilutional coagulopathy until about 80% of her blood volume has been replaced with crystalloid. Colloids such as albumin, dextran, hydroxyethyl starch, and modified fluid gelatin stay in the vascular space longer, but are associated with poorer outcomes than crystalloids.

 Fluid flows twice as fast through a 14-gauge catheter as it does through an 18-gauge.

Raise the woman's legs and administer oxygen. Antishock garments constrict the vasculature of the lower extremities, raising blood pressure around vital organs, and are especially useful in low-resource settings.

Blood Transfusion

A healthy pregnant woman can usually tolerate a blood loss of 1,500 cc before requiring a transfusion of blood products. Blood typing, Rh, and antibody screening should be evaluated in the antenatal period. Two to 4 units of packed red blood cells are transfused initially to enhance oxygen-carrying ability of the circulating volume and to increase intravascular volume by increasing osmolality. One unit of red blood cells will raise the hematocrit by approximately 3% and the hemoglobin by about 1g/dl. In many settings, whole blood is no longer used In a hemorrhagic emergency, uncrossmatched O-type Rh-negative PRBCs are readily available at most hospitals. After about 5 units of PRBCs, a unit of fresh frozen plasma is usually given, and platelets are usually given in packs of 5–6 U to correct thrombocytopenia. Platelet preparations contain some RBCs, necessitating anti-D immunoglobulin (RhoGAM, WinRho) administration for the Rh-negative woman after the hemorrhage is resolved.

Retained Placenta

Recent research shows that most placentas separate from the uterine wall within 1 min after the birth of the infant and deliver within an average of 8–9 min. The risk of PPH doubles if third stage lasts more than 10 min. A retained placenta, defined as undelivered 30 min after the baby's birth, occurs in less than 3% of vaginal deliveries (Smith & Brennan, 2006). The likelihood of PPH escalates dramatically if third stage is greater than 30 min.

Invasive Placenta
If not bleeding, priority 3; if bleeding, priority 1

In some cases, the placenta has invaded beyond the normal cleavage plane and grown into the uterine wall (*placenta accreta*), into the uterine muscle (*placenta increta*), or entirely through the uterine wall (*placenta percreta*). Percreta is often associated with placental implantation over a uterine scar, especially in conjunction with placenta previa. Although placenta percreta with bladder invasion may cause hematuria during pregnancy, the first clinical manifestation of invasive placenta is usually life-threatening hemorrhage that occurs when the provider attempts manual removal of the placenta.

Though it is still a rare condition, the incidence of invasive placenta has increased with the rising rate of cesarean section. In 1950, the rate of invasive placenta was 1 in 30,000. Today 1 delivery in 2,500 involves placenta accreta, conveying a 7% risk of maternal mortality (Russo-Stieglitz & Resnik, 2007). Every cesarean delivery increases the risk of invasive placenta further, as do advanced maternal age, placenta previa (especially when associated with a scarred uterus), high parity, and prior invasive placenta. Women who have had two or more cesarean deliveries and anterior or central placenta previa have nearly a 40% risk of developing placenta accreta (Russo-Stieglitz & Resnik).

Placenta accreta is suspected when the placenta appears contiguous with the bladder wall on ultrasound examination and exhibits specific findings on color Doppler ultrasonography. Some women with placenta accreta will have an elevated MSAFP level on second-trimester screening.

Placenta accreta has become one of the most common indications for peripartum hysterectomy. In some cases, placenta percreta is managed by leaving the placenta in situ, sometimes dosing the woman with methotrexate until beta-HCG levels fall to zero.

Uterine Inversion
Priority 1
Uterine inversion occurs when the entire uterus turns inside out and protrudes through the cervical os (incomplete), into the vagina (complete), or beyond the vulva (prolapsed). The result is usually life-threatening hemorrhage and shock. A rare complication, uterine inversion is often associated with an invasive fundal placenta. Conventional wisdom holds that this condition may be iatrogenic, caused by cord traction without fundal counterpressure or with an uncontracted uterus. Following uterine replacement, vigorous massage and uterotonic administration should be employed.

Table 12. Postpartum Hemorrhage Priorities

Get help

ABCs

Begin fundal massage

Trendelenberg positioning

Start two large bore IV lines

Baseline labs—CBC, PT, PTT fibrinogen

IV crystalloid

Oxygen 10 L by non-rebreather mask

Uterotonics

Treat for shock

Look for traumatic bleeding and repair if possible

Look for retained products and remove if possible

Insert Foley

Transport at earliest opportunity if unstable

The inverted uterus appears as a blue-gray mass jutting from the vagina, often with the placenta still attached. Replace the uterus rapidly, without removing the placenta, by taking the uterus into the palm of your hand and pressing on the inverted fundus from inside the uterus, restoring it to its proper location. This is similar to placing your fingers at the toe of an inverted sock and pushing to turn the sock right side out. Follow with uterotonic medications to induce contraction and prevent recurrence. If the prolapsed uterus will not reduce, the physician may try magnesium sulfate, terbutaline, nitroglycerin, or general anesthesia to facilitate replacement, or may resort to surgery.

Late Postpartum Hemorrhage
Usually priority 2

Late PPH is excessive bleeding occurring between 24 hr and 12 weeks postpartum. It follows 0.5–2% of births in developed countries (Smith & Brennan, 2006). It appears to result from subinvolution related to retained products or infection or from persistent diffuse atony.

Bleeding from late PPH is not usually as heavy as that which immediately follows delivery. Retained products or abnormal uterine lining can be identified on sonographic examination as an echogenic mass in an enlarged uterine cavity or as a mixed-echo pattern. Treatment includes uterotonic agents as with primary PPH. Broad-spectrum antibiotic therapy is instituted if endometritis is suspected, as indicated by fever, uterine tenderness, or foul-smelling discharge. Surgical procedures (D&C, suction curettage) may be indicated for removal of retained products.

Disseminated Intravascular Coagulation (DIC)
Priority 1

DIC, also called consumption coagulopathy and defibrination syndrome, is a life-threatening derangement of the clotting cascade creating both thrombosis and hemorrhage. DIC is initiated by underlying disease or trauma, such as placental abruption, eclampsia, intrauterine fetal demise, amniotic fluid embolism, septic shock, or trauma. DIC is likely to cause serious morbidity, including bleeding (64%) renal dysfunction (25%), hepatic dysfunction (19%), respiratory dysfunction (16%), shock (14%), thromboembolism (7%), central nervous system involvement (2%), and fetal distress in the pregnant woman (Leung, 2007).

During DIC, the body forms and dissolves fibrin clots throughout the circulation, causing simultaneous uncontrolled bleeding and clotting. DIC begins when an event triggers the formation of innumerable microscopic clots, which use up the clotting factors. The body responds by attempting to dissolve the unneeded clots. The byproducts of widespread clot formation and dissolution interfere with the ability of the blood to coagulate, and the woman begins to hemorrhage.

The woman with DIC will present with bleeding from body orifices and breaks in the skin, including venipuncture sites, nose, mouth, GI tract, and vagina. Bruising, purpura, and petechiae are commonly noted on the skin.

Acute DIC is diagnosed when laboratory values indicate increased thrombin generation (fibrinogen is decreased) and increased fibrinolysis (FDPs and D-dimer are elevated). Fibrinogen levels are considerably elevated during pregnancy—a fibrinogen level that would be normal for a nonpregnant woman can indicate serious coagulopathy in pregnancy. D-dimer (monoclonal antibody) tests may be performed to determine whether levels of serum fibrin degradation products are increased.

The first priority is to treat the underlying disease while providing hemodynamic support. Clients who are hemorrhaging, have significant thrombocytopenia, are at high risk for bleeding, or require invasive procedures are usually treated with platelets, fresh frozen plasma or cryoprecipitate.

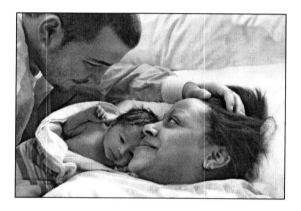

Figure 47. Quick action and good management can lead to a good outcome following postpartum hemorrhage.

Care Following Resuscitation

During and after significant hemorrhage, hospital providers will closely monitor the woman's level of consciousness, vital signs, and urine output, which should be greater than 30 cc/hr. Serial blood work may include CBC, coagulation, and arterial blood gas values. Pulse oximetry monitors heart rate, oxygen saturation, and perfusion status. Repeated lung auscultation is necessary because of the risk of subsequent pulmonary edema or adult respiratory distress syndrome. Few clients experiencing PPH require invasive procedures such as a central arterial or venous line; those that do are generally managed in the intensive-care unit.

In the days following postpartum hemorrhage, women tend to become edematous from crystalloid overload coupled with the fluid-retaining effects of oxytocin. Within a few days, the woman with healthy kidneys will eliminate the excess fluid.

BIBLIOGRAPHY

Ailsworth, K., Anderson, J., Atwood, L.A., Bailey, R.E., & Canavan, T. (2006). *ALSO: Advanced life support in obstetrics* (4th ed.). Leawood, KS: American Academy of Family Practice Physicians.

Carroli G., & Bergel E. (2004). Umbilical vein injection for management of retained placenta (Cochrane Review). *The Cochrane Library* (3). Chichester, UK: John Wiley & Sons.

Cunningham, F., Grant, N., Leveno, K., Gilstrap, L., Hauth, J., & Wenstrom, K. (2005). *Williams obstetrics* (22nd ed.). New York: McGraw-Hill.

Gabbe, S.G., Niebyl, J.R., & Simpson, J.L., Eds. (2007). *Obstetrics: Normal and problem pregnancies* (5th ed.). New York: Churchill Livingstone.

Gilbert, E.S. (2007). *Manual of high risk pregnancy and delivery* (4th ed.). St Louis: Mosby.

Gruenberg, Bonnie U. (2005). *Essentials of prehospital maternity care.* Upper Saddle River, NJ: Prentice Hall.

Jacobs, A.J. (2007). Causes and treatment of postpartum hemorrhage. In B.D. Rose (Ed.), *UpToDate.* Wellesley, MA: UpToDate.

Leung, L.L.K. (2007). Clinical features, diagnosis, and treatment of disseminated intravascular coagulation in adults. In B.D. Rose (Ed.), *UpToDate.* Wellesley, MA: UpToDate.

Makai, G., & Laufer, M.R. (2007). Evaluation and management of lower genital tract trauma in women. In B.D. Rose (Ed.), *UpToDate.* Wellesley, MA: UpToDate.

Resnik, R. (2007). Diagnosis and management of placenta accreta. In B.D. Rose (Ed.), *UpToDate.* Wellesley, MA: UpToDate.

Roberts, D.J. (2007a). Histopathology of placental disorders. In B.D. Rose (Ed.), *UpToDate.* Wellesley, MA: UpToDate.

Roberts, D.J. (2007b). Placental anatomy and examination. In B.D. Rose (Ed.), *UpToDate.* Wellesley, MA: UpToDate.

Russo-Stieglitz, K., & Lockwood, C.J. (2007). Placenta previa and vasa previa. In B.D. Rose (Ed.), *UpToDate.* Wellesley, MA: UpToDate.

Russo-Stieglitz, K., & Resnik, R. (2007). Diagnosis and management of placenta accreta. In B.D. Rose (Ed.), *UpToDate.* Wellesley, MA: UpToDate.

Simpson, K.R., & Creehan, P.A. (2007). *AWHONN's perinatal nursing* (3rd ed.). Hagerstown, MD: Lippincott Williams & Wilkins.

Smith, J.R., & Brennan, B.G. (2006). *Postpartum hemorrhage* (eMedicine, topic 3568). Retrieved May 10, 2008, from http://www.emedicine.com/med/ topic3568.htm

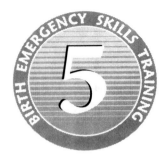

Pain, Syncope, Difficulty Breathing, and Altered Level of Consciousness

OBJECTIVES

▶ Describe the typical presentation of appendicitis in the pregnant woman and nontypical variations.

▶ Provide differential diagnoses for the client who presents with third-trimester abdominal and back pain.

▶ Identify the signs and symptoms of deep-vein thrombosis and pulmonary embolism; discuss treatment modalities.

▶ Discuss the clinical signs of pulmonary edema and list three possible etiologies.

PELVIC AND ABDOMINAL PAIN

AACT and ReACT
ALERT—Be alert ▶ Exercise hypervigilant attention
ANALYZE—Think about possible causes
CONSIDER—Use OLDCART ▶ Gather data
TREAT—Make first response ▶ Proceed to definitive care
ReACT | ReAssess ▶ ReConsider ▶ Re-Treat

✍ AACT—Alert

Most pregnant women feel abdominal discomfort during pregnancy. Usually these aches and pains prove inconsequential, but any complaint of abdominal pain should be taken seriously. Many gastrointestinal, gynecologic, urologic, or obstetric problems that necessitate surgical intervention present with abdominal pain.

When the pregnant uterus becomes an abdominal organ at about 12 weeks' gestation, it compresses and displaces the abdominal viscera while the overlying abdominal wall slackens. This rearrangement of organs may change pain perception and may alter or delay signs of peritonitis. Pain from elsewhere in the body may refer to the abdomen, confusing the clinical picture. Many etiologies of abdominal pain present nonspecifically; nausea, vomiting, abdominal pain, indigestion, and bowel irregularity are common symptoms of abdominal pathology and of normal pregnancy. Leukocytosis is not always meaningful, for white blood cell count may be as high as 16,000 during pregnancy and can climb to 20,000–30,000 in labor. Close monitoring and serial examinations are often necessary to make the correct diagnosis.

Peritonitis is a sign of significant abdominal pathology caused by peritoneal inflammation. The woman with peritonitis avoids movement and keeps the knees flexed. Any bump, cough, or palpation of the abdomen elicits severe pain. Rebound tenderness and abdominal wall rigidity (involuntary guarding) is also a sign of peritonitis.

✍ AACT—Analyze

▶ What is the source of the pain?
▶ Differential diagnoses

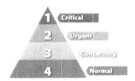

Pain, syncope, difficulty in breathing, and altered level of consciousness can be priority 1, 2, 3, or 4. Determining acuity is an important aspect of management.

Ligament Pain
Priority 4

Round ligaments run from the lateral aspect of the uterus to the pubic bone bilaterally to provide support. During the second trimester, the uterus becomes an abdominal organ and falls forward, stressing these ligaments and causing crampy spasms on either or both sides of the uterus and up to the level of the umbilicus. The right side is more commonly affected because of the dextrorotation of the uterus in pregnancy. Fetal movement, Braxton Hicks contractions, sneezing, sudden movement, physical exertion, and prolonged standing can trigger or exacerbate round-ligament pain.

The pain is physiologically benign, but is often sharp and severe. Splinting the painful area with the hand, flexing the hip on the affected side, applying heat, and wearing a maternity belt can improve symptoms.

Appendicitis
Priority 2 to 1

Appendicitis is the most common nonobstetrical surgical emergency during pregnancy, occurring in about 1 pregnancy per 1,000 (Ratcliffe, Baxley, Cline, & Sakornbut, 2008). While pregnancy does not make appendicitis more likely to occur, diagnosis may be delayed in the pregnant woman, resulting in a higher rate of perforation. Until recently, it was thought that the uterus displaces the appendix to the right iliac crest by 24 weeks, but research has shown no such change in location. Appendicitis presents initially as dull, poorly localized periumbilical pain in both pregnant and nonpregnant women, but later localizes to sharp focal pain in the right lower quadrant. The client with appendicitis may also complain of fever, chills, nausea and vomiting, involuntary guarding, and rebound tenderness (test for increased pain with cough). CBC with differential will show leukocytosis above the physiological baseline of pregnancy with an increased number of bands and predominance of neutrophils.

If appendicitis is suspected, rapid surgical intervention is essential. An infected appendix is more likely to rupture in the pregnant client than in the nonpregnant woman, probably because of delay in diagnosis. Though unruptured appendicitis carries a fetal loss rate of 5–10%, a ruptured appendix brings 20–30% mortality to the fetus (Ratcliffe, et al., 2008). Careful physical examination is essential, but ultrasound, MRI, or helical CT is sometimes employed to aid diagnosis.

~ Differential Diagnoses

Ruptured ovarian cyst, adnexal torsion, pelvic inflammatory disease (PID), ovarian cancer, abruption placenta, Chorioamnionitis, uterine fibroid degeneration, labor, ruptured ectopic pregnancy, Crohn's disease, diverticulitis, and ureteral stone.

Urinary-Tract Infection

Priority 3 for uncomplicated UTI to priority 2 or 1 for pyelonephritis with septicemia

Pregnancy predisposes women to urinary-tract infections, which can range from asymptomatic to critical. Pregnancy hormones relax smooth muscle in the ureters, which can kink and allow urine to pool and support bacterial growth. Sometimes urinary-tract infection mimics or triggers preterm labor.

Cystitis, or bladder infection, presents with frequent urination, lower pelvic cramping (especially while voiding), a burning sensation with urination, and sometimes a low-grade fever. Urine may be cloudy, bloody, or bad-smelling. Cystitis may have no symptoms at all and be recognized only through laboratory results.

Pyelonephritis, or kidney infection, is often preceded by cystitis and occurs in about 2% of pregnancies. Symptoms include sudden onset of high fever, shaking chills, hematuria, nausea, vomiting, urinary pain and urgency, flank or low-back pain, costovertebral angle (CVA) tenderness, and malaise. During pregnancy the right side is most likely to be affected because the intestines push the uterus to the right and compress the right ureters and kidney. Untreated pyelonephritis can cause preterm labor or maternal septicemia and shock.

Hydronephrosis and Renal Calculi

Subacute is priority 3; acute presentation is usually priority 2

Hydronephrosis is fluid buildup in the kidneys when urine flow is obstructed in the urinary tract. During pregnancy, this condition most commonly results from smooth-muscle relaxation of the ureter due to progesterone and HCG, coupled with compression of the ureter at the pelvic brim by the heavy uterus, obstructing urine flow. Physiologic hydronephrosis and hydroureter of pregnancy are seen in 90% of pregnancies and are usually asymptomatic (Delzell & Lefevre, 2000).

The woman with symptomatic hydronephrosis often presents similar to the client with pyelonephritis or renal calculi, exhibiting severe flank pain that may be acute or chronic, but usually without fever. If hydronephrosis threatens kidney function, the client may require percutaneous or stent drainage. Rarely, hydronephrosis can exacerbate hypertension or cause renal failure.

Hydronephrosis can persist for months, sometimes causing intractable pain for the pregnant woman. Many clients are managed on narcotic medications and taught techniques to reduce pressure on the kidneys and ureters, such as urinating while positioned on hands and knees in a bathtub. Pain from hydronephrosis may increase if the condition worsens or if she develops a urinary-tract infection.

Kidney stones (nephrolithiasis) cause pain when they pass from the renal pelvis into the ureter. Most cases of renal colic present in the second or third trimester of pregnancy. Renal calculi may form more easily in pregnancy because of increased excretion of calcium and urinary stasis, and existing stones are more likely to become symptomatic secondary to the increased urine flow and dilated urinary tract. As in nonpregnant women, kidney stones present with a flank-loin-abdomen distribution of severe pain often accompanied by dysuria, hematuria, and nausea. Pain comes in waves as the stone moves in the ureter and causes ureteral spasm. Paroxysms of severe pain often last 30–60 min. Pain from upper ureteral stones tends to radiate to the flank, and pain from lower ureteral obstruction radiates to the labia. The location and character of the pain may change as the stone migrates. Kidney infection may accompany nephrolithiasis, causing fever and malaise. Uncommonly, kidney stones can lead to premature labor or preeclampsia. Urinary obstruction with concurrent infection is unusual, but when present, it carries a high risk of spontaneous abortion and premature labor.

Dietary modification is helpful in preventing stones. The woman should increase fluids and decrease foods high in oxalates, purines, and sodium. High-oxalate foods include chocolate, nuts, green leafy vegetables, coffee, spinach, beets, and tea. A low-purine diet decreases red meats, beef, chicken, fish, and peanuts. Analysis of the stone's composition will determine which specific long-term dietary changes should be made.

Whereas calculi can affect either side, physiologic hydronephrosis is usually more pronounced on the right. Management is conservative and includes hydration, analgesics, and straining the urine for stones. About 70–80% of stones will pass on their own (Ratcliffe, et al., 2008). Antibiotic therapy is initiated if pyelonephritis is present. Ultrasound scan identifies nephrolithiasis in 60–95% of cases (Ratcliffe , et al.). Renal arterial resistance index and sometimes a one-shot IV pyelogram are used to aid diagnosis. Rarely, ureteral stent placement or nephrostomy tubes may be necessary.

~ *Differential Diagnoses*
  Appendicitis, bowel obstruction, cholecystitis.

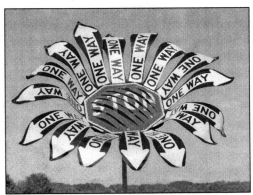

Figure 48. Which way to the correct diagnosis? Nausea, vomiting, abdominal pain, indigestion, and bowel irregularity are symptoms of many abdominal disorders and may accompany normal pregnancy.

Ruptured Ovarian Cyst
Priority 1
  Ovarian cysts are a common finding in pregnancy, and seldom cause complications or pain. Rupture of an ovarian cyst may occur spontaneously or secondary to minor trauma such as intercourse or a fall. The woman may have mild, chronic lower abdominal pain that suddenly becomes acute. Rebound tenderness and guarding may be present, and ultrasound may reveal fluid in the cul-de-sac. A ruptured ovarian cyst necessitates surgical treatment.

Adnexal Torsion
Priority 1
  Adnexal torsion is an uncommon emergency, but 20% of adnexal torsions occur during pregnancy, usually during the first trimester (Scott-Conner & Perry, 2006). In most cases, the woman has an ovarian mass, usually a dermoid cyst, occurring most commonly on the right side. The woman who has undergone treatment for infertility may have large, hyperstimulated ovaries—sometimes approaching the size of softballs—that are especially prone to torsion.
  Adnexal torsion presents with severe, colicky, unilateral lower abdominal and pelvic pain that may come and go. Symptoms include severe pain, nausea, vomiting, and fever, but physical examination does not always yield concrete information about the source of the problem. The clinician may elicit cervical-motion tenderness or rebound tenderness, or may palpate a tender adnexal mass. Ultrasound can identify the presence of an ovarian cyst, and color

Doppler may document absent ovarian flow in the central ovarian parenchyma. Ultrasound may show peritoneal fluid and an adnexal mass. Laparoscopy or laparotomy is performed either to remove the tube and ovary or to untwist the infundibulopelvic ligament.

~ *Differential Diagnoses*

Ectopic pregnancy, appendicitis, endometrioma, degenerating fibroid.

Degenerating Uterine Fibroids
Priority 2

Many pregnant women have uterine fibroids, which usually remain stable or decrease in size with advancing gestation. Between 12 and 20 weeks' gestation, a fibroid may outgrow its blood supply and degenerate, causing acute onset of significant localized abdominal pain, nausea, vomiting, low-grade fever, and leukocytosis. Hemorrhagic infarction of a large leiomyoma can cause all these symptoms as well as uterine bleeding. On ultrasound scan, a degenerating myoma has a mixed echogenic or echolucent appearance. Fibroid degeneration is a self-limited process. Treatment often involves a 48-hour regimen of indomethacin or narcotic analgesia.

~ *Differential Diagnoses*

Appendicitis, pyelonephritis, cholecystitis, placental abruption.

Chorioamnionitis
Priority 2 or 1

Chorioamnionitis occurs when disease-causing microorganisms ascend from the vagina into the upper reproductive tract to infect fetal membranes. The most significant risk factor is prolonged rupture of the membranes, but this infection frequently develops during a prolonged labor with many vaginal examinations. Intrauterine infection is associated with many if not most preterm births and appears to be an independent risk factor for cerebral palsy. Women who have undergone cerclage are at higher risk for chorioamnionitis. Chorioamnionitis may initiate uteroplacental bleeding, placental abruption, or a precipitous delivery.

Signs and symptoms of chorioamnionitis include fever >100.4° F (>37.8°C), maternal tachycardia >120 bpm, fetal tachycardia >160 bpm, purulent or foul-smelling amniotic fluid or vaginal discharge, uterine tenderness, increasing maternal leukocytosis >15,000–18,000 cells/μL and a generalized feeling of illness. The fetus usually shows signs of distress, such as tachycardia, before the mother becomes symptomatic. Maternal complications include endometritis, localized pelvic infections requiring drainage, intra-abdominal infections, and thrombosis of pelvic vessels/pulmonary emboli.

Few mothers die from chorioamnionitis, but the fetal and neonatal mortality rate is high. In the 1970s, 50% of newborns with group B streptococcus (GBS) infections died. Today sepsis from GBS kills 10% of infected newborn infants (Ratcliffe, et al., 2008). Although beta hemolytic strep prophylaxis has reduced the incidence of GBS sepsis, ampicillin chemoprophylaxis has contributed to escalating rates of similarly life-threatening ampicillin-resistant *E. coli* neonatal sepsis. Because of this, penicillin rather than ampicillin is now recommended for GBS prophylaxis.

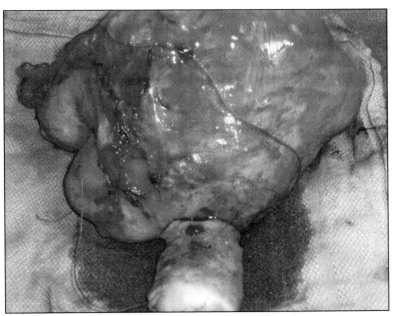

Figure 49. Fibroid uterus. In the nonpregnant woman, pain and bleeding from uterine fibroids can necessitate hysterectomy. Courtesy of Dr. Ayodeji Bakare.

Risk of neonatal infection increases as the duration of ruptured membranes lengthens. Serious neonatal complications of chorioamnionitis include septic shock, pulmonary hypertension, respiratory failure, and meningitis. Signs of sepsis in the infant include tachypnea, expiratory grunt, retractions, cyanosis, tachycardia, pale or mottled appearance, abdominal distention, vomiting, diarrhea, hypothermia or hyperthermia, petechiae, behavioral abnormalities, and seizures. Bulging fontanel or nuchal rigidity is not a consistent sign of meningitis in a newborn. Infectious pneumonia should be suspected in the infant born without respiratory distress who becomes symptomatic in the first hours of life.

Maternal white blood cell (WBC) counts or C-reactive protein (CRP) levels are often used to diagnose chorioamnionitis. The CRP level may be more accurate, especially if corticosteroid therapy has elevated WBC count. Amniotic fluid collected via amniocentesis may be evaluated for leukocyte count, Gram stain, pH, glucose concentration, endotoxin, lactoferrin, or cytokine levels. Low glucose concentration in amniotic fluid is a very sensitive marker for chorioamnionitis.

Chorioamnionitis is always an emergency and is potentially life-threatening to both mother and fetus. Treatment for chorioamnionitis includes antibiotic therapy, often clindamycin and an aminoglycoside (usually gentamicin), sometimes along with ampicillin.

~ *Differential Diagnoses*

PID may also occur in pregnancy and is most commonly caused by chlamydia or gonorrhea. It can be life-threatening to the fetus and cause serious maternal morbidity.

The woman with epidural anesthesia may become febrile in the absence of sepsis. Epidural anesthesia can also lead to fetal tachycardia and neonatal temperature >37.8 °C.

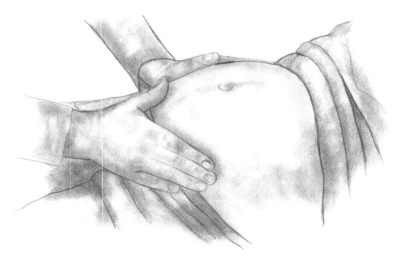

Figure 50. Palpating for tenderness. Chorioamnionitis presents with abdominal tenderness.

Cholecystitis/Cholelithiasis

Usually priority 3 progressing to priority 2

Cholelithiasis is the formation of gallstones, a condition that is often asymptomatic. Gallstones are rock-like accretions that form within the gallbladder. In the United States, 75–80% of gallstones are formed from cholesterol when there is an imbalance or change in the composition of bile (Lee & Chiang, 2006). Gallbladder sludge is crystallization within bile without stone formation which may progress to stones or persist independently.

Ninety-five percent of cholecystitis cases are caused by cholelithiasis (Dunphy, Winland-Brown, Porter, & Thomas, 2007). Pregnancy hormones encourage gallstone formation by changing the composition of bile and encouraging bile stasis. Biliary colic is usually caused when the gallbladder contracts after a fatty meal, pushing a stone against a duct and increasing pressure in the gallbladder. The pain subsides when the contraction stops and the stone falls back into the gallbladder. The gallbladder appears to empty more slowly in pregnancy, leading to biliary sludge (31%) and gallstone formation (2%). About 28% of women with gallbladder pathology will develop pain (Lee & Chiang, 2006).

The pain is often described as intense and dull. Acute cholecystitis presents with deep, gnawing right-upper-quadrant or epigastric pain, sometimes radiating to the shoulder, back, or chest; anorexia; nausea; vomiting; and fever. The pain begins within an hour or two postprandially and persists for 1–5 hr. The woman may be tender to palpation over the right upper quadrant, or have pain when pressed on the right midclavicular line on inspiration (Murphy's sign). The pain becomes increasingly worse over the span of a few hours; then as the gallbladder relaxes, the stones shift position and pain subsides. Pale or gray stools may occur if the bile duct is completely obstructed. Leukocytosis, increased bands, and sometimes elevated liver enzymes are present. Ultrasound scans can identify gallstones and biliary sludge, inflammation of the gallbladder, and dilation of the common bile duct.

Expectant management of cholecystitis is the safest approach in the pregnant client, but surgery may be indicated if pancreatitis, common bile duct obstruction, or cholangitis occurs. Severe cholecystitis can lead to abscess and gangrene or to perforation of the gallbladder with peritonitis caused by bile spilling into the abdominal cavity. Laparoscopic cholecystectomy (removal of the gallbladder), the most common laparoscopic procedure in pregnancy, is preferably performed in the second trimester. Although the risk of fetal loss to surgical intervention is low, surgery should be delayed until after delivery wherever possible.

~ Differential Diagnoses
Appendicitis, hepatitis, pancreatitis, right-sided pneumonia, intra-abdominal abscess, and acute fatty liver of pregnancy.

Pancreatitis
Priority 2 to 1
Pancreatitis occurs in 1 in 3,300 pregnancies (Cunningham, et al., 2004). It is usually associated with cholecystitis if a gallstone lodges within the ampule of Vater, blocking drainage of the pancreatic duct. Pain is typically sudden and severe, starting in the upper abdomen and radiating to the back, improved by leaning forward. Nausea, vomiting, decreased bowel sounds, and elevated amylase and lipase are typical findings. Rarely, flank ecchymosis, rebound tenderness, or ascites is present. If ultrasound shows gallstones as the cause of pancreatitis, surgery is usually performed. For other etiologies of pancreatitis, expectant management is the treatment of choice, and symptoms usually resolve in about 5 days with bowel rest, nasogastric suction, pain medication, and IV hydration.

~ Differential Diagnoses

Gastric or duodenal ulcer, bowel obstruction, ectopic pregnancy, biliary colic, appendicitis, diverticulitis.

Bowel Obstruction

Small-bowel obstructions occur in about 1 pregnancy in 1,500, often caused by adhesions from prior surgery, neoplasms, volvuli, intussusception, or hernia, or the pressure from a third-trimester uterus (Sinclair, 2004). Symptoms include diffuse, poorly localized pain (small-bowel obstruction being more painful than colonic obstruction), nausea, persistent vomiting of malodorous material, extreme constipation, and abdominal distention with tympany to percussion. Pain typically comes in waves—every 4–5 min for upper-bowel obstruction, every 10–15 min for lower-bowel. The clinician may palpate a loop of bowel and auscultate abnormal bowel sounds. Fetal mortality secondary to maternal bowel obstruction is 36% in the second trimester and 64% in the third; and maternal mortality is 20% (Sinclair, 2004). Diagnosis is confirmed by examination and abdominal scan, and surgery involves midline vertical abdominal incision.

~ Differential Diagnoses

Gastric or duodenal ulcer, pancreatitis, ectopic pregnancy, biliary colic, appendicitis, diverticulitis.

Acute Fatty Liver of Pregnancy

Acute Fatty Liver of Pregnancy (AFLP) is a rare, but serious, complication characterized by the accumulation of microvesicular fat within hepatocytes. AFLP usually presents in the third trimester with nausea and vomiting, right-upper-quadrant pain, jaundice, malaise. Laboratory values may show moderate elevations in serum aminotransferase levels (although usually not above 1,000 IU/L) with minimal elevations in bilirubin, as well as elevations in prothrombin time and activated partial thromboplastin time. Liver biopsy will show microvesicular fat. The disease carries high risk of both fetal and maternal mortality, and untreated it will progress to fulminant hepatic failure with jaundice, encephalopathy, disseminated intravascular coagulation (DIC), and fetal demise.

Treatment involves delivery of the fetus and supportive measures in the ICU for maternal coma, respiratory or renal failure, coagulopathy, or hemodynamic instability. The maternal mortality rate is approximately 12% (Bacq, 2008). Symptoms often resolve with delivery; but in some cases, liver disease continues to advance until liver transplantation is required.

~ Differential Diagnoses

Severe preeclampsia, HELLP syndrome, hepatitis.

Intrahepatic Cholestasis of Pregnancy

Intrahepatic cholestasis of pregnancy (ICP) occurs in otherwise healthy women only during pregnancy or use of oral contraceptives. In cases associated with pregnancy, it resolves after delivery without any increased risk of liver disease. ICP is characterized not by pain, but by severe generalized pruritus (itching) and skin lesions related to maternal liver dysfunction. ICP usually presents late in pregnancy. Pruritus is worse on the palms and the soles of the feet, but it resolves rapidly postpartum. The diagnosis is made when otherwise unexplainable pruritus occurs with abnormal laboratory values: gamma-glutamyl transpeptidase (GGT), alanine aminotransferase (ALT), aspartate aminotransferase (AST), or fasting serum total bile acids. Postpartum hemorrhage is more likely because of poor vitamin K absorption. If prothrombin time is abnormal, parenteral vitamin K is sometimes given.

As ICP progresses, jaundice or dark urine may occur, but not hepatic failure, hemolysis, thrombocytopenia, or DIC. Although the disorder does not appear to cause long-term harm to the mother, the fetus is at increased risk for stillbirth. Close fetal surveillance in the form of twice-weekly non-stress tests and AFI is usually recommended for the client with ICP. The fetus is usually delivered with documented lung maturity at 37 weeks unless nonreassuring fetal testing, meconium, or severe maternal symptoms necessitate earlier delivery.

~ Differential Diagnoses

Dry skin, drug reaction, uremia, iron deficiency, leukemia, thyroid disorders, diabetes.

Other Obstetrical Causes of Abdominal Pain

In early pregnancy, abdominal pain is often the initial symptom of ectopic pregnancy, spontaneous abortion, or septic abortion. Later in pregnancy, pain may be the only sign of placental abruption, placenta percreta, HELLP syndrome, or uterine rupture. These conditions are discussed at length elsewhere in this book.

Other Pain

Pregnant women can have intestinal gas or diarrhea cramps just as the rest of the population does. Acute diarrhea is usually caused by viruses, bacteria, or parasites. Constipation can cause persistent abdominal pain. Any woman who has had uterine or abdominal surgery may have adhesions—scar tissue—that bind and anchor her organs painfully as they try to expand and shift position. Abdominal pain in a pregnant woman can indicate placental abruption, uterine rupture, preeclampsia, preterm labor, ectopic pregnancy, or trauma. Gastroesophageal reflux disease (GERD) is very common in pregnancy. Left-upper-quadrant pain can result from diseases of the spleen.

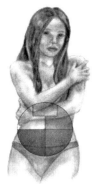

Figure 51. Where is the pain? Location can be an important clue to diagnosis.

Table 13. Etiologies To Consider for Abdominal Pain	
Epigastric Pain	
Consider gastric or duodenal ulcer, early appendicitis, hiatal hernia, HELLP syndrome, heartburn, gallbladder disease, pancreatitis—or rarely, myocardial infarction.	
Right-Upper-Quadrant Pain (RUQ)	**Left-Upper-Quadrant Pain (LUQ)**
Consider abruption, uterine rupture, cholecystitis, hepatitis, HELLP syndrome, constipation, pneumonia, diverticulitis, diarrhea, intestinal gas, fetal position, appendicitis. Right-flank pain radiating to the RUQ may be caused by renal calculi, hydronephrosis, or gallbladder.	Consider abruption, uterine rupture, heartburn, ulcers, constipation, diarrhea, diverticulitis, or enlarged spleen (such as with infectious mononucleosis).
Right-Lower-Quadrant Pain (RLQ)	**Left-Lower-Quadrant Pain (LLQ)**
Consider abruption, uterine rupture, round-ligament pain, intestinal gas, appendicitis, ectopic pregnancy, postsurgical adhesions, kidney stones, diverticulitis, inguinal hernia, endometriosis lesions, ovarian cysts and tumors, ovarian torsion, fibroids, cystitis.	Consider abruption, uterine rupture, round-ligament pain, colon pain, intestinal gas, ectopic pregnancy, postsurgical adhesions, kidney stones, diverticulitis, inguinal hernia, endometriosis lesions, ovarian cysts and tumors, ovarian torsion, fibroids, cystitis.

Somatization Disorder

Somatization or functional disorders can cause psychogenic pelvic pain. Because providers are unable to find a physical reason for the pain, these clients are often labeled attention-seekers, addicts, or malingerers. The holistic provider, however, recognizes that the nervous system, the endocrine system, the immune system, and all other body functions are interconnected. This is why emotional reactions can raise blood pressure or trigger vomiting or diarrhea.

Often, if a woman has experienced emotional trauma or suffers other psychological imbalance, blocked or diverted emotions apparently emerge as physical complaints that have no identifiable physical origin. Most frequently, the complaints involve chronic pain and problems with many seemingly unrelated body systems. These symptoms are very real to the client and may even be disabling. Treatment often involves psychological therapy, but medications such as selective serotonin reuptake inhibitors and alternative treatments such as acupuncture, myofascial release, and Reiki may be of benefit.

AACT—Consider and Treat

Priorities:
- OLDCART history
- Airway, breathing, and circulation, vital signs
- If vital signs unstable, provider or EMS should start IV line of saline or lactated Ringer's with appropriate lab draw, administer high flow oxygen, position for comfort and optimal vital signs, and transport rapidly to facility with the capacity for immediate surgery
- If client is stable, consult or transfer care as indicated, and arrange for transport as recommended by a physician
- Chart essential data and history for the receiving facility

DYSPNEA IN PREGNANCY

AACT—Alert

Sixty to 70% of healthy pregnant women complain of shortness of breath at some point in the pregnancy (Weinberger, 2007). During the first trimester, many women report a sensation of air hunger, which typically increases during the second trimester. High levels of progesterone increase respirations to the point of mild respiratory alkalosis, causing the feeling of breathlessness.

It can be difficult for the clinician to differentiate between progesterone-induced hyperventilation and respiratory pathology. Shortness of breath can be related to anemia or a cardiac problem, but most pathological dyspnea in pregnancy is related to asthma, lower respiratory infection, or pulmonary embolism.

Rapid onset of dyspnea may indicate acute asthma, anaphylaxis, pulmonary edema, or pulmonary embolism. Slow onset is associated with pneumonia or infections. The client with asthma will usually have a wheeze or cough, features that distinguish it from dyspnea of pregnancy.

Although dyspnea of pregnancy is gradual and persistent, pulmonary embolism usually has a sudden onset and may be accompanied by pleuritic chest pain (pain with breathing) and hemoptysis. Acute respiratory distress syndrome (ARDS) occurs rarely, usually in association with severe preeclampsia, amniotic fluid embolism, or use of tocolytic agents.

✍ AACT—Analyze and Consider

Venous Thromboembolism
Priority 2 to 1

Venous thromboembolism (VTE) includes deep-vein thrombosis (DVT), a blood clot that forms in the veins of the lower extremities or pelvis, and pulmonary embolism (PE) when a clot dislodges and travels to block the pulmonary arteries. VTE complicates between 1 in 500 and 1 in 2,000 pregnancies and is the *leading cause of maternal mortality in developed countries*, responsible for about 20% of direct maternal deaths (Schwartz, Malhotra, & Weinberger, 2007).

During pregnancy the risk of pulmonary embolism is increased five- to six-fold due to venous stasis, endothelial injury, and a hypercoagulable state (Virchow's triad). Thromboembolism can occur in any trimester, but it is most common postpartum, especially after cesarean delivery. Delivery is associated with vascular injury and hemostasis at the site of uteroplacental interface, increasing VTE in the immediate postpartum period. Risk factors include varicosities, inherited thrombophilia, antiphospholipid antibody syndrome, obesity, older age, personal or family history of thromboembolic events, recent surgery, trauma, immobility, and high parity.

A thrombus may form in a superficial or deep vessel. Deep-vein thrombosis is more serious. It is most likely to involve the left leg because of compression of the left iliac vein by the right iliac artery, pressure of the pregnant uterus on the inferior vena cava, and changes in venous capacitance. Most DVTs in pregnancy form in the iliofemoral vein; relatively few arise in the calf. The woman will present with pain, heat, redness, and swelling in one of her legs and perhaps a palpable rigid, distended leg vein; and the affected leg may be considerably more swollen and mottled than the other. The provider should suspect DVT if the circumference of one leg is more than 2 cm greater than that of the other. She may be febrile. Homan's sign (pain on dorsiflexion of the foot) may not be positive with deep-vein thrombosis. DVT can also occur in the iliac veins of the pelvis, causing pain in the lower abdomen. Untreated, as many as 24% of women with DVTs will go on to develop pulmonary embolism, and 15% of those will die (Howell, Grady, & Cox, 2007).

The clinical diagnoses of both DVT and PE are notoriously nonsensitive and nonspecific. Many cases of PE are essentially asymptomatic; only 20% display the classic triad of hemoptysis, pleuritic chest pain, and dyspnea. Pulmonary embolism may present with tachypnea (89%), dyspnea (81%), pleuritic chest pain (72%), apprehension (59%), cough (54%), tachycardia (43%), hempoptysis (34%), and/or temperature >37c (34%) (Howell, et al., 2007). Some women with PE present with only vague apprehension, chest discomfort, or shortness of breath, which may be attributed to the usual discomforts of pregnancy and postpartum. Diagnosis is especially elusive in pregnant women, because lower-extremity swelling and leg discomfort are common in advanced pregnancy, mimicking DVT.

Diagnosis of VTE during pregnancy can be complicated by physiologic changes associated with pregnancy and by reluctance of parents and physicians to expose the fetus to even small amounts of ionizing radiation. Doppler ultrasound is a noninvasive, relatively inexpensive test that can be highly sensitive and specific for DVT. All tests positive for proximal DVT should prompt immediate treatment. It is important to diagnose DVT accurately so that acute treatment can be initiated and the client can be screened for underlying thrombophilia, but objective testing confirms DVT in fewer than 10% of women presenting with signs and symptoms (Schwartz, et al., 2007).

Arterial blood gases in both PE and normal pregnancy show respiratory alkalosis. D-dimer, a breakdown product of cross-linked fibrin, is normally elevated in pregnancy, increasing with gestational age and reaching approximately 685 ng/ml at delivery and immediately postpartum. D-dimer alone is not enough to rule out or rule in the diagnosis of PE.

The clinical severity of PE can be highly variable. Acute pulmonary embolism is often fatal—its mortality rate is approximately 30% without treatment (Schwartz, et al., 2007). Without treatment, approximately one third of clients who survive an initial PE of any severity die of a future embolic episode.

✍ AACT—Treat

When a client presents with suspected VTE, initial care should focus on stabilizing her and getting her to definitive care. Death from pulmonary embolism is most likely to occur within a few hours of onset, but prompt treatment with anticoagulants decreases mortality to 2–8%.

Suspected DVT involves consultation with a physician and expeditious transport to a facility capable of diagnosis and treatment. The woman should be transported with the leg elevated and no pressure on the affected vein. Do not massage the leg and use caution when palpating the swelling—rubbing the leg may dislodge the clot and send it to the lungs.

If you suspect your client has a pulmonary embolism, move quickly, prioritizing airway, breathing, and circulation and optimal placental perfusion. Rapid transport is essential for the client with a suspected pulmonary embolism, preferably via EMS. Oxygen by nasal cannula at 4 L/min is suitable for the client in minor distress; but with dyspnea, high-flow oxygen by mask is indicated. Administer IV fluids carefully, infusing no more than about 500 ml during the initial resuscitation period to avoid fluid overload that can precipitate right ventricular failure. If cardiovascular collapse occurs, resuscitate as appropriate. Paramedics will initiate cardiac monitoring and will intubate and support respirations if she is unable to maintain her airway.

Definitive Care

In the hospital, the pregnant woman with thromboembolic disease is diagnosed similarly to her nonpregnant counterpart. Doppler ultrasound examination of the lower extremities, helical computed tomographic (CT) scan, and low-dose radioisotope ventilation perfusion (V/Q) scan are often employed, but pulmonary angiography is avoided unless necessary.

There are no definitive tests for pulmonary embolism. The ventilation-perfusion (V/Q) scan is the most accurate diagnostic modality, but it can show false negatives. Bloodwork, chest X rays, and EKGs are usually unremarkable.

Pulmonary embolism can lead to severe hypoxemia or respiratory failure requiring intubation and mechanical ventilation. Massive PE is characterized by persistent hypotension necessitating hemodynamic support. To save the life of a hemodynamically unstable woman, the physician may consider thrombolysis, surgical embolectomy, or transvenous catheter embolectomy despite possible risks to the fetus.

If noninvasive testing is equivocal, the physician may opt for contrast venography with appropriate shielding. Alternatively, MRI may be performed if there is contraindication to venography, client refusal of contrast, or strong clinical suspicion of pelvic thrombosis. Magnetic resonance imaging (MRI) is highly accurate in diagnosing thigh and pelvic vein DVT in the nonpregnant pregnant, but has not yet been well studied in pregnancy. MRI is likely to take the place of venography as the gold standard for the diagnosis of pregnancy-associated DVT. Helical (spiral) CT scanning using IV contrast (CT angiography) is also useful for diagnosing pulmonary embolism. The estimated fetal radiation exposure from the combination of a chest radiograph, V/Q scanning, and pulmonary arteriography is 0.5 to 1% of the dose considered teratogenic.

When diagnosis of DVT or PE is made, therapeutic anticoagulation is initiated with low-molecular-weight heparins, such as enoxaparin and dalteparin, or unfractionated heparin. Heparin is considered safe for pregnant and lactating women because it does not cross the placenta and is not secreted in breast milk. LMW heparins are at least as effective as unfractionated heparin, and side effects such as thrombocytopenia; osteoporosis, bleeding and allergy are less common.

The woman on LMW heparin is at risk for epidural hematoma at the time of epidural catheter placement or removal, so many clients are changed to subcutaneous unfractionated heparin 2 weeks before expected delivery to allow regional anesthesia for labor and delivery. Epidural anesthesia should not be attempted within 24 hr of the last LMW heparin injection. If the PTT is markedly prolonged, protamine sulfate is used to reverse the effects of heparin at the time of delivery

Heparin is typically restarted 6 hr after a vaginal delivery or 12 hr after cesarean if no major bleeding has occurred. Heparin should be continued or switched to warfarin in the postpartum period. Warfarin (Coumadin) is avoided during pregnancy because it crosses the placenta and increases the risk of miscarriage and stillbirth, causes fetal anomalies, and can produce maternal and fetal hemorrhage near term. Warfarin is, however, considered safe for nursing women because it does not accumulate substantially in breast milk. Warfarin may be prescribed 4–6 weeks after delivery for a total course of anticoagulation lasting 3–6 months. Occasionally, inferior vena cava filters are used if anticoagulation is contraindicated or PE recurs despite adequate anticoagulation.

Compression stockings increase femoral-vein flow velocity in late pregnancy. The prophylactic regimen of choice in pregnant women at high risk for VTE is

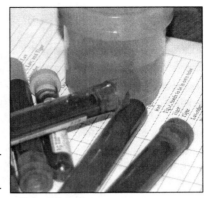

Figure 52. Laboratory tests are indispensable for diagnosing and treating dyspnea in the pregnant client.

subcutaneous low-dose heparin in doses of 5,000–10,000 units continued until delivery. The woman with a history of idiopathic VTE or documented hypercoagulable state should be prophylaxed with subcutaneous adjusted-dose heparin.

Pulmonary Edema
Priority 1

Pulmonary edema can develop antepartum, intrapartum, or postpartum. Normal pregnancy involves increased cardiac output, faster heart rate, and decreased systemic vascular resistance and colloid osmotic pressure, which can lead to pulmonary edema if the fluid balance is altered. Pregnancy-related pulmonary edema is usually associated with use of tocolytic medications, underlying cardiac disease, iatrogenic fluid overload, or preeclampsia.

Tocolytics are more likely to cause pulmonary edema if used in combination, especially when IV magnesium sulfate is used with subcutaneous terbutaline. Occasionally, tocolytic–related pulmonary edema progresses to acute respiratory distress syndrome (ARDS). Pulmonary edema may also herald the onset of peripartum cardiomyopathy, a life-threatening condition that can arise at the end of pregnancy or postpartum.

Pulmonary edema presents with basilar crackles (rales) that do not clear after a cough, usually bilaterally. When fluid or mucus collects in the lung bases, alveoli collapse and the walls of the alveoli stick together. When the woman takes a breath, the alveolar walls are forced open with a popping sound. Fine crackles are usually late-inspiratory, soft, high-pitched, and very brief. The sound is similar to that of a lock of hair rolled between the fingers near the ears. Coarse crackles are early inspiratory, louder, and low-pitched, and they last longer than fine crackles. The sound is similar to the snap of opening Velcro. Sometimes pulmonary edema presents with wheezing. Other symptoms of pulmonary edema include dyspnea (76%), chest pain (24%), cough (17%), and fever (14%) (Poole & Spreen, 2005). Severe cases involving heart failure may include expectorating pink foam (Ernst, 2007).

Although pulmonary edema is potentially life-threatening, it responds quickly to treatment. First, address the underlying cause. Sit the woman upright to encourage fluid pooling in the dependent body parts. Diuretic therapy with furosemide (Lasix) may be employed to relieve intravascular volume overload. Besides increasing elimination of excess fluid, furosemide also acts initially as a vasodilator, opening peripheral vessels to shunt excess fluid from the lungs to the extremities. Morphine sulfate, in doses of 2–5 mg intravenously also increases venous capacitance and reduces the workload of the heart, while increasing the stroke volume and cardiac output. Morphine relieves anxiety as well. Almost all cases in the obstetrical client resolve within 12–24 hr with morphine, furosemide, and oxygen supplementation (Poole & Spreen, 2005).

Asthma

Priority 3, 2, or 1

✍ AACT—Consider

Asthma is the most common chronic condition in pregnancy, involving inflammation of the airways and an abnormal accumulation of eosinophils, lymphocytes, mast cells, macrophages, dendritic cells, and myofibroblasts. An "asthma attack" occurs when smooth muscle of the bronchioles and bronchi contract, decreasing the size of the air passages and vascular congestion, bronchial wall edema, and thick secretions further obstruct the flow of air. Between exacerbations, most clients are free from symptoms.

Asthma complicates 4–6% of pregnancies, remaining stable in about one third of pregnant women, worsening in about one third, and improving in about one third (Coleman & Rund, 1997). Occasionally, asthma is diagnosed for the first time during pregnancy, so the clinician should suspect asthma when evaluating any pregnant client complaining of wheezing, cough, or dyspnea. Perinatal mortality is no higher for stable asthmatic women than for women without the disease. Severe or poorly controlled asthma, however, can lead to preeclampsia, IUGR, and premature delivery. Steroid-dependent women with severe asthma are more likely to develop gestational diabetes, congenital anomalies, and hypertension.

Asthma can be triggered by allergy, upper-respiratory-tract infection, gastroesophageal reflux, sinusitis, exercise, aspirin, nonsteroidal anti-inflammatory agents, tobacco smoke, chemical fumes, humidity, and emotional upset. Exacerbations are most likely to occur early in the third trimester, usually triggered by viral infection or nonadherence to inhaled corticosteroid medication. Only 10% of asthmatics experience bronchoconstriction during labor and delivery (Coleman & Rund, 1997).

Pregnant women with asthma are usually managed on the same medications they used before pregnancy, including bronchodilators and steroids. Albuterol (Proventil), metaproterenol (Alupent), or isoetharine (Bronkosol) are all Category B and considered safe for pregnant women.

If your client is having an asthma attack, rapidly address the ABCs and POP. The bronchoconstriction of an asthma attack often produces audible wheezing. A wheeze is a continuous, coarse whistle produced by air moving across a narrowed or obstructed passage within the respiratory tree. Expiratory wheezing represents a 50% reduction in peak expiratory flow rate. Some clients with asthma present with coughing rather than wheezing; and if bronchospasm is severe, wheeze may be absent due to decreased airflow.

Other symptoms of asthma exacerbation include cough, chest tightness, and nocturnal awakenings. Physical examination may show tachypnea, pulsus paradoxicus (pulse that is weaker during inhalation and stronger during exhalation), wheezes, diffuse rhonchi (gurgles). The expiratory phase of respiration is often longer than the inspiratory phase.

Assess the severity of the dyspnea. The woman with a severe asthma attack may have decreased breath sounds and no wheeze, due to lack of air exchange. Use of accessory muscles to breathe (sternocleidomastoid, abdominal, pectoral), agitation, confusion, lethargy, cyanosis, and exhaustion herald impending respiratory arrest. "Tripodding" is an instinctive posture adopted by people in respiratory distress to minimize airway resistance, upright with hands on knees or thrust forward, torso inclined slightly forward, and the neck extended to the "sniffing" position

✍ AACT—Treat

Consult a physician or transfer to the hospital as indicated. Consider EMS for transport if respiratory distress is significant. Provide oxygen—high flow for moderate or severe distress, low flow for mild distress. Establish IV access with normal saline. Frequently assess the client, the severity of the attack, and the client's response to treatment.

In the ambulance or at the hospital, cardiac monitoring and pulse oximetry are initiated. Oxygen is titrated to maintain oxygen saturation higher than 95%. An inhaled beta-2 agonist is usually given as three doses over 60–90 min. Systemic steroids such as prednisone take effect within 4–6 hr of the start of therapy and shorten the hospital stay. Arterial blood gas (ABG) analysis can be used to identify respiratory acidosis. Fetal monitoring is employed near or above the threshold of viability. Hand-held peak-flow meters can compare measurements to a known baseline to assess the severity of the attack. Very few women require intubation or mechanical ventilation. The physician may consider alternative pharmacological regimens to reduce the likelihood of future attacks and educate the client about triggers to avoid.

~ Differential Diagnoses

Anaphylaxis, drug reaction, airway obstruction, amniotic fluid embolism, congestive heart failure (CHF) related to peripartum cardiomyopathy, physiologic dyspnea of pregnancy.

Pneumonia

Priority 3 to 2

Pneumonia is the most common cause of nonobstetric infection in the pregnant woman. Pneumonia can occur at any stage of gestation, but is most likely to occur midway through the third trimester. Women with a history of tobacco or cocaine use, anemia, or respiratory disease are at highest risk, and delay in diagnosis may result in severe complications.

Pneumonia presents similarly in pregnant and nonpregnant clients and often follows upper-respiratory-tract infection and cough. Fever above 38.3°C (101°F) is often seen, and the woman may or may not report dyspnea. Pneumonia increases the risk of preterm labor, especially between 20 and 36 weeks' gestation.

Most cases of pneumonia are caused by *Streptococcus pneumoniae, Haemophilus influenzae, Mycoplasma pneumoniae, Legionella, Chlamydia pneumoniae,* or influenza A. Alterations in immune status make the pregnant woman especially vulnerable to pneumonia and make viral, fungal, and tuberculous infections particularly pathogenic. The elevated intragastric pressure of pregnancy increases risk of aspiration pneumonia as well. Chest radiographs are recommended for the client with a history suggestive of pneumonia. Typical labs include CBC with differential, chemistry panel, blood cultures at two sites, and sputum Gram stain and culture. Therapy for bacterial pneumonia is determined by the safety profile and effectiveness against typical and atypical pathogens.

~ *Differential Diagnoses*

Bronchitis, appendicitis, pyelonephritis.

Hyperventilation and Hyperventilation Syndrome

✍ AACT—Consider

Hyperventilation

Priority 1, 2, 3, or 4, depending on etiology

Hyperventilation is a condition of decreased carbon dioxide levels in the blood causing respiratory alkalosis. Rapid breathing, however, may be a symptom of underlying pathology such as myocardial infarction, uremia, sepsis, shock, hypoxia, liver failure, or medication reaction/overdose or overdose. Diabetic ketoacidosis can cause deep, rapid respirations. Pulmonary embolus can cause rapid, shallow breathing. Tachypnea can also be a normal response to pain.

Hyperventilation Syndrome

Priority 4—not exactly normal, but benign

"Hyperventilation syndrome" occurs when stress, anxiety, depression, or anger triggers rapid respirations that skew the balance of carbon dioxide in the blood. The client has a sensation of being unable to breathe, despite the increased respirations, and may develop numbness in hands, feet, and face. Severe cases include carpopedal spasms, involuntary muscular contraction of the hands and feet that occur when the low carbon dioxide levels cause hypocalcemia. Panic leads to rapid breathing, which reinforces the panic.

✍ AACT—Treat

When your client is breathing rapidly, attempt to find the cause. Give oxygen. If the problem is hyperventilation syndrome, the problem is a decreased carbon dioxide level, not too much oxygen. Oxygen will not compound the problem, and if the tachypnea is pathological, oxygen may be beneficial. Attend to ABCs with POP, monitor lung sounds, and reassure the client. Consult a physician or transfer to the hospital as indicated. Pulse oximetry, electrocardiogram, a complete metabolic panel and other tests will help the hospital provider determine etiology.

SYNCOPE IN PREGNANCY

Priority depends on etiology

Syncope commonly occurs in pregnant women, and most episodes are benign and self-limiting. Fainting takes place when blood flow to the brain is temporarily reduced, and it is often related to redistribution of blood volume, hypoglycemia, overheating, or a vagal response.

When a healthy nonpregnant person stands, 500–1000 ml of blood pools in the lower extremities, decreasing venous return to the heart and thereby decreasing cardiac output and blood pressure. The body quickly responds with the baroreceptor reflex, which increases sympathetic tone and reduces parasympathetic outflow. Peripheral vascular resistance, venous return, and cardiac output increase, limiting drop in blood pressure until it is clinically insignificant. Postural (orthostatic) hypotension is diagnosed when 2–5 min of standing is followed by a 20 mmHg or greater fall in systolic pressure, 10 mmHg or greater fall in diastolic pressure, and symptoms of cerebral hypoperfusion (Kaufmann, Kaplan, & Freeman, 2004). Orthostatic syncope occurs when blood collects in the veins of the legs or abdomen, and cardiac output and arterial pressure fall.

Progesterone causes decreased vascular tone, which can increase the pooling of blood in dependent areas with prolonged standing or changing from supine to standing. In the second half of pregnancy, pressure from the gravid uterus can decrease blood flow through the vena cava when the woman is supine or seated upright. Dehydration can increase this effect by reducing blood volume. When the ambient temperature is high, heat syncope can result from vasodilation, peripheral pooling, and volume depletion.

Neurocardiogenic (vasovagal) syncope is one of the most common causes of fainting in the pregnant and nonpregnant populations. It is an abnormal autonomic response causing peripheral vasodilation and increased vagal tone, leading to reduced cardiac filling and bradycardia. Neurocardiogenic syncope may be induced by prolonged standing, venipuncture (experienced or witnessed), heat exposure, painful or noxious stimuli, fear of bodily injury, or exertion. Some individuals, however, have recurrent episodes without an identifiable cause (Olshansky, 2004). It is usually preceded by lightheadedness, diaphoresis, pallor, blurry or darkening vision, nausea, or hot flashes (Kaufmann, et al., 2004).

Cardiogenic syncope results from the failure of the heart to pump enough blood to perfuse the brain. Bradycardia may be related to a cardiac conduction problem, medication reaction or overdose, head injury, poisoning, severe hypoxia, or a vagal response. Tachycardia can cause the heart to pump inefficiently. Very fast rates such as those related to supraventricular tachycardia (SVT) may not allow the heart to fill between beats, reducing cardiac output. This may result in an apical heart rate considerably faster than the radial pulse. The amplitude (strength) of the pulse may vary from beat to beat (pulsus alternans), even though the apical rhythm is regular.

Table 14. Symptoms Associated with Changes in Consciousness Can Aid Diagnosis

Headache
Think stroke, hypoglycemia, carbon monoxide poisoning, trauma, tumor
Chest pain
Think cardiogenic shock
Shortness of breath
Think hypoxia, cardiogenic shock
Thirst
Think heat stroke, diabetic ketoacidosis
Frequent urination
Think diabetic ketoacidosis, urosepsis
Numbness
Think spinal trauma, stroke
Unilateral weakness or paralysis
Think stroke, hypoglycemia, cardiogenic shock

Decreased cardiac return can also cause fainting. Saunas, tanning beds, hot tubs, and other extremes of heat (all of which should be avoided in pregnancy) dilate peripheral vessels and decrease venous return, causing fainting when the woman stands upright. Straining during exercise, coughing, bowel movement, and urination increases the pressure in the chest and abdomen, decreasing cardiac return and thereby reducing blood flow to the brain, precipitating syncope.

Although most syncope is benign, the provider must consider pathological causes, such as ruptured ectopic pregnancy, seizure disorder, hemorrhage, stroke, PE, arrhythmia, Wolff-Parkinson-White syndrome, or cardiomyopathy. Many medications and some herbal remedies contribute to syncope.

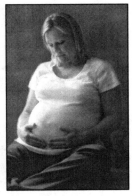

Figure 53. Mental status changes—altered level of consciousness may indicate serious illness.

Syncope is self-limiting. The woman should be turned on her side with her legs elevated, and consciousness should rapidly return. If the woman remains unresponsive, the situation is undoubtedly more serious. Injury from falling is a concern, especially if fainting occurs when driving or climbing stairs. Sometimes syncope can resemble a seizure, presenting with brief tonic-clonic activity. The syncopal client rapidly regains consciousness with positioning to increase cerebral blood flow. A seizure is followed by a postictal state, however, and will not show the hypotension and bradycardia that often accompanies syncope.

Syncope may warrant evaluation by a physician, but the best treatment is prevention. The woman with presyncopal symptoms should be taught to flex her leg muscles periodically after prolonged standing, to sit for a minute before rising from a supine position, and to rest in a lateral recumbent position. She should drink fluids until her urine runs clear and possibly increase her salt intake if she is chronically hypotensive. Prescription support stockings reduce pooling of blood in the lower legs. Counsel her to maintain optimal blood sugar with high protein snacks and to avoid simple carbohydrates and caffeine. Stimulation of the carotid sinus can cause syncope, so the woman should avoid wearing tight clothing around the neck. If she feels as if she might faint, she should immediately lie on her side and elevate her legs. If she remains in this position for about 15 min, sipping water and perhaps snacking, chances are good that she will feel better upon rising.

- ▶ *Alert and oriented x 4* **means**
  - ▶ **Person**—Does she know her name?
  - ▶ **Place**—Does she know where she is?
  - ▶ **Time**—Does she know the date?
  - ▶ **Purpose**—Does she know what she was doing when the event occurred?

Table 15. Glasgow Coma Scale (Used to assess the degree of coma)		
Eye opening	Spontaneously	4
	To verbal command	3
	To pain	2
	No response	1
Best motor response	Obeys commands	6
	Localizes to pain	5
	Withdraws to pain	4
	Abnormal flexion	3
	Abnormal extension	2
	No response	1
Best verbal response	Oriented, converses	5
	Disoriented	4
	Inappropriate words	3
	Incomprehensible sounds	2
	No response	1
A perfect GCS score is 15. The worst possible score is not 0, but 3.		

Altered Level of Consciousness
Usually priority 1 or 2

✍ AACT—Consider

There are many potential causes for altered level of consciousness or unresponsiveness in the pregnant client. Changes in consciousness can range from a subtle shift in personality to unresponsiveness. Choking can obstruct the airway and cause loss of consciousness. Anaphylactic, cardiogenic, septic, or hemorrhagic shock can also cause the client to become stuporous or unconscious. Status epilepticus can occasionally present with subtle rhythmic twitching of some of the digits of either hand or horizontal jerking of the eyes.

Trauma, including head injuries, shock, and hypoxia, commonly cause unconsciousness, sometimes in conjunction with a precipitating medical event such as hypoglycemia. If one pupil is dilated and unresponsive to light, suspect severe head injury or stroke. Cushing's triad (progressive hypertension, bradycardia, and slowing respirations) is a pre-morbid sign of critically rising intracranial pressure, usually due to head trauma or stroke. Head injury is not usually associated with hypotension–if her blood pressure is low and she has an obvious head injury, seek alternative explanations such as internal bleeding.

Table 16. States of Consciousness

Alertness

Normal state of arousal.

Sleep

Non-pathological decreased mental status from which the client can be readily aroused to full consciousness.

Confusion

Adequate arousal, but with clinical evidence of cognitive dysfunction and disorientation

Delirium

Confusion with agitation and hallucinations.

Lethargy

Arousal is diminished but is maintained spontaneously or with repeated light stimuli. May drift slowly into unconsciousness if unstimulated.

Obtundation

Decreased arousal with purposeful responses to touch or verbal stimuli, drowsiness between unconscious states.

Stupor

Severely impaired arousal with purposeful responses to vigorous stimuli, drifts immediately into unconsciousness when vigorous stimulation ceases.

Coma

Markedly depressed consciousness. Poorly responsive or unresponsive to vigorous physical stimuli.

Persistent vegetative state

Vital functions intact, awareness absent.

Women with diabetes can experience alterations in consciousness related to blood-sugar levels, especially when insulin dependent. Pregnant diabetic women can experience wide swings in blood sugar from significantly hyperglycemic to seriously hypoglycemic, sometimes within the span of hours. Unstable blood glucose is most often seen in women who are learning to use insulin or who are noncompliant with treatment. Hypoglycemia usually has a rapid onset and may be caused by too much insulin, inadequate food intake after insulin dose, exertion, malnutrition, alcoholism, sepsis, cancer (especially pancreatic), or hypothermia.

Symptoms of hyperglycemia are increased urination, thirst, hunger, and fatigue, progressing to coma, deep (Kussmaul's) respirations, and an acetone scent to the breath. Diabetic ketoacidosis (DKA) occurs when there is insufficient insulin to allow glucose to move from the blood into the cells. The cells become starved for glucose and begin to break down primary fats for energy, resulting in acidosis. DKA evolves over 12–48 hr. It is treated with insulin, IV fluids, careful attention to electrolytes (including calcium, phosphorous, potassium, and magnesium), and determining the cause. Glucocorticoids and beta-2 agonists will worsen hyperglycemia.

Poisoning may be accidental or intentional. Excessive alcohol consumption can cause a life-threatening coma. Sympathomimetics like cocaine and methamphetamine can cause tachycardia, hypertension, dilated pupils, delirium, stroke, or cardiac arrest. Cholinergics, found in pesticides (organophosphates, carbamates) and nerve agents (sarin, somin), cause headache, dizziness, bradycardia, weakness, coma, seizures, and SLUDGE (Salivation, Lacrimation, Urination, Defecation, Gastrointestinal upset, and Emesis). Atropine in large doses will reverse the effects.

The woman with acute opiate toxicity from an overdose of heroin or prescription narcotic medications will have respiratory depression and pinpoint pupils. The IV drug abuser may have visible track marks. Narcan (naloxone) 2 mg administered very slowly by IV push will completely reverse the symptoms of opiate overdose. The client will suddenly become fully conscious, but the chronic abuser is likely to become combative and develop projectile vomiting.

Suspect stroke or brain tumor in any client with altered level of consciousness. Associated symptoms include severe headache, vomiting, hemiparesis or hemiplegia, aphasia, unequal pupils, facial droop, slurred speech, drooling, unequal handgrips, seizures, incontinence, ataxia, vision problems, and vertigo.

If you are familiar with the woman, it may be easier to determine the cause. If you encounter an unresponsive pregnant woman not previously known to you, obtain history from witnesses or bystanders. How long has the woman been unconscious? Has she been using medication, chemicals, or illicit drugs? Are there environmental clues such as unusual odors, other people with similar symptoms, suicide notes, weapons, or drug bottles? If the person appears to have fallen, did she become unconscious and then fall, or did she fall and then lose consciousness? What begins as simple fainting may become a head injury with cervical spine damage.

✍ AACT—Treat

Treatment should follow clinical findings. Consult or transfer as indicated, summon EMS when appropriate, and transport as necessary. Initial care includes

Airway

- Opening the airway using the chin-lift/head-tilt or jaw-thrust maneuver
- Removing any airway obstruction
- Maintaining an open airway if the woman is unable to maintain it herself. The tongue can obstruct the airway in the unconscious person, and suctioning may be necessary to clear secretions and vomitus.
- Intubation if indicated.
- Maintaining the woman in the left lateral position, if there is no trauma, to let secretions flow out of the mouth and away from the airways and to maximize placental perfusion.

Breathing

- Assessing rate, rhythm, lung sounds and tidal volume
- Assisting ventilations if breathing is ineffective
- Rescue breathing (if the woman is not breathing) using mouth-to-mouth, mouth-to-mask, or bag-valve-mask
- Administering oxygen by nasal cannula or mask

Circulation

- Assessing pulse rate, rhythm, and quality
- Optimizing placental perfusion
- Starting an IV line of normal saline. If blood pressure is low due to hypovolemia, institute appropriate fluid replacement.
- Initiating cardiac monitoring and treating as indicated
- Giving naloxone (usually done by EMS) to clients who are unresponsive from an unknown etiology

Check glucose with a glucometer and administer carbohydrates if the woman is conscious (20 g, obtainable from approximately 12 oz of orange or apple juice, 15 oz of milk, 14 oz of carbonated soft drink, or sugar paste). If she is unconscious, give IV D-50 or IM glucagon.

Carbon Monoxide Poisoning

Usually priority 2, but priority depends on condition

Carbon monoxide is a leading cause of poison-related mortality and morbidity in industrialized countries. Carbon monoxide is an odorless, colorless gas formed by the incomplete combustion of organic compounds. Carbon monoxide toxicity may occur when exhaust systems malfunction, when ventilation is obstructed or when equipment designed for the outdoors is used in confined areas. Possible sources include gas water heaters, kerosene space heaters, charcoal grills, propane stoves, and propane-fueled forklifts. In Florida during the 2004 hurricane season, a substantial number of people suffered carbon monoxide toxicity from gasoline-powered backup generators operating outdoors, but near residential air conditioners, which drew carbon monoxide indoors. House fires generate carbon monoxide along with other toxins such as cyanide. Many successful suicides involve carbon monoxide exposure. Fumes from some spray paints, solvents, degreasers, and paint removers are converted to carbon monoxide in the liver.

Carbon monoxide is an abortifacient and a teratogen. It binds with maternal hemoglobin with an affinity 200–250 times greater than that of oxygen, and fetal hemoglobin has an even stronger attraction. Fetal carbon monoxide levels can be significantly higher than those of the mother, and the fetus can suffer severe damage even if maternal symptoms are moderate. Exposure can result in immediate or delayed pregnancy loss, physical malformations, and neurological impairment. Risk is greater when the woman is exposed to carbon monoxide for an hour or more. Smokers may have baseline levels of carboxyhemoglobin as high as 10%, and are more susceptible to toxic effects from other sources of carbon monoxide.

The nervous system and heart are very susceptible to damage from carbon monoxide poisoning, but other organs are also affected. When the hemoglobin is saturated with carbon monoxide, it cannot pick up oxygen, and the woman becomes hypoxic at the cellular level. Intracellular uptake of carbon monoxide may also be a mechanism for injury. Some women develop cognitive deficits to incapacitating movement disorders up to 40 days after exposure. Undetected exposure can be fatal.

Persons with carbon monoxide poisoning often overlook or fail to notice the symptoms, may include headache, dizziness, nausea, flu-like malaise, exertional dyspnea, chest pain, ventricular dysrhythmias, disorientation, lethargy, hallucinations, agitation, lack of coordination, abdominal pain, syncope, seizure, and coma. Cherry-red skin color is rare; most carbon monoxide poisoning victims are pale and cyanotic. Small infants may present with only vomiting and may show symptoms before the rest of the family. Clients who present with these symptoms should be questioned about the use of gas- or oil-fueled appliances and the presence of similar symptoms in other household members, in pets, or in neighbors.

Emergency treatment priorities include stabilization of airway, breathing, and circulation; removal from the toxic environment; application of 100% oxygen; cardiac monitoring; and rapid transport. The pregnant woman with high carboxyhemoglobin levels or serious symptoms may require treatment with hyperbaric oxygen at a regional facility. Hyperbaric oxygen accelerates the clearance of carbon monoxide from the body, correcting hypoxia and preventing central nervous system damage.

Heat-Related Illness
Priority 1, 2, or 3, depending on severity

Extremes of heat can cause alteration in level of consciousness. Heat syncope can occur following exposure to a hot environment, secondary to venous pooling and volume depletion. The client will usually make a full recovery if moved to a cool environment, allowed to rest on her side, and encouraged to take oral fluids.

Heat exhaustion results from a warm ambient environment and excessive fluid loss with insufficient rehydration. The client with heat exhaustion may show tachycardia; muscle weakness; muscle cramps; thirst; anxiety; headache; nausea and vomiting; and hot, red skin. Often the client can be treated at home by moving her to a cool environment, placing her in the left lateral position with legs elevated, and encouraging her to take at least 1 L of fluids an hour. If recovery is not rapid or fetal heart tones are not reassuring, transport.

Heat stroke is a serious illness that carries a mortality rate of 10% and may damage multiple organ systems (Dunphy, et al., 2007). Core body temperature soars to > 104.9°F, and sweating is no longer present. The client's respirations are rapid, and she may become confused or lose consciousness. Nausea, vomiting, hypotension, oliguria, and seizures may occur. Heat stroke requires rapid transport by ambulance, with ice packs in the groin and axillae, rapid infusions of normal saline, and airway management as indicated by the woman's condition.

Seizures
Usually priority 2 or 1

When a pregnant woman is found seizing, the clinician's first thought is often eclampsia. Although it is important to consider this possibility, remember that some pregnant women have preexisting seizure disorders and can seize at any time. Any given person has a 9% lifetime risk of experiencing at least one seizure and a 3% risk of developing epilepsy (Pohlmann-Eden, Beghi, Camfield, & Camfield, 2006). Seizures can also accompany head injury, alcohol withdrawal, or stroke. Some seizures due to vascular abnormalities occur only during pregnancy.

About 20% of clients with a seizure disorder show a worsening of seizures during pregnancy (Ratcliffe, et al., 2008). Some physiologic changes of pregnancy—electrolyte balance, respiration, and intracellular volume—may lower the seizure threshold, and fatigue and emotional stress may contribute to more frequent seizures. It may be difficult to maintain therapeutic levels of anticonvulsant medications during pregnancy because of nausea, vomiting, changes in blood volume, or a client's reluctance to take the medications.

Women with seizure disorders have a higher risk of spontaneous abortion and perinatal mortality. Some seizures occur without warning, causing shoulder dislocations and broken bones. Most anticonvulsants have the potential to cause anomalies in the infant; but because maternal seizures can cause fetal acidosis, fetal and maternal hypoxia, and placental abruption, most women are maintained on anticonvulsants throughout pregnancy, and it is not advisable to change these medications for the purpose of reducing teratogenic risk in established pregnancy. Women taking carbamazepine or valproate should take 4 mg/day of folic acid, starting before conception (Schachter, 2006). Women taking phenobarbital, carbamazepine, phenytoin, topiramate, or oxcarbazepine should take oral vitamin K 10–20 mg/day in the last month of pregnancy.

Table 17. Kinds of Seizure

Grand Mal Seizures (May Be Preceded by Aura)

Loss of consciousness

Tonic-clonic movement

Incontinence

Clenched teeth, tongue biting

Postictal phase

Petit Mal Seizures

Loss of consciousness (10–30 seconds)

Eye or muscle fluttering

May lose muscle tone

Psychomotor Seizures

Characterized by distinctive auras (such as metallic taste)

No loss of consciousness

May become disoriented

May have sudden, brief personality change or violent outbursts

Focal Seizures (Partial or Jacksonian Seizures)

Usually no change in awareness or alertness

May include rhythmic muscle contractions in one area of the body, lip smacking, head turning, eye movements, or seemingly purposeful movements

May include sensory abnormalities such as numbness or tingling

Less commonly, changes in speech, thought, personality, or mood; sensation of déjà vu; or hallucinations

May start with localized twitching of a limb and progress to grand mal seizure

Grand mal seizures may begin with an aura, usually a strange light or unpleasant smell. The tonic phase is often accompanied by apnea secondary to laryngeal spasm, and lasts for about 10–20 seconds. As muscles stiffen, air forced through vocal cords may cause a strange groan. As she loses consciousness, she falls to the floor, muscles tense and extended. The clonic phase involves rhythmic jerking of the limbs as phases of atonia alternate with repeated violent flexor spasms at a rate of 4–8 tremors per second. Bladder or bowel incontinence may occur as the seizure subsides. The postictal state includes a variable period of unconsciousness during which the woman becomes quiet and breathing resumes, often deep and snoring. Consciousness returns gradually, accompanied by confusion or agitation.

Consult or transfer as indicated, and summon EMS for transport. Initial care includes

▶ ABC's and POP, maintaining an open airway

▶ Making no attempt to restrain the woman; helping her to the floor

▶ Clearing the area of dangerous objects and loosening any clothing that might compress her neck

▶ Removing her glasses

▶ Refraining from forcing anything into her mouth

▶ After the seizure, turning her on her left side and suctioning if necessary

▶ Staying with the woman until she is fully awake

▶ Oxygen via mask

▶ Spinal stabilization if trauma is evident

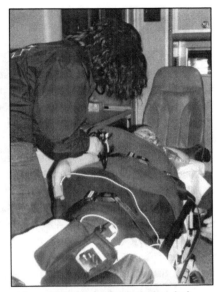

Figure 54. Transporting to the hospital. The client who is postictal after a seizure of unknown etiology requires rapid transport to the hospital.

▶ IV of normal saline 0.9 % at a KVO rate

▶ Managing seizures. If they do not stop within 5 min, EMS may administer diazepam 5–10 mg IV slowly (not faster than 1 ml/min) or as local protocols dictate.

▶ Determining glucose level. If the client is severely hypoglycemic, administer 25 g 50% dextrose IV.

If the woman may have eclampsia (look for high blood pressure or history of hypertension with this pregnancy, brisk reflexes, generalized swelling, or presence of severe headache, epigastric pain and/or visual disturbances before seizure)

▶ Transport rapidly in the left lateral recumbent position.

▶ Avoid bright or flashing lights, sirens, jostling, or any other excessive sensory stimulation.

▶ Monitor urinary output if possible.

▶ If the woman may have eclampsia, EMS may administer magnesium sulfate. Loading dose is 4–6 g in 100 ml of lactated Ringer's or normal saline over 30 min. Infusion is usually run at 2 g/hr. Assess for decreased patellar reflexes and respiratory depression.

Magnesium sulfate may stop labor contractions. It may be reversed by calcium chloride IV over 5 min.

▶ Monitor, vital signs, fetal heart tones, level of consciousness, patellar reflexes, respiratory rate, and oxygenation status. EMS providers should monitor cardiac rhythm.

▶ Monitor for pulmonary edema.

BIBLIOGRAPHY

Ailsworth, K., Anderson, J., Atwood, L.A., Bailey, R.E., & Canavan, T. (2006). *ALSO: Advanced life support in obstetrics* (4th ed.). Leawood, KS: American Academy of Family Practice Physicians.

Coleman, M.T., & Rund, D.A. (1997). Non-obstetric conditions causing hypoxia during pregnancy: Asthma and epilepsy. *American Journal of Obstetrics and Gynecology, 177* (1), 1–7.

Colwell, C. (2007). Management of shock in adult trauma. In B.D. Rose (Ed.), *UpToDate*. Wellesley, MA: UpToDate.

Delzell, J.E., Jr., & Lefevre, M.L. (2000). Urinary tract infections during pregnancy [Electronic version]. *American Family Physician, 61* (3), 713–721. Retrieved May 10, 2008, from http://www.aafp.org/afp/20000201/713.html

Dunphy, L., Winland-Brown, J.E., Porter, B., & Thomas, D. (2007). *Primary care: The art and science of advanced practice nursing* (2nd ed.). Philadelphia:, F. A. Davis.

Funai, E.F., Gillen-Goldstein, J., & Roqué, H. (2007). Changes in the respiratory tract during pregnancy. In B.D. Rose (Ed.), *UpToDate*. Wellesley, MA: UpToDate.

Howell, C., Grady, K., & Cox, C. (Eds.). (2007). *Managing obstetric emergencies and trauma: The MOET course manual* (2nd ed.) London: RCOG Press.

Hunt, C.M., & Sharara, A.I. (1999). Liver disease in pregnancy. *American Family Physician, 59* (4), 829–836. Retrieved December 3, 2004, from http://www.aafp.org/afp/990215ap/829.html

Kaufmann, H., Kaplan, N.M., & Freeman, R. (2004). Mechanisms and causes of orthostatic and postprandial hypotension. In B.D. Rose (Ed.), *UpToDate*. Wellesley, MA: UpToDate.

Lee, F.M., & Chiang, W.K. (2006). Cholelithiasis (eMedicine, topic 97). Retrieved May 10, 2008, from http://www.emedicine.com/emerg/topic97.htm

Lockwood, C.J., & Bauer, K.A. (2007). Inherited thrombophilias in pregnancy. In B.D. Rose (Ed.), *UpToDate*. Wellesley, MA: UpToDate.

Morris, S., & Stacey, M. (2003). ABC of Resuscitation: Resuscitation in pregnancy. *British Medical Journal, 327* (7246), 1277–1279.

Newberry, L. (Ed.). (2003). *Sheehy's emergency nursing: Principles and practice* (5th ed.). St. Louis: Mosby.

Olshansky, B. (2004). Neurocardiogenic (vasovagal) syncope and carotid sinus hypersensitivity. In B.D. Rose (Ed.), *UpToDate*. Wellesley, MA: UpToDate.

Pearlman, M., Tintinalli, J., & Dyne, P. (2004). *Obstetric and gynecologic emergencies: Diagnosis and management*. New York: McGraw-Hill.

Pohlmann-Eden, B., Beghi, E., Camfield, C., & Camfield, P. (2006). The first seizure and its management in adults and children [Electronic version]. *British Medical Journal, 332* (7537), 339–342. Retrieved May 10, 2008, from http://www.bmj.com /cgi/content/full/332/7537/339

Poole, J.H., & Spreen, D.T. (2005). Acute pulmonary edema in pregnancy. *Journal of Perinatal & Neonatal Nursing, 19* (4), 316–331.

Queenan, J., Hobbins, J., & Spong, C. (Eds.). (2005). *Protocols for high-risk pregnancies* (4th ed). Hoboken, NJ: Wiley-Blackwell.

Ratcliffe, S.D., Baxley, E.G., Cline, M.K., & Sakornbut, E.L. (2008). *Family medicine obstetrics* (3rd ed.). Philadelphia: Mosby Elsevier.

Schachter, S.C. (2006). Management of epilepsy and pregnancy. In B.D. Rose (Ed.), *UpToDate*. Wellesley, MA: UpToDate.

Schwartz, D.R., Malhotra, A.M., & Weinberger, S.E. (2007). Deep vein thrombosis and pulmonary embolism in pregnancy. In B.D. Rose (Ed.), *UpToDate*. Wellesley, MA: UpToDate.

Scott-Conner, C.E.H., & Perry, R. (2006). *Acute abdomen and pregnancy* (eMedicine, topic 3522). Retrieved May 10, 2008, from http://www.emedicine.com/ med/topic3522.htm

Sharma, S. (2006a). *Pulmonary disease and pregnancy* (eMedicine, topic 3252). Retrieved March 8, 2008, from http://www.emedicine.com/ med/topic3252.htm

Tapson, V.F. Treatment of acute pulmonary embolism. In B.D. Rose (Ed.), *UpToDate*. Wellesley, MA: UpToDate.

Weinberger, S.E. (2007). Dyspnea during pregnancy. In B.D. Rose (Ed.), *UpToDate*. Wellesley, MA: UpToDate.

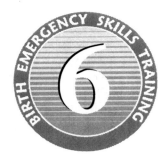

Hypertensive Disorders

OBJECTIVES

▶ Describe the typical clinical manifestations of chronic hypertension, gestational hypertension, HELLP syndrome and preeclampsia, and eclampsia.

▶ Explain the rationales of management for hypertensive disorders in pregnancy.

▶ Summarize the maternal and fetal effects of hypertension in pregnancy.

▶ Describe how the provider can assess the severity of chronic hypertension, gestational hypertension, and preeclampsia.

AACT and ReACT
ALERT—Be alert ▶ Exercise hypervigilant attention
ANALYZE—Think about possible causes
CONSIDER—Use OLDCART ▶ Gather data
TREAT—Make first response ▶ Proceed to definitive care
ReACT | **ReAssess ▶ ReConsider ▶ Re-Treat**

AACT—Alert

Hypertension in pregnancy falls into one of the following disease entities.

▶ **Preeclampsia** is defined as the new onset of hypertension and proteinuria after 20 weeks' gestation (but typically after 34 weeks) in a previously normotensive woman. The woman with preeclampsia may develop eclampsia (grand mal seizures in a woman with gestational hypertension or preeclampsia). Preeclampsia is categorized as either mild or severe based on symptoms.

▶ Chronic or preexisting hypertension (affecting 3% of pregnancies) is defined as systolic pressure ≥140 mmHg, diastolic pressure ≥90 mmHg, or both, that is documented before pregnancy, presents within the first 20 weeks of pregnancy, or persists more than 12 weeks after delivery.

▶ **Gestational hypertension** is defined as hypertension (usually mild) without other signs of preeclampsia after 20 weeks' gestation, resolving by 12 weeks postpartum. Previously, hypertension was defined as a systolic increase of 30 mmHg or a diastolic increase of 15 mmHg, but this concept is outdated. If hypertension persists longer than 12 weeks postpartum, the diagnosis is chronic hypertension that was obscured by the initial antepartum physiologic decrease in blood pressure. Preeclampsia develops in 15–25% of women initially diagnosed with gestational hypertension (Magloire & Funai, 2007).

▶ **Preeclampsia superimposed on chronic hypertension**, defined as new-onset proteinuria after 20 weeks' gestation in the woman with preexisting hypertension. If a woman has preexisting hypertension with proteinuria, she is diagnosed with preeclampsia if blood pressure tops systolic ≥160 mmHg or diastolic ≥110 mmHg after 20 weeks, especially if platelets are low and liver enzymes are elevated.

First Thought, Worst Thought

What is the most likely cause of high blood pressure?
Gestational hypertension.
What is the worst it could be?
Severe preeclampsia.

Accurate measurement is essential. Ensure the cuff is properly fitted to the woman's arm. The length of the cuff should be 1.5 times the woman's upper arm circumference, or the cuff bladder should encircle at least 80% of the arm. A cuff that is too small will yield a falsely elevated reading, and one that is too large will record a false low. Have the woman sit for at least 10 min before taking her pressure. Document position with each blood pressure. If the initial blood pressure is elevated then recheck in 10 min.

In early pregnancy, blood pressure is highest in the upright or sitting position, lower in the supine position, and lowest in the side-lying position, but third trimester pressures are influenced by how the uterus compresses the inferior vena cava and the aorta in any given posture. Inferior vena caval compression by the pregnant uterus can cause transient hypotension when the woman is supine. Blood pressure readings taken in the left lateral position may yield falsely low values unless the cuff is carefully positioned at the level of the heart.

Hypertension is still a leading cause of maternal and fetal mortality. When a pregnant woman becomes hypertensive, the provider must determine whether the problem is preeclampsia, which has a different course and prognosis from gestational or chronic hypertension; determine whether hypertension is mild or severe, which affects outcome; and assess fetal condition, which can deteriorate.

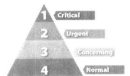 *Hypertension can be priority 2, 3, or 4. Hypertensive disorders are classed as mild or severe by the degree of blood-pressure elevation by clinical symptoms that indicate injury to kidneys, brain, liver, and cardiovascular system.*

Gestational Hypertension

Priority 3, 2, or 1

Gestational hypertension has recently replaced the term *pregnancy-induced hypertension.* Gestational hypertension affects about 6% of pregnancies, but unless it is severe, it does not usually increase risk to mother or fetus (Magloire & Funai, 2007). Gestational hypertension is defined as elevated blood pressure (systolic ≥140 mmHg, diastolic ≥90 mmHg) after 20 weeks, on two occasions at least 6 hr apart without significant proteinuria. About half of women with gestational hypertension eventually develop preeclampsia; some of these will develop chronic hypertension after delivery, and some will become normotensive postpartum (Ailsworth, et al., 2006).

It is unclear whether gestational hypertension is an early or mild stage of preeclampsia or the two conditions are separate entities. There are differences in demographics; preeclampsia is associated with primigravidas, but gestational hypertension is not. Differentiating between the conditions can be difficult. One in 10 women with clinical or histological signs of preeclampsia will not develop proteinuria.

Severe gestational hypertension is characterized by pressure ≥160 mmHg systolic, or ≥110 mmHg diastolic for at least 6 hr without proteinuria or history of chronic hypertension. Perinatal outcomes of severe gestational hypertension are similar to those of severe preeclampsia: increased risk of preterm delivery, IUGR, and placental abruption.

When pregnancy is complicated by hypertension, the provider should monitor fetal wellbeing through serial biophysical profiles or nonstress tests with amniotic fluid index, assessments of growth, and sometimes through umbilical artery Doppler velocimetry if the fetus is growth restricted. There is no evidence that routine fetal surveillance improves neonatal outcome in mild hypertension, but serial NSTs, amniotic fluid index (AFI) measurements, cord Dopplers, and/or evaluations of fetal growth are indicated if hypertension is severe.

Severe hypertension is treated with antihypertensive medication to reduce the risk of a maternal brain hemorrhage. Antihypertensive medications are not usually used in mild gestational hypertension, for they do not improve outcomes and can mask the onset of severe disease.

The woman with mild gestational hypertension should see her provider every week. Delivery at 39–40 weeks' gestation reduces risk to the baby. During labor, the provider should remain vigilant for signs of developing preeclampsia. Most women become normotensive within the first postpartum week, but hypertension may persist until 12 weeks postpartum.

If your client develops new-onset hypertension at a routine prenatal visit
- ▶ Recheck blood pressure in 10 min
- ▶ Dip urine for protein

If the BP is 140/90 or greater, but less than 160/100, and there are no other symptoms
- ▶ Consult as appropriate
- ▶ Consider sending client to antepartum unit for evaluation
- ▶ Consider nonstress test with AFI or biophysical profile

If client is sent home
- ▶ Increase fluid intake
- ▶ Recommend bed rest in right and left lateral positions. Left lateral is optimal for perfusion, but immobility increases risk of thrombosis; so the woman should be encouraged to position herself on both right and left sides and change position often.
- ▶ Decrease, but do not eliminate, salt intake
- ▶ Increase protein in diet
- ▶ Monitor fetal kick counts
- ▶ Instruct her to report severe headache, visual changes, sudden weight gain, or upper abdominal pain
- ▶ Have her return for reassessment of blood pressure in 3–4 days
- ▶ Laboratory tests may include BUN, ALT, AST, uric acid, creatinine, CBC, platelet, fibrinogen, PT, PTT, D-Dimer, and 24-hour urine for protein, and creatinine clearance

If BP is ≥ 160/100, refer to an appropriate site for evaluation.

Chronic Hypertension
Priority 1, 2, or 3

Chronic hypertension is defined as blood pressure greater than 140/90 mm Hg on two occasions in the first half of pregnancy. Because blood pressure usually decreases during first two trimesters, the client with preexistent hypertension may be normotensive early in pregnancy. It is also be difficult to differentiate between mild preeclampsia and preexisting hypertension in the woman who presents late to care. Although hypertension related to preeclampsia normalizes after delivery, blood pressure remains elevated with preexisting hypertension.

When chronic hypertension is mild to moderate, antihypertensive therapy does not improve fetal outcomes and will not prevent preeclampsia. In fact, decreasing the blood pressure in these women may decrease placental perfusion and actually endanger the fetus. Pharmacologic treatment, usually with methyldopa, labetalol, and/or nifedipine, is appropriate if blood pressure is persistently ≥ 150–180 systolic or ≥ 100–110 mm Hg diastolic (Ailsworth, et al., 2006). ACE inhibitors and angiotensin II receptor antagonists cause IUGR, oligohydramnios, neonatal renal failure and death. Beta-blockers are associated with IUGR, and thiazide diuretics can cause derangement of the fluid balance if preeclampsia should develop.

Preeclampsia
Priority 3, 2, or 1, depending on severity

Preeclampsia (once called toxemia) involves gradual or abrupt onset of hypertension, proteinuria, and generalized edema, usually after 34 weeks, but sometimes much earlier or postpartum. Far more complex than simple hypertension, preeclampsia involves systemic abnormal vascular tone that can lead to poor perfusion and eventually tissue ischemia of the placenta and maternal cardiovascular, renal, neurologic, hepatic, and hematologic systems. Chronically poor placental perfusion can cause fetal growth restriction. Because preeclampsia is characterized by poor placental perfusion, lowering the blood pressure may increase physiologic dysfunction and exacerbate fetal hypoxia.

Preeclampsia affects 3–14% of all pregnancies worldwide (5–8% in the United States) and may be superimposed on underlying chronic hypertension (August & Sibai, 2008). The groundwork for this disease is laid early in pregnancy when abnormalities in maternal vasculature cause abnormally shallow implantation. Dietary, immunological, genetic, and hemodynamic factors have been implicated, but researchers do not fully understand the disease or its etiology.

Risk factors include African American heritage, multiple gestation, maternal age less than 18 or greater than 35, long interval between pregnancies, lower socioeconomic class, nulliparity (or first baby with a new partner), family history of preeclampsia, underlying chronic hypertension, collagen vascular disease or renal disease, obesity and antiphospholipid syndrome. Severe preeclampsia in a prior pregnancy carries a 25–65% recurrence rate (August & Sibai, 2008). Diabetes present in early pregnancy elevates risk due to underlying vascular disease, high plasma insulin levels, and abnormal lipid metabolism.

Preeclampsia is a progressive disorder, and in its mild or early form symptoms can develop subtly and appear benign. Rising blood pressure is usually the first sign of evolving preeclampsia, but pressures typically do not reach the diagnostic threshold until near term. Less frequently, preeclampsia appears suddenly late in the second trimester. Preeclampsia before 20 weeks is usually related to molar pregnancy.

A poorly perfused liver may produce fewer blood proteins, the lack of which allows fluid to escape from blood vessels and cause edema. The presence of edema is no longer a diagnostic criterion for preeclampsia, for many women without preeclampsia have edema, and one third of women with preeclampsia do not. On the other hand, abrupt weight increase of greater than 5 lb in a week with facial edema may be associated with preeclampsia. Pulmonary edema can develop secondary to elevated pressure in the pulmonary vessels, capillary leak, left heart failure, or volume overload from IV crystalloids.

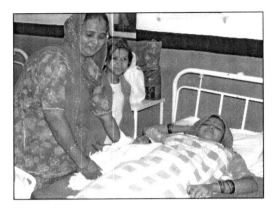

Figure 55. Preeclampsia affects 3–14% of all pregnancies worldwide. Preeclampsia may develop antepartum, intrapartum, or postpartum.

Preeclampsia may also present with headache, blurred vision, scotomata, and occasionally with cortical blindness. One in 400 mildly preeclamptic and 2% of severely preeclamptic women will progress to eclamptic seizures (August & Sibai, 2008). Stroke is a rare but serious complication of severe preeclampsia and eclampsia. The woman may also experience placental abruption or DIC.

Typically in preeclampsia, hematocrit rises as blood volume contracts and fluid extravasates into the tissues. In HELLP syndrome, hemolysis occurs and may drop the hematocrit. These two processes can coexist, resulting in a hematocrit that appears normal. Microthrombi may develop, causing thrombocytopenia. The woman with preeclampsia has a glomerular filtration rate (GFR) 30–40% less than her normotensive counterpart, and serum uric acid rises (August & Sibai, 2008). Prothrombin time, partial thromboplastin time, and fibrinogen concentration are usually unchanged unless the disease is severe. Creatinine levels above 0.9 mg/dl in pregnancy are abnormal and indicate worsening preeclampsia. Abnormal values are more easily recognized if the woman at high risk for preeclampsia has baseline laboratory tests drawn early in pregnancy, including platelet count, creatinine concentration, liver function tests, and 24-hour urine collection for protein and creatinine clearance.

Right-upper-quadrant or epigastric pain and elevated liver enzymes may herald liver damage. In severe preeclampsia, vasospasm, precipitation of fibrin, hemorrhage, ischemic lesions, and microvesicular fat deposition can damage or even rupture the liver. Liver damage also elevates hormone and toxin levels (the liver metabolizes both) and interferes with clotting and other vital processes.

⌂ AACT—Consider

The diagnosis of preeclampsia is clinical, based on the new onset of hypertension and proteinuria after 20 weeks' gestation in a previously normotensive woman. Gradually rising blood pressure and proteinuria in pregnancy are usually due to preeclampsia, particularly in a primigravida. Suspect preeclampsia in any pregnant woman with hypertension and characteristic signs/symptoms, even if proteinuria is absent. Preeclampsia is diagnosed by obtaining an elevated blood pressure on two occasions at least 6 hr, but no more than 7 days, apart.

Kidneys damaged by restricted blood flow are poor filters that allow proteins to escape the bloodstream while allowing toxins to remain; in some cases kidneys may fail altogether. Another diagnostic criterion for preeclampsia is ≥300 mg of protein in a 24-hour urine specimen or two dipsticks greater than or equal to 1+ (30 mg/dl) 6 hr apart (Ailsworth et al, 2006). Proteinuria, however, occurs late in the course of preeclampsia, and some women with severe preeclampsia have no proteinuria. Obtain a fresh, clean voided midstream urine specimen uncontaminated by vaginal secretions and dip urine for protein. Dipsticks can be inaccurate with highly acidic urine, dehydration, bacteriuria, or nonalbumin proteinuria. A dipstick positive for protein should be confirmed using a urine protein-to-creatinine ratio on a random sample or with a 24-hour urine collection.

Although preeclampsia is typically associated with a rise in the uric acid level above 5.5–6 mg/dl, serum uric acid level is a poor predictor of development of the disease. Uric acid tends to remain below this level in preexisting hypertension unless there is superimposed preeclampsia.

Half of women with gestational hypertension are later diagnosed with preeclampsia (Ailsworth, et al., 2006). Preeclampsia is more likely to develop in those who become hypertensive before the third trimester.

Severe Preeclampsia

Priority 1

Women with early-onset severe preeclampsia have a 25–65% recurrence rate in future pregnancies (August & Sibai, 2008).

The woman who develops early-onset severe preeclampsia, recurrent preeclampsia, gestational hypertension, or preeclampsia with onset as a multipara is at greater risk for hypertension, ischemic heart disease, and stroke later in life. Preeclampsia that develops in primigravidas late in pregnancy with no repetition in subsequent pregnancies does not appear to confer this increased cardiovascular risk.

Expectant management of women with mild preeclampsia may include blood-pressure readings, nonstress tests (NSTs), urine dip for protein twice a week, weekly preeclampsia laboratory profile (CBC, ALT, AST, LDH, uric acid, and creatinine), weekly 24-hr urine collection for protein and creatinine clearance, weekly amniotic fluid indices (AFIs) or biophysical profiles (BPPs), and sonographic evaluation of fetal growth every three weeks.

Clinical Features of Severe Preeclampsia

Signs and symptoms of severe preeclampsia include severe hypertension, persistent headache, visual changes, IUGR, oligohydramnios, epigastric or right upper abdominal pain, abnormal liver function tests, decreased urine output, thrombocytopenia, and hemoconcentration or hemolysis. The woman with mild preeclampsia may be managed at home on bed rest, but *severe* preeclampsia is an emergency. Preeclampsia is classed as mild or severe by the degree of blood-pressure elevation and proteinuria and by clinical symptoms that indicate injury to kidneys, brain, liver and cardiovascular system.

Women with preexisting renal disease are at greater risk for severe preeclampsia with onset earlier in gestation than the typical presentation. On the other hand, increasing hypertension and proteinuria in a woman with kidney disease may reflect a worsening of the underlying disease in response to the demands of pregnancy.

Severe preeclampsia may be manifested as eclampsia or HELLP syndrome. Severe preeclampsia may be gradual or fulminant and may include

▶ Hypertension—systolic pressure ≥160 mmHg, diastolic pressure ≥110 mmHg
▶ Significant proteinuria
▶ Oliguria: urine is dark, concentrated, and scanty
▶ Visual disturbances: blurred or double vision, flashing lights, or blindness
▶ Hyperreflexia: reflexes greater than +2, presence of clonus
▶ Epigastric pain: liver ischemia, swelling, or rupture can cause epigastric pain or tenderness in the right upper quadrant
▶ Nausea and vomiting
▶ Pulmonary edema
▶ Poor blood clotting
▶ Fetal distress or poor growth; oligohydramnios
▶ Headache—progressive and does not respond to over-the-counter remedies.
▶ Seizures (eclampsia)
▶ Anxiety, malaise, or restlessness

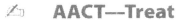 **AACT—Treat**

Managing the Woman with Preeclampsia

ABCs with POP
AIRWAY—Taking care with the spine
BREATHING
CIRCULATION—With attention to bleeding
Placenta Optimally Perfused

- ▶ ABC-POP
- ▶ Assess with the OLDCART method
- ▶ Reduce environmental stimulation
- ▶ Establish IV access and draw labs

Remember at all times that the woman with preeclampsia can decompensate rapidly, moving from mild, ambiguous symptoms to full-blown eclampsia, organ damage, and fetal death in a very short time. Keep potential complications in mind while treating her, and monitor for the earliest indication of decompensation, such as signs of abruption or central nervous system dysfunction. Monitor her level of consciousness.

If you must deliver the child of a woman with preeclampsia outside the hospital, remain vigilant for changes in her condition and take steps to keep her stimulation level and blood pressure as low as possible. Position her on her side for delivery, and do not coach forceful pushing or prolonged breath-holding with each contraction. Open-glottis pushing moves the baby down more gradually and improves placental oxygenation and maternal blood pressure. Administer low-flow oxygen to maximize fetal oxygenation.

The woman with preeclampsia may not have the intravascular reserve to tolerate blood loss after delivery. She remains at risk for eclamptic seizures for 48 hr after delivery and occasionally may seize within 2 weeks postpartum.

The only cure for preeclampsia is delivery of the fetus. Most clients with preeclampsia recover quickly after delivery, with decreased blood pressure, diuresis, and general clinical improvement. Some authorities advocate immediate induction, regardless of gestational age. Others advocate for expectant management until the fetus demonstrates lung maturity, maternal or fetal distress develops, or a gestational age of 34 weeks is achieved. Delivery is generally not indicated for women with mild preeclampsia until 37–38 weeks and should be accomplished by 40 weeks (Ailsworth, et al., 2006).

Prevention of Preeclampsia

Calcium supplementation has been shown to reduce the risk of hypertension and preeclampsia for high-risk women and for women with insufficient dietary calcium. When otherwise healthy nulliparous women take calcium supplements, neonatal mortality and certain maternal complications decrease. Low-dose aspirin confers low to moderate protection against developing preeclampsia, especially in women at high risk for developing the disorder.

~ Differential Diagnoses

Differential diagnoses include acute fatty liver, systemic lupus erythematosus, gestational or autoimmune thrombocytopenia, cerebral hemorrhage, migraine, hepatitis, cholestasis, pancreatitis, renal disease, acute fatty liver, exacerbation of systemic lupus erythematosus, gestational thrombocytopenia, autoimmune thrombocytopenia, chronic hypertension, and gestational hypertension.

HELLP Syndrome
Priority 1

The medical community has yet to agree on whether HELLP syndrome is a separate category of preeclampsia or a variant of severe preeclampsia, but it occurs in 20% of pregnancies complicated by preeclampsia (Bacq & Sibai, 2007). The acronym describes the physiologic abnormalities, diagnosed primarily by laboratory findings, that define the syndrome: Hemolysis, Elevated Liver enzymes, and Low Platelets.

Sometimes HELLP syndrome will develop before signs of preeclampsia appear. The majority of cases are diagnosed between 28 and 36 weeks' gestation, but about 30% present postpartum and occasionally as much as a week after delivery (Bacq & Sibai, 2007).

The woman may present with the same symptoms as the preeclamptic—epigastric pain, chest pain or right-upper-quadrant pain, headache, nausea and vomiting, and malaise—but sometimes with very few physical manifestations. Hypertension ≥140/90 and proteinuria are present in about 85% of cases, but either or both may be absent in women with otherwise severe HELLP syndrome (August & Sibai, 2008). The right upper quadrant and epigastrium will be tender to palpation.

Because the presentation can be subtle, the clinician should draw a complete blood count, platelet count, and liver enzymes on any woman with right-upper-quadrant or epigastric pain, nausea, or any sign of preeclampsia.

Magnesium sulfate is given to prevent seizures. The woman with HELLP should receive magnesium sulfate from the time of admission to the hospital until 24–48 hr postpartum. Corticosteroids accelerate lung maturation in fetuses less than 34 weeks and tend to improve platelet counts and other laboratory values, but do not improve maternal outcomes. Hypertension may be controlled with labetalol, hydralazine, nifedipine, or in severe cases with sodium nitroprusside.

Fresh frozen plasma, platelets, and packed red blood cells are used to treat coagulation defects and hemorrhage. Hemorrhage is unlikely if platelet counts are ≥50,000/μl, but platelet transfusions are beneficial if the count is less than 20,000/μl or if the woman is bruising or bleeding from puncture sites. If cesarean delivery is planned, then some authorities have recommended platelet transfusion, as necessary, to achieve a preoperative platelet count greater than 40,000/μl.

If HELLP presents after 28 weeks, delivery is usually accomplished 24–48 hr after the first dose of dexamethasone or betamethasone. Mode of delivery is influenced by parity, cervical ripeness, fetal maturity, and the severity of the disease. Cesarean delivery may be performed for unfavorable cervix, fetal compromise or customary obstetrical indications such as breech, but may be complicated by coagulation and blood pressure issues. Vaginal delivery is desirable for women in labor or with ruptured membranes and a vertex presenting infant, regardless of gestational age. Labor can be induced in women with favorable cervixes or pregnancies >30–32 weeks. Cesarean delivery can be considered in very preterm gestations (<30–32 weeks), however.

Some women with HELLP worsen in the immediate postpartum period, developing hepatic rupture, renal failure, pulmonary edema, ascites, pleural effusion, postpartum hemorrhage, or DIC.

~ Differential Diagnoses

Right-upper-quadrant pain: cholecystitis, hepatitis, acute fatty liver of pregnancy, gastroesophageal reflux, gastroenteritis, and pancreatitis.

Urinalysis abnormalities: pyelonephritis, hemolytic uremic syndrome, and ureteral calculi.

Thrombocytopenia: gestational thrombocytopenia, HIV, immune thrombocytopenic purpura, systemic lupus erythematosus, antiphospholipid syndrome, hypersplenism, DIC, congenital thrombocytopenias, and medications.

Eclampsia

✍ AACT—Alert, Analyze, Consider

Eclampsia is not the endpoint of preeclampsia. It is one of several clinical expressions of severe preeclampsia. Eclampsia consists of one or more generalized convulsions or coma in a preeclamptic woman without other neurologic disease.

Goals of management include stabilizing the mother, preventing recurrent seizures, treating severe hypertension, and delivering the fetus.

Eclampsia may be preceded by increasingly severe preeclampsia, may appear unexpectedly in a woman with mild preeclampsia, or may develop suddenly in a woman with minimally elevated blood pressure and no proteinuria. Most women who develop eclampsia show marked edema, persistent headache, blurred vision, photophobia, right-upper-quadrant or epigastric pain, altered mental status, significantly increased blood pressure, or increased proteinuria before seizing. The usual presentation of eclampsia is tonic-clonic seizures lasting less than 1 min, but partial seizures can also occur, and some clients will move directly into coma without observed seizure. Coma can also result from a brain hemorrhage or brain swelling without hemorrhage.

Convulsions can occur antepartum (53%), during labor (19%), or postpartum (28%) (Norwitz, 2006). As many as one quarter of all postpartum eclamptic seizures occur between 48 hr and 4 weeks after delivery. Eclampsia is both more common and more lethal in locations with limited resources and inadequate prenatal care. Mortality in the United States is about 3 per 1,000 eclamptics, but in Mexico the death rate approaches 14% (Norwitz). Women in developing countries who receive prenatal care are less likely to die from complications of severe preeclampsia, eclampsia and HELLP syndrome.

The eclamptic convulsion is typically of the tonic-clonic type, 60–90 seconds in duration and accompanied by apnea. After the seizure, the postictal

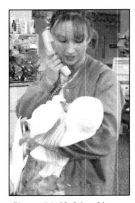

Figure 56. Multitasking. When a client is acutely ill, the provider must juggle many simultaneous tasks.

client will appear deeply asleep, often with snoring respirations, and gradually returns to consciousness confused and agitated.

During the convulsion, the fetus will usually become bradycardic from hypoxia, hypercarbia, and uterine hyperstimulation, but this is not an indication for immediate cesarean delivery. As the mother becomes postictal, the fetus will become tachycardic and will show decreased variability and sometimes decelerations. If the mother is appropriately managed with magnesium sulfate, positioning, oxygen, and antihypertensives, the fetus will usually recover. Within 10–15 min after the convulsion, the fetal heart rate is usually reassuring unless the placenta has abrupted. It is advantageous to delay delivery until fetal status has improved. A tertiary-care facility has the capacity for rapid surgery and a NICU capable of managing the sickest of newborns.

Eclamptic seizures are best controlled by magnesium sulfate. Diazepam and phenytoin can depress respirations, especially when combined with magnesium sulfate, and are not as effective at controlling eclamptic seizures (Ailsworth, et al., 2006). If not treated promptly, about 10% of women will have recurrent seizures (Norwitz, 2006). Because the convulsion is usually of short duration, the provider should focus on preventing the next seizure rather than stopping the current one.

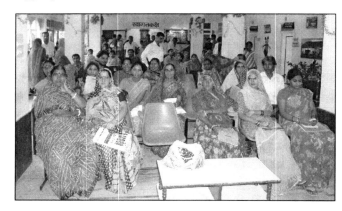

Figure 57. Prenatal clinic in Jaipur, India.

Up to 70% of women with eclampsia suffer complications including abruption (7–10%), DIC (7–11%), aspiration pneumonia (2–3%), and cardiopulmonary arrest (2–5%) (Norwitz, 2006). Most of these complications resolve after delivery with proper treatment, but brain damage from hemorrhage or hypoxia may cause lifelong neurological impairment. The fetal prognosis is primarily dependent upon gestational age at delivery.

If your client has an eclamptic seizure:
▶ Call for EMS
▶ Do not attempt to restrain the woman; help her to the floor if not reclining
▶ Clear the area of dangerous objects and loosen any clothing that might compress her neck
▶ If she wears glasses, remove them
▶ Do not force anything into her mouth
▶ Ensure an open airway and prevent aspiration
▶ Suctioning may be necessary to maintain the airway
▶ Give oxygen to ensure adequate oxygenation
▶ Initiate cardiac monitoring

After the seizure ends
▶ ABC-POP
▶ Suction her mouth as needed
▶ Give high-flow oxygen after breathing resumes
▶ If breathing does not resume, support respirations
▶ Do not leave her unattended
▶ Position the woman on her left side in the CPR recovery position
▶ Establish IV access; draw preeclampsia labs if practical
▶ Monitor the woman and fetus for signs of abruption
▶ Auscultate the lungs for evidence of aspiration or pulmonary edema

Definitive Care

At the hospital, a 6 g loading dose of magnesium sulfate is infused over 15–20 min, followed by a maintenance dose of 2 g/hr. Aggressive antihypertensive therapy with hydralazine or labetalol should be started if pressures exceed 105–110 mmHg diastolic or are ≥160 mmHg systolic. Pharmacologic treatment of mild hypertension does not improve outcomes and is not recommended.

When the woman has been stabilized, a physician will make a decision about mode of delivery. Gestational age, cervical ripeness, presence of labor, and fetal position and wellbeing influence whether the birth will be vaginal or cesarean. The definitive treatment of eclampsia is delivery, but it may be advantageous for small medical centers to stabilize the woman on magnesium sulfate, then transfer to a tertiary-care center.

~ Differential Diagnoses

Seizures may result from cerebrovascular accident, hypertensive encephalopathy, brain tumor, hypoglycemia, uremia, meningitis, encephalitis, epilepsy, methamphetamine or cocaine use, or trauma.

BIBLIOGRAPHY

Ailsworth, K., Anderson, J., Atwood, L.A., Bailey, R.E., & Canavan, T. (2006). *ALSO: Advanced life support in obstetrics* (4th ed.). Leawood, KS: American Academy of Family Practice Physicians.

August, P., & Sibai, B. (2008). Clinical features, diagnosis, and long-term prognosis of preeclampsia. In B.D. Rose (Ed.), *UpToDate*. Wellesley, MA: UpToDate.

Bacq, Y. (2008). Acute fatty liver of pregnancy. In B.D. Rose (Ed.), *UpToDate*. Wellesley, MA: UpToDate.

Bacq, Y., & Sibai, B. (2007). HELLP syndrome. In B.D. Rose (Ed.), *UpToDate*. Wellesley, MA: UpToDate.

Chamberlain, G., & Steer, P. (1999). ABC of labour care: Obstetric emergencies. *British Medical Journal, 318* (7194), 1342–1345.

Cunningham, F., Grant, N., Leveno, K., Gilstrap, L., Hauth, J., & Wenstrom, K. (2005). *Williams obstetrics* (22nd ed.). New York: McGraw-Hill.

Gabbe, S.G., Niebyl, J.R., & Simpson, J.L., Eds. (2007). *Obstetrics: Normal and problem pregnancies* (5th ed.). New York: Churchill Livingstone.

Heppard, M., & Garite, T. (2002). *Acute obstetrics: A practical guide* (3rd ed.). St. Louis: Mosby.

Magloire, L., & Funai, E.F. (2007). Gestational hypertension. In B.D. Rose (Ed.), *UpToDate*. Wellesley, MA: UpToDate.

Norwitz, E.R. (2006). Eclampsia. In B.D. Rose (Ed.), *UpToDate*. Wellesley, MA: UpToDate.

Norwitz, E.R. (2007). Predicting preeclampsia. In B.D. Rose (Ed.), *UpToDate*. Wellesley, MA: UpToDate.

Queenan, J., Hobbins, J., & Spong, C. (Eds.). (2005). *Protocols for high-risk pregnancies* (4th ed). Hoboken, NJ: Wiley-Blackwell.

Sinclair, C. (2004). *A midwife's handbook*. St. Louis: Saunders.

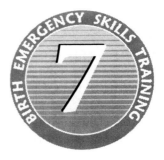

Trauma, Shock, and Cardiac Arrest

OBJECTIVES

- ▶ Identify the presenting symptoms and signs of shock and describe immediate and specific management.
- ▶ Discuss how physiological changes of pregnancy affect traumatic injury and how management of the pregnant victim of trauma differs from that of the nonpregnant client.
- ▶ Identify modifications that improve blood flow when administering CPR to the pregnant client.
- ▶ Identify three etiologies of shock that may be seen in the intrapartum setting.

TRAUMA IN PREGNANCY

The out-of-hospital midwife does not provide definitive care for the victim of significant trauma, but is nonetheless likely to encounter injured women from time to time. A client may suffer a fall, or the midwife may happen upon a motor vehicle accident or assault victim. Obstetrical providers often may volunteer in remote areas or assist pregnant women at disaster sites. Basic knowledge of trauma management may be lifesaving for the victim.

Trauma, the leading nonobstetric cause of maternal death in the United States, complicates 1 in 12 pregnancies (Gabbe, Niebyl, & Simpson, 2007). (The three most common *obstetric* causes of maternal death are thromboembolism, hypertensive disorders, and hemorrhage.) The most common causes of trauma in pregnancy are motor vehicle accidents (42%); falls (34%); assault to the abdomen—often by domestic partner (18%); and other causes, including penetrating trauma such as bullet and stab wounds (6%) (Ailsworth, et al., 2006). Eighty-five percent of traumatic maternal deaths result from head injury or shock (Ailsworth, et al.). If the mother dies, the fetus usually dies. If the mother survives the trauma, placental abruption may occur and put the fetus at risk for hypoxia or death. Major maternal trauma involving multiple fractures and life-threatening injury is often fatal for the fetus.

The severity of the trauma does not always predict the likelihood of adverse fetal outcome; about 50% of fetal losses occur after relatively minor maternal trauma (ACOG, 1998). Even women who suffer seemingly uncomplicated trauma in pregnancy have higher rates of preterm birth, low birth weight, and abruption, probably from subclinical chronic abruption.

Three causes are responsible for most of the trauma suffered by pregnant women.

Motor vehicle accidents are the most common cause of significant trauma in pregnancy. Unrestrained occupants in MVAs are 6 times more likely to die, but not all women wear seatbelts. Fetal mortality often occurs in motorcycle accidents, when victims are ejected from motor vehicles, and when pedestrians are struck by motor vehicles.

Domestic violence is a problem in all races, ages, and socioeconomic groups. Abuse often escalates in pregnancy. Stab wounds and gunshot wounds are a relatively common cause of significant trauma in pregnancy, and homicide is a leading cause of trauma-related maternal mortality. Typically, the gravid uterus is the target of the attack. About 25–30% of pregnant women are physically or sexually abused, but only 3–8% of these abuses are identified (Gilbert, 2007).

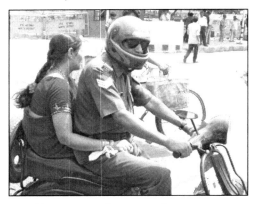

Figure 58. Vulnerable to trauma. Women who suffer seemingly uncomplicated trauma in pregnancy have higher rates of preterm birth, low birth weight, and abruption.

Falls account for 34% of trauma to pregnant women and commonly result from alterations in balance or orthostatic hypotension (Ailsworth, et al., 2006). Most falls occur in the third trimester.

Mechanism of Injury

Mechanism of injury is the combined strength and nature of forces that caused the trauma, which direction they were applied, and what body parts they affected. Gunshot wound severity depends on the type of gun used, range, and whether there is an exit wound. In the case of blunt trauma, the skin may appear almost undamaged, but serious injury could occur internally. In penetrating trauma, the duller the object, the more force it takes to penetrate.

In an MVA, damage to the vehicle often predicts injury to the occupant. Damage to the windshield can indicate head injury if hair is embedded in the glass, but it may be caused instead by another body part, the airbag, or a loose object in the vehicle. Dents or cracks in the lower dashboard indicate possible knee, hip, or femur injuries.

Side impacts cause about 27% of automotive fatalities because forces are transferred directly to the occupant, usually without the benefit of airbags (Bledsoe, Porter, & Cherry, 2003). Intrusion into the passenger compartment usually means significant injury to the occupant. Rear-end crashes tend to be less severe, but are often associated with whiplash injuries. If the steering wheel is bent beneath the airbag, look for chest and abdominal injuries. Unbelted drivers tend to bounce around the vehicle's interior and sustain injury with each impact, especially in a rollover accident.

Table 18. Mechanisms of Trauma Likely To Result in Serious Injury

Falls of 15 ft or more

Rearward displacement of front of car by 20 in or greater

Rearward displacement of front axle

Passenger compartment intrusion of 20 in or more

Driver's compartment intrusion of 15 in or more

Ejection from any moving vehicle (including ATV, motorcycle, moped, or truck bed)

Rollover without restraint

Gross deformity of contact point (for example, steering wheel)

Death of any occupant in the same car

Pedestrian hit at 15 m.p.h. or more

Vehicular damage so severe that hydraulic tools are needed to extricate patient

Penetrating injury to head, neck, or torso

Suspected spinal cord injury

Newton's First Law of Motion states that an object in motion will remain in motion until acted on by another force. A vehicle in motion will remain in motion unless something—a pole, another vehicle, the brakes, another vehicle—causes it to stop. People in the vehicle will continue to move at the original speed until a seat belt, the steering wheel, or the windshield causes them to stop. The organs of the body will continue to move at the original speed until stopped by the supporting structures within the body. An abrupt stop—as when a car strikes a tree—does more damage than a slow stop—as when a car runs off the road into a sandlot. If two vehicles hit head-on, forces are additive.

In trauma, hemorrhage can quickly become life-threatening if it occurs in the thoracic cavity, peritoneal cavity, retroperitoneal space (often from a pelvic fracture), muscle or subcutaneous tissue (usually from a long-bone fracture), or major external wounds (Colwell, 2007).

Vulnerability to Trauma

Pregnant women who die from trauma usually succumb to the injury itself, most commonly head injury or hemorrhage. Fetal death is likely to result not from trauma itself, but from maternal shock or placental abruption.

During the first trimester, the uterus is well protected within the bony pelvis. The fetus is small and cushioned by a thick uterus and abundant fluid. In the second trimester, the uterus rises to a more vulnerable position in the abdomen, but the fetus is still protected. Abdominal trauma is more common in pregnant women than in their nonpregnant counterparts. Pregnant women are at increased risk of retroperitoneal hemorrhage due to dilated pelvic vessels.

During the third trimester, even small injuries can be catastrophic. Toward the end of pregnancy, the uterus becomes larger and thinner-walled, and it is increasingly vulnerable to blunt trauma, penetration, or rupture. The well-perfused uterus bleeds copiously when injured and can be a major source of blood loss in trauma. The third-trimester fetus occupies more space within the uterus and is surrounded by a proportionally smaller fluid volume.

Fetal injuries can vary. Maternal pelvic fracture can injure the fetal head and brain if the fetus has descended into the pelvis. Penetrating trauma can puncture any part of the fetus. Blunt trauma is more likely to damage the uterus and placenta and indirectly affect the fetus than to cause direct harm to the unborn child.

Direct trauma, shearing forces, or maternal shock can cause the placenta to detach from the uterine wall. Maternal catecholamines, such as adrenaline released by stress or injury, can constrict vessels and decrease placental perfusion, causing fetal hypoxia.

Physiological changes associated with pregnancy greatly affect a woman's response to trauma. In the second and third trimesters, cardiac output increases by 40%, and uterine blood flow increases from 60–600 ml/min to keep the fetus oxygenated (Bridges, et al., 2003). Blood vessels in the pregnant uterus remain maximally dilated and have no mechanism for increasing perfusion when cardiac output is decreased. A drop in cardiac output can quickly result in decreased placental blood flow, and as a result the fetus may become severely compromised even when the mother's condition is stable. A pregnant woman also has a reduced oxygen reserve caused by diaphragm elevation and an increase in oxygen consumption associated with the fetus, placenta, and uterus.

The blood volume of a pregnant woman increases by 50% through the course of her pregnancy, creating dilutional anemia—her blood has more liquid and therefore fewer red cells by volume than that of a nonpregnant woman. Despite her greater blood volume, the pregnant trauma victim may appear hypovolemic in the absence of serious injury because of the mild tachycardia and hypotension considered normal in pregnancy. The systolic blood pressure of a young healthy pregnant woman may normally range from 80 to 90.

An injured mother's body seeks to protect itself at the expense of blood flow to the fetus. Catecholamines can constrict vessels and shunt blood away from the placenta to perfuse maternal vital organs. She may not appear shocky until her blood loss is great enough to endanger the fetus. Once shock becomes obvious, fetal mortality may be as high as 80% (Chang, 2006).

Obstetric Complications of Trauma

Preterm labor or preterm rupture of the membranes can follow even minor trauma. All women beyond 18–20 weeks who have experienced trauma should be monitored at length for the presence of contractions, and those of earlier gestational age should be observed and evaluated. Continuous fetal heart-rate monitoring is used only beyond 23–24 weeks' gestation, for no obstetric intervention will change the outcome with a pre-viable fetus (Grossman, 2004). Screening modalities for compromised pregnancies are limited.

Placental Abruption

Toward the end of pregnancy, the placenta is a massively perfused, comparatively rigid organ attached to the elastic uterine wall. If the uterus is subjected to abrupt accelerations or decelerations, even without blunt trauma, the placenta may shear off the uterine wall Most placental abruptions are seen within 24 hr of the accident; but it is important to remember that abruption can occur more than 5 days after trauma and follow even very minor injuries. Up to 30–50% of patients with significant injuries from trauma and up to 5% of patients with minor injuries will suffer placental abruption (Chang, 2006). Even minor abdominal trauma without obvious injury can cause fetal death from abruption. The location of the placenta does not affect risk.

Suspect abruption in women with abdominal injury, particularly if accompanied by abdominal or uterine tenderness, contractions, or vaginal bleeding. Abruption is diagnosed through clinical signs such as pain, contractions, and nonreassuring fetal heart patterns. Approximately 50–80% of placental abruptions are not identifiable on ultrasound; but ultrasonography can evaluate fetal wellbeing, placental location, gestational age, and amniotic fluid index (Grossman, 2004). Laboratory assessments may be unremarkable despite pathology. Abruption leading to nonreassuring fetal heart-rate patterns and death can occur despite relatively mild maternal trauma or discomfort. In pregnancy, normal fibrinogen values are greater than 200 mg/dl. A fibrinogen value <200 mg/dl or thrombocytopenia indicates possible disseminated intravascular coagulation (DIC) and may be a sign of abruption.

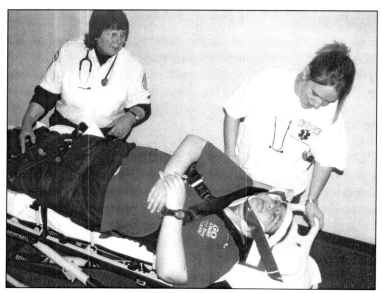

Figure 59. Avoid supine hypotensive syndrome. When the woman requires supine spinal immobilization, the backboard should be tilted to a 15° angle (raise the right side of the board 4 in).

Fetomaternal hemorrhage occurs when the fetal circulation bleeds into the maternal vasculature, causing fetal anemia, fetal death, and Rh iso-immunization. The Kleihauer-Betke (KB) test measures the percentage of fetal red blood cells in maternal blood. Many providers routinely order this test with any maternal trauma. The amount of RhoGAM required depends on the number of fetal cells found. A large fetomaternal hemorrhage may need multiple doses of RhoGAM.

Uterine rupture secondary to trauma is rare, but carries nearly 100% fetal mortality.

Penetrating trauma such as gunshot or stab wounds may directly injure the fetus. Maternal pelvic fracture may also cause direct injury to the fetus.

Hemorrhage: Maternal hemorrhage decreases placental perfusion. A pregnant woman may lose 1,000–1,500 ml of blood before showing signs of shock. Once hemorrhage has progressed to shock, the mother may survive the ordeal, but the baby will usually die. Fetal blood loss can result in fetal anemia or death, and fetal blood may enter the maternal system and cause her to make antibodies against the baby's blood.

Aspiration: Slowed gastric emptying and the physical pressure of a large uterus on the organs of digestion increase the chance that the woman will aspirate stomach contents. If she is unable to maintain her own airway, be aggressive with intubation.

AACT and ReACT
ALERT—Be alert ▶ Exercise hypervigilant attention
ANALYZE—Think about possible causes
CONSIDER—Use OLDCART ▶ Gather data
TREAT—Make first response ▶ Proceed to definitive care
ReACT | **ReAssess ▶ ReConsider ▶ Re-Treat**

✍ AACT—Treat

Management of the pregnant trauma victim includes ABC's-POP while protecting the cervical spine.

Cervical Spine

Always consider the possibility of neck injury. In the adrenaline rush following an accident, severe injuries may be asymptomatic. People have been known to emerge from a vehicle with a stable neck fracture, only to sever the spinal cord with a turn of the head. The cervical spine can be injured by whiplash injuries, head trauma, diving injuries, or hanging.

Airway

Open, protect, and secure the airway while protecting the cervical spine. A secure airway enables oxygenation and protects against aspiration.

Breathing

Administer oxygen and assist ventilation when breathing is inadequate. Reduced oxygen reserve and increased oxygen consumption put the pregnant woman and her fetus at increased risk for hypoxemia, so oxygen therapy should be aggressive.

Circulation

Control bleeding, establish IV access with a large-bore catheter, and administer a fluid bolus as indicated. Every liter of estimated blood loss should be replaced by three liters of lactated Ringer's, if available, or 0.9% normal saline. Lactated Ringer's is the solution of choice for trauma because it is more physiologic and less acidic than normal saline, but saline is also useful as a volume expander.

Control external hemorrhage by applying direct pressure. Scalp lacerations can bleed heavily. If the vessel that is causing the bleeding can be visualized, it may be clamped. A tourniquet is used to control bleeding only if it is quite literally "life or limb"—the tourniquet may cause eventual loss of the limb due to lack of circulation. Damage to the distal extremity can be minimized by periodically loosening the tourniquet to allow tissue perfusion. Tourniquets may also be used to stop bleeding in the case of traumatic amputation.

Bloodwork includes type and cross-matched packed red blood cells, baseline hemoglobin or hematocrit, coagulation studies, a platelet count, and chemistry panel.

Disability—assess the victim neurologically. Is she alert and oriented? Does she have movement and sensation in all limbs?

Exposure—remove clothing and examine for further injury, taking care to protect her from the environment.

Fetal Stabilization

The fetus is best served by making maternal stabilization your priority. Pregnant victims of major trauma should be treated generally like other trauma victims, but with accommodations for the physiological and anatomic changes of pregnancy.

POP—Placenta Optimally Perfused

Perform a rapid primary survey of the fetus using the mnemonic "FETAL."

FETAL: Assess for
FETAL heart rate or presence of fetal movement.
ESTIMATED gestational age based on maternal or family report, abdominal measurement, or proximity of the uterus to the umbilicus. Is she sure there is only one fetus?
TRAUMA—observe for evidence of direct injury or penetrating trauma to uterus.
ABDOMINAL palpation for tenderness and presence of uterine contractions.
LOSS of amniotic fluid or vaginal bleeding.

The pregnant trauma victim should be positioned in the left lateral position rather than supine whenever possible. If she lies supine, her blood pressure may precipitously drop by 30%, causing symptoms of shock and making it unclear whether injury or position is behind them. This response may be even more pronounced in hemodynamically compromised victims. When the woman requires supine spinal immobilization, the backboard should be tilted to a 15°

angle (raise the right side of the board 4 in). High-flow oxygen by mask should be initiated at the earliest opportunity. If she cannot support her own ventilations or maintain her airway, she should be intubated.

The EMS professional is well equipped to immobilize and stabilize a trauma victim. The emergency medical technician (EMT) is trained in life support to the basic or intermediate level. The paramedic is certified in advanced life support and uses many of the same lifesaving medications and procedures as the emergency-room physician.

Remain alert for the possibility of internal hemorrhage that could compromise the fetus long before signs are apparent in the mother. If internal injuries are suspected or if significant bleeding is present, bilateral large-bore IV lines should be established with isotonic crystalloid solution, preferably lactated Ringer's. Fluid resuscitation should be aggressive. Assess for uterine tenderness, vaginal bleeding, contractions, and fetal movement, and monitor fetal heart tones. Initiate cardiac monitoring when appropriate. Obstetric clients beyond 20 weeks' gestation who suffer multiple trauma should be transported to a facility that can provide comprehensive trauma and obstetrical care even if the woman appears stable.

Any treatment required to save the mother's life or treat her critical status should be undertaken regardless of her pregnancy, including any necessary diagnostic imaging. After 24 weeks' gestation, efforts to save the fetus by cesarean delivery should be considered.

Any pregnant woman with an Rh-negative blood type (such as AB negative) will need to receive an injection of anti-D immunoglobulin (RhoGAM) if any fetal cells have entered her system. RhoGAM is commonly administered to Rh-negative women after any episode of vaginal bleeding or suspected abruption. A blood test (Kleihauer-Betke) can quantify the amount of fetal cells that entered the maternal blood stream in case of trauma. If the obstetrical provider fails to administer RhoGAM, the mother may produce antibodies that can cause hemolysis in a subsequent Rh-positive fetus.

Many providers discharge women with fewer than 6 contractions per hour, no vaginal bleeding, no abdominal pain, and a normal fetal heart-rate tracing after 4 hr of monitoring. If the woman has frequent or painful contractions, vaginal bleeding, nonreassuring fetal heart pattern, tense uterus, abdominal pain, or low platelets or fibrinogen, she will probably be admitted for 24 hr of observation. Abruption can occur up to six days after the accident, but the risk of abruption is very low if the woman is asymptomatic during the first 4 hr.

SHOCK

Shock is systemic decrease in tissue perfusion and oxygenation. Initially, shock can be reversible, but prolonged shock results in end-organ damage, failure of multiple organ systems, and death. Sixty percent to 90% of people with cardiogenic shock will die, and about 35–40% of people who develop septic shock die within one month (Gaieski & Manaker, 2008). Shock is second only to brain injury as a cause of death from trauma. Hypovolemic shock can often be reversed with rapid recognition and treatment.

Shock is a progressive three-stage decline provoked by an initial event that causes a systemic circulatory disruption and, if not reversed, ending with end-organ damage and death.

Compensated Shock (Pre-shock, "Warm Shock")

At the onset of the insult, the body's compensatory mechanisms maintain homeostasis. A pregnant woman may lose 30% of her blood volume before her vital signs reflect hypovolemia. Tachycardia, peripheral vasoconstriction, and perhaps an orthostatic decrease in blood pressure may be the only indication of early hypovolemic shock.

Table 19. Clinical Clues to Diagnosis

Scleral icterus (whites of eyes are yellow)—think liver disease

Dry conjunctivae and mucous membranes—think hypovolemia

Pinpoint pupils, slow or absent respirations—think narcotic overdose

Dilated, fixed pupils—think hypoxemia

Nystagmus—think drug or alcohol overdose

Neck—Jugular venous distention; delayed carotid upstroke *(pulsus parvus et tardus)*; carotid bruits; meningeal signs

Crackles (rales) in lung sounds—think pulmonary edema, congestive heart failure

Consolidation in lungs—think pneumonia

Squeaky extra cardiac sound—think pericardial friction rub of pericarditis

Abdominal distention—think bowel obstruction or internal bleeding

Rebound tenderness and guarding—think peritonitis

Uncompensated Shock

Priority 1

Compensatory mechanisms are overwhelmed and organs begin to malfunction. When there is not enough blood to perfuse the whole body, the nonvital organs are sacrificed to preserve the vital organs. Stimulation of the sympathetic nervous system causes tachycardia and compensatory vasoconstriction to raise blood pressure and shunt blood flow to vital organs. (Early distributive shock, however, may present with warm, flushed skin.) Reduced urine output is a sign of renal blood flow shunting to other vital organs. Other clinical signs of uncompensated shock include poor skin turgor; lack of axillary sweat; dry mucous membranes; tachypnea; restlessness; and cool, pale, clammy skin. Hypotension is subtle at first, then profound as compensatory mechanisms fail. Pulse pressure, and the difference between the systolic and the diastolic pressures may narrow to <25 mmHg. The client in compensatory shock may initially have respiratory alkalosis, becoming acidotic as shock becomes more profound.

End-Organ Dysfunction

Increasing lactate production causes increasing metabolic acidosis, which coupled with hypoxia cause the peripheral vasculature to dilate and cause cardiovascular collapse. Progressive end-organ dysfunction results in irreversible organ damage. Urine output declines and ceases. Mental status changes from restlessness to agitation, confusion or delirium, stupor, and coma. Acidosis increases organ damage, cardiac output declines, cellular metabolism becomes deranged, organs fail, and the woman dies.

Classification of Shock

There are three basic categories of shock: hypovolemic, cardiogenic, and distributive.

Hypovolemic Shock
Priority 1

Hypovolemic shock can result from fluid loss related to hemorrhage, diarrhea, vomiting, heat stroke, insensible losses, burns, or "third-spacing." Insufficient intravascular fluid reduces preload, causing *decreased* cardiac output.

Shock may exist even if vital signs are within normal range, making diagnosis difficult.

Diaphoresis may appear before alteration in vital signs. Cool extremities, weak peripheral pulses, pallor and capillary refill >2 seconds may indicate peripheral vasoconstriction. Mild tachypnea may be a sign of compensation for metabolic acidosis. Decreased urine output may indicate insufficient renal perfusion, and a high urine specific gravity may be the body attempting to

 Having confusion about perfusion? Systemic tissue perfusion depends on systemic vascular resistance (SVR) and adequate cardiac output (CO). SVR, the amount of resistance the heart must push against, is determined by vessel diameter, vessel length, and blood viscosity. CO, the amount of blood the heart is able to pump, is determined by heart rate and stroke volume. Stroke volume (the amount of blood pumped per beat) is determined by preload (the pressure stretching the left ventricle after passive filling and atrial contraction), amount of blood, myocardial contractility, and afterload (impedance to blood flow).

retain fluids. See Chapter 3, Antepartum, Intrapartum, and Postpartum Bleeding for treatment of hemorrhagic shock.

Cardiogenic Shock
Priority 1

Cardiogenic shock is failure of the heart to pump adequately, causing *decreased* cardiac output. Cardiogenic shock can be related to cardiomyopathy, myocardial infarction, arrhythmias, valvular malfunctioning, pulmonary embolism, pericardial tamponade, tension pneumothorax, severe pulmonary hypertension severe constrictive pericarditis, and myocardial depression from advanced septic shock. In cardiogenic shock, the left ventricle is unable to pump enough blood to meet the body's demands. The heart rate rises to compensate. As the left heart fails, blood backs up and congests the pulmonary vasculature, causing pulmonary edema and tachypnea. If the right heart fails as well, jugular veins distend, the liver congests, and generalized edema occurs. Inadequate oxygen delivery leads to cellular damage, multiorgan failure, and death.

Peripartum Cardiomyopathy
Priority 1

Peripartum cardiomyopathy is an idiopathic condition that develops during the last month of pregnancy and up to 6 months postpartum. Clinical signs include jugular venous distention, tachycardia, decreased oxygen saturation, third heart sound, pulmonary rales, orthopnea, fatigue, palpitations, hemoptysis, chest pain, arrhythmias, and dyspnea. She may awaken abruptly in the night, feeling short of breath (paroxysmal nocturnal dyspnea). Treatment includes diuretics, vasodilators, digoxin, and close monitoring. Peripartum cardiomyopathy carries a 5–25% mortality risk and tends to recur in subsequent pregnancies (Ailsworth, et al., 2006).

Amniotic Fluid Embolism
Priority 1

Amniotic fluid embolism is a devastating complication, carrying a mortality rate of 61%, but only 15% of survivors were neurologically intact (Howell, et al., 2007). While rare, occurring in fewer than 1 in 8,000 pregnancies, this condition accounts for 13% of maternal deaths in France, and over 30% in Singapore (Howell, et al.).

AFE is most common during the intrapartum period, but can also occur during pregnancy or immediately postpartum. AFE occurs when small amount of amniotic fluid enters the maternal circulation, triggering what may be an anaphylactic reaction; pulmonary embolism from fetal skin, hair, and vernix contained in the fluid,; or the result of vasoactive substances introduced into the maternal circulation. Uterine manipulation or trauma may be associated with AFE, but the majority of women who suffer the syndrome have no risk factors. More than 80% of women with AFE will present with cardiorespiratory arrest, and half of these cannot be resuscitated (Baldisseri, 2007).

Signs and symptoms of AFE include fetal distress, then maternal cardiovascular collapse (23%), maternal hypotension, shortness of breath, fetal bradycardia shortly before delivery (14%). Maternal loss of consciousness/seizure shortly before delivery (35%), maternal loss of consciousness/seizures immediately following delivery (14%), or maternal cardiovascular collapse following cesarean delivery (14%) (Howell, et al., 2007).

Diagnosis of AFE is made on clinical signs and symptoms—confirmation is only possible if fetal cells are found in the maternal lungs after death from sudden cardiovascular collapse. Differential diagnoses include uterine atony, placental abruption, uterine rupture, preeclampsia/eclampsia, septic shock, pulmonary embolism, air embolism, myocardial infarction, stroke, anaphylaxis, drug reaction, or aspiration of gastric contents. Treat as with shock, DIC, and/or cardiac arrest until a physician assumes care.

Distributive (Vasodilatory) Shock
Priority 1

Distributive or vasodilatory shock is related to loss of systemic vascular resistance and is often associated with increased cardiac output. Etiologies include septic shock, toxic shock syndrome, anaphylaxis, drug or toxin reactions, and neurogenic shock after a spinal cord injury.

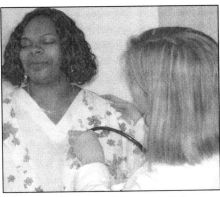

Figure 60. Auscultating lung sounds. Pulmonary edema can present with tachypnea, cough with foamy sputum, and crackles.

Septic Shock
Priority 1

Septic shock is a major cause of death in obstetric clients, usually related to septic abortion, chorioamnionitis, pyelonephritis, pneumonia and postpartum infections.

Septic shock is caused by endotoxin-producing aerobic gram-negative bacilli, gram-positive bacteria, and mixed or fungal infections. Anaerobes such as *Bacteroides* species, *Fusobacterium*, peptostreptococci, or *Clostridium* are usually involved in mixed infections (Gonik & Leonardi, 2008). Microbes from the normal genitourinary and gastrointestinal flora may become pathogens following tissue trauma or use of broad spectrum antibiotics. Septic shock may occur during pregnancy because of overwhelming infection caused by gram-positive bacteria, viruses, or fungi. Gram-negative bacteria such as *Escherichia coli*, *Klebsiella* species, *Pseudomonas aeruginosa*, and *Serratia* species cause most cases of septic shock. The microorganisms produce endotoxins that activate complement systems and cytokines, initiating an inflammatory response. The mediators of sepsis are responsible for vasodilation, low peripheral vascular resistance, and hypotension. Furthermore, blood flow is poorly distributed, resulting in inadequate perfusion of certain organs, leading to cellular damage, multiorgan failure, and death.

Pyelonephritis is one of the most common causes of septic shock in pregnant women, more often occurring in the right kidney due to pressure from the dextrorotated uterus. Vaginal, perineal, and fecal floral organisms (most commonly *E. coli*) often ascend the urinary tract to cause infection. Symptoms may include fever (>38°C), shaking chills, costovertebral angle tenderness, flank pain (especially on the right), anorexia, nausea, and vomiting. Some women will develop hypothermia as low as 34°C.

Chorioamnionitis presents with maternal fever >100.4°F (>38°C), maternal tachycardia (>120 bpm) and fetal tachycardia (>160 bpm), leukocytosis >15,000–18,000 cells/μL, contractions, uterine tenderness, and purulent or foul vaginal discharge. If two or more of these signs are present, the risk of neonatal sepsis is increased.

Postpartum endometritis following cesarean is a most common cause of septic shock (accounting for 15–85% of septic shock in obstetric clients) and less commonly after vaginal delivery (1–4% of obstetric septic shock) (Gonik & Leonardi, 2008). Onset is typically within five days of delivery. The woman with endometritis develops fever, uterine tenderness, foul lochia, and leukocytosis, sometimes accompanied by abdominal distention and decreased bowel sounds. Lochia culture is not usually helpful because it tends to show a mixed flora, and it is difficult to culture the uterus through the cervix without contaminating the swab with vaginal organisms. Retained products of conception with infection presents similarly, often including a boggy, tender uterus and dilated cervix.

Necrotizing fasciitis is a devastating, fast-advancing "flesh-eating" infection, usually caused by group A beta-hemolytic streptococci. Gas-forming organisms form crackly pockets of subcutaneous air. Toxins destroy skin and the soft tissues beneath it, including fat and superficial and deep fascia, and create large areas of tissue necrosis that must be debrided.

Sepsis progresses along a continuum, beginning with bacteremia (presence of viable bacteria in the blood). Severe sepsis is systemic inflammatory response with organ dysfunction, hypoperfusion, or hypotension, indicated by acidosis, oliguria, or decreased mental status. Septic shock occurs when hypotension and hypoperfusion continue in spite of fluid resuscitation, and there is no way to predict which women will decline from shock to multiple organ system failure.

At first, the woman with sepsis may have malaise, nausea, vomiting, shaking chills, fever, tachycardia, and diarrhea—and sometimes with mental status changes. Endotoxins directly affect the respiratory center in the brain and cause tachypnea or dyspnea, sometimes followed by acute respiratory distress syndrome (ARDS). The fetus is less affected by the direct effects of endotoxin than the mother, presumably due to inability of the immature fetal immune system to mount an inflammatory response. Initially, blood pressure may be normal due to peripheral vasoconstriction, which also results in cold extremities, oliguria, and peripheral cyanosis. As shock progresses, cardiac output and systemic vascular resistance become inadequate to maintain systemic perfusion, and the woman becomes cold, clammy, bradycardic, and cyanotic. Metabolic acidosis, electrolyte imbalances, and disseminated intravascular coagulation (DIC) may ensue.

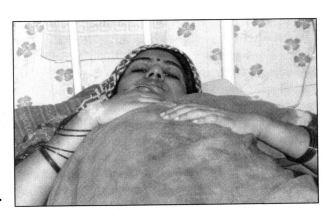

Figure 61. Risk of infection. Pregnant women who have inadequate prenatal care are at greatly increased risk for septic shock.

White blood cell count may be decreased initially, followed by marked leukocytosis. Initial catecholamine release elevates blood glucose, followed by hypoglycemia from liver dysfunction. Tachypnea may cause initial respiratory alkalosis, followed by metabolic acidosis from increasing lactic acid concentration.

Ultrasound and computed tomography (CT) imaging can identify an intra-abdominal abscess, retained products of conception, microabscesses in the myometrium, or septic pelvic vein thrombophlebitis.

The fetus is best treated by saving the mother. Treatment of septic shock includes immediate resuscitation, determining the underlying cause, and antimicrobial therapy. At least two sets of blood cultures are drawn, as well as cultures from other suspected sites, such as urine, sputum, wound, or endometrium. Amniotic fluid may be cultured via amniocentesis. Hypovolemia is corrected with crystalloids and colloids, then vasoactive agents such as dopamine, ephedrine or norepinephrine are indicated after fluids are replaced. Oxygen therapy is crucial—septic clients have increased oxygen requirements, but at a cellular level their tissues are less able to use it. Some clients may require intubation and mechanical ventilation.

Antibiotics that cover a variety of aerobic and anaerobic gram-negative and gram-positive bacteria are started immediately. Often therapy includes ampicillin (2 g Q 4 hr), gentamicin (1.5 mg/kg Q 8 hr), and clindamycin (900 mg Q

8 hr) or metronidazole (15 mg/kg initially then 7.5 mg/kg Q 6–8 hr). Therapy may be adjusted when culture results become available.

D&C is promptly performed after initiating antibiotics and stabilizing the woman in cases of septic abortion or retained products of conception. The woman in septic shock from chorioamnionitis with a viable fetus needs expeditious delivery. Cesarean delivery may be appropriate after initial maternal resuscitation, but a woman in unstable septic shock may not survive the surgery. In some cases hysterectomy may be necessary.

Anaphylaxis
Priority 1 or 2, depending on severity
Anaphylaxis is a severe, systemic allergic reaction involving urticaria (hives), hypotension, bronchospasm or the rapid swelling of skin, mucosa and submucosal tissues. This swelling can rapidly progress to airway obstruction. The first time the individual encounters the allergen, the body does not react, but makes an immunological memory. The next time the individual is exposed to the allergen, the immune system overreacts.

Common allergens that can trigger anaphylaxis include nuts, legumes (especially peanuts), fish and shellfish, milk, eggs, latex, intravenous radiocontrast dye, aspirin and nonsteroidal anti-inflammatory drugs, and hymenoptera venom (from bees, wasps, ants, et al.). Penicillin and cephalosporin may cause anaphylaxis in an individual with no prior exposure; conversely, up to 85% of clients reportedly allergic to penicillin do not react on subsequent exposure (Krause, 2006).

Anaphylactic symptoms appear within 1–15 min of exposure to the allergen—or rarely, within the hour. The faster a reaction develops, the more severe it is likely to be. An anaphylactic reaction may progress so rapidly that it leads to collapse, apnea, seizures, and coma within 1–2 min and may quickly become fatal.

Symptoms can include
▶ Urticaria (hives), erythema, pruritus, or swelling. Lesions are red and raised, may be small or may become confluent, with irregular borders and sometimes central blanching.
▶ Congestion, sneezing, cough, hoarseness, or a sensation of tightness in the throat.
▶ Airway obstruction, upper airway edema.
▶ Swelling of the tongue or oropharynx may block the airway. Stridor (high-pitched breathing sound) indicates narrowing of the upper airway. Most anaphylactic deaths are due to complete airway obstruction.
▶ Itchy, red, tearing eyes.
▶ Dyspnea, bronchospasm. Wheezing indicates bronchospasm or mucosal edema narrowing the lower airways.
▶ Abdominal cramping, nausea, vomiting, or diarrhea.

- Tachypnea, tachycardia, or hypotension. Hypotension is secondary to systemic vasodilation. If vascular tone is lost, compensatory tachycardia occurs. Increasingly permeable capillaries leak fluid into the interstitial space, causing edema with hypovolemia from third-spacing.
- Anxiety, restlessness, tremor, decreased level of consciousness.
- Cardiovascular collapse or respiratory arrest.

✍ AACT—Treat

Anaphylaxis can be life-threatening. Do not attempt to treat severe reactions or to "wait and see." Transfer the woman to the emergency department or call EMS.

- Consider giving 50 mg of diphenhydramine (Benadryl) if the reaction is mild and the woman can swallow.
- If the woman has bronchospasm, consider giving an inhaled bronchodilator such as albuterol (Proventil) if available.
- Place her on her left side unless dyspnea forces her to sit upright.
- If her symptoms are life-threatening, give epinephrine 0.3 ml of 1:1,000 subcutaneous. Repeat if ineffective. Give Benadryl 25–50 mg IM.
- Administer high-flow oxygen, support the airway, and assist respirations as indicated.
- Establish bilateral large-bore IVs of isotonic crystalloid solution (normal saline, Ringer's lactate). Infuse 1 L at a rapid rate if the woman is unstable, or at keep vein open (KVO) rate for stable vital signs.

Care provided by EMS and the emergency department may include aggressive airway management including intubation or even cricothyrotomy as indicated, cardiac monitoring, large volumes of isotonic crystalloid solutions, epinephrine to counteract vasodilation, inhaled beta-agonists for bronchospasm, antihistamines such as diphenhydramine (Benadryl), vasopressors, or corticosteroids.

Shock may occur without a rash, history of exposure, or any obvious signs of anaphylaxis, so the provider should consider this diagnosis for clients who present with inexplicable shock.

Cardiac Arrest in Pregnancy
Priority 1

Cardiac arrest in pregnancy is a rare, but devastating occurrence (Morris & Stacey, 2003). The three most common *obstetric* causes of maternal death are thromboembolism, pregnancy-induced hypertension, and hemorrhage. Most cardiac arrests in pregnant women result from multisystem trauma, intracranial hemorrhage, myocardial infarction, sepsis, overdose, anaphylaxis, aspiration of gastric contents, or massive pulmonary embolism.

Even if the cause of the cardiac arrest is survivable, the odds of successful resuscitation for the mother and fetus are low, especially if cardiac arrest occurs outside the hospital. Non-pregnant adults suffer irreversible brain damage after three to four minutes of cardiac arrest, but pregnant women become hypoxic more quickly (Morris & Stacey, 2003).

The best way to increase survival rates from cardiac arrest is to prevent it or at least delay the arrest until the woman has arrived at the hospital. Perfectly performed CPR on a nonpregnant client results in cardiac output that is only 25–33% of normal. The fetus's best chance for survival without deficit is delivery by cesarean section within 4–5 min of maternal cardiac arrest. When arrest occurs outside the hospital, the woman and fetus are usually beyond resuscitation by the time they arrive at the emergency department.

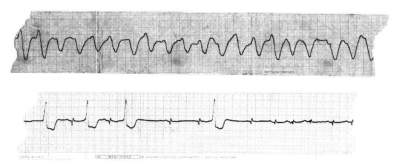

Figure 62. Maternal cardiac arrest. Maternal cardiac arrest often results in the death of both mother and fetus.

Anatomical changes of pregnancy work against successful resuscitation of the woman in cardiac arrest. Increased oxygen requirements and reduced chest compliance makes ventilation more difficult. Flared ribs, raised diaphragm, increased body fat, and breast enlargement make performing chest compression on a pregnant woman challenging. Vomiting and subsequent aspiration are common; cricoid pressure decreases the risk.

External chest compression during CPR is more difficult because of reduced chest compliance in pregnancy. Because the diaphragm is pushed up by the abdominal contents, the heart is also higher, necessitating a slight adjustment in hand position for maximum effectiveness in compressions. However, there are no guidelines for hand position on the sternum specific for pregnant women.

The uterus reaches the level of the maternal umbilicus by approximately 20 weeks' gestation and is large enough to compress the vena cava if the woman is supine or, less commonly, lying on her right side. This compression can decrease cardiac output and placental blood flow. Stroke volume, as an example, can decrease to only 30% of normal in the supine pregnant woman. Therefore, displacing the uterus to the left, off the vena cava, is critical to maximizing effectiveness of CPR.

Although babies have been resuscitated after as much as 30 min of maternal cardiac arrest, survival with intact neurological function is more likely if the infant is delivered within the first 4–5 minutes. In some instances, emptying the uterus by performing a cesarean delivery is required to save the mother's life. The American Heart Association (AHA) recommends cesarean delivery after 4 min of CPR. In nonpregnant women, irreversible brain damage begins after 4–6 min without oxygen. The pregnant woman has less functional respiratory reserve and becomes anoxic more quickly than the nonpregnant client in respiratory arrest. If the uterine fundus ≥4 fingerbreadths above the umbilicus, resuscitation efforts may become effective if the uterus is emptied and aortocaval compression is relieved.

Table 20. The ABCs of Resuscitation

Airway

Open the airway quickly with the head tilt-jaw thrust or head tilt-chin lift maneuver.

Suction the airway if vomitus is present.

Remove loose foreign bodies from the mouth.

If you have an oral airway, you may insert it.

Breathing

If the woman is not breathing adequately, begin intermittent positive pressure using mouth-to-mouth or mouth-to-airway until a self-inflating bag and mask are available.

Ventilate with the head and neck in a sniffing position, without a pillow under the head.

Continue ventilating with 100% oxygen via bag and mask.

Apply cricoid pressure to block aspiration until the airway has been protected by a cuffed tracheal tube.

Circulation

Begin chest compressions as per AHA guidelines

(Morris & Stacey, 2003)

When cardiac arrest occurs, the priority is restoring maternal circulation. Proceed as with AHA guidelines for adult CPR with certain modifications. Open the airway, while immobilizing the cervical spine if trauma is suspected. Check the mouth for foreign bodies. Assess for breathing for no more than 10 seconds. If breathing is absent, circulation is absent. Gasping or agonal breathing may occur in the minutes after cardiac arrest. These respiratory attempts do not provide adequate gas exchange, and are a sign of impending death. Treat the woman with ineffective breathing as with apnea and support respirations. Start compressions as per AHA guidelines.

In the supine woman greater than 20 weeks' gestation, one rescuer should manually displace the gravid uterus from the midline by lifting it with two hands to the left and toward the woman's head while CPR is in progress to improve cardiac return. Alternatively, employ a 25–30° left lateral tilt. Tilt should not exceed 30°, or the woman will shift onto her side, rendering compressions ineffective. A pillow wedged under the right flank and hip to displace the uterus to the left can take the place of an extra pair of hands. The client can also be tilted onto the rescuer's knees or onto the back of an up-turned chair to provide a stable position for CPR.

The trachea should be intubated at the earliest possible opportunity. Often EMS personnel are trained and equipped to accomplish this on scene.

Do not waste time looking for fetal heart tones; their presence or absence will not change treatment. Palpate for pulses during CPR compressions. If you can feel a carotid pulse but not a femoral pulse, placental perfusion may be inadequate. While performing CPR, take steps to counteract the root problem. If the arrest is secondary to a magnesium sulfate overdose, give calcium chloride. If hypovolemic shock precipitated arrest, infuse lactated Ringer's or normal saline rapidly through bilateral IV lines.

Transport includes left lateral positioning or tilt, aggressive airway management, oxygenation, and IV fluid replacement, in conjunction with rapid transport and any treatments appropriate to her particular condition. When the pregnancy is greater than 24 weeks, chances for survival are much greater for mother and fetus if she arrests in the ED rather than in the field.

Paramedics have the capacity to intubate, defibrillate, and administer most of the same resuscitation medications that would be given in the emergency room. The advanced cardiac life support (ACLS) guidelines for pregnancy are the same as for the nonpregnant client. If the client is in cardiac arrest, benefits outweigh risks if the medication restores circulation, even if it is potentially dangerous.

Cardiac Problems
Priority 1, 2, or 3

Pregnancy can exacerbate preexisting heart conditions, and some cardiovascular disorders present for the first time during pregnancy. Hypertension, valvular disease, arrhythmias, cardiomyopathies, aortic dissection (especially in clients with Marfan syndrome), and ischemic heart disease can occur during pregnancy. Previously benign congenital heart anomalies may become symptomatic during pregnancy. The woman with a cardiac disorder may decompensate suddenly even if closely monitored by her physician. Pregnancy places women with artificial valves or atrial fibrillation at increased risk for embolism, and heparin or Lovenox may be prescribed.

Pregnant women have 50% more blood circulating through their vessels. Cardiac output increases further between 28 and 34 weeks, when blood volume expands rapidly; during labor; and immediately postpartum. Every contraction of labor increases cardiac output by about 20%. For days or weeks postpartum, fluid shifts can cause sudden fluctuations in cardiac output and can cause the woman to decompensate.

The growing uterus shifts the heart up and forward, frequently causing a 15° left axis deviation on electrocardiograms by the end of pregnancy. The electrocardiogram may also show flattened or inverted T waves in lead III, and Q waves in lead III and AVF (Podrid, 2007).

Arrhythmias in the pregnant woman are generally treated as they are in the nonpregnant state, but with a few differences. Adenosine is relatively safe in pregnancy and is the first-line drug for treating supraventricular tachycardia (SVT), although it can trigger heart block or bradyarrhythmias that could compromise the fetus. Verapamil is also useful for treating this condition. Amiodarone can cause birth defects, so it should be avoided in the first trimester and used in the second and third trimesters only for arrhythmias unresponsive to all other measures; check with medical control before using this drug. Lidocaine is generally safe in pregnancy, but uterine artery constriction can occur at high blood levels. Procainamide, which has not been shown to injure the fetus, is the first-line drug for undiagnosed wide-complex tachycardia. Cardioversion poses little risk to the fetus and should be used when necessary.

BIBLIOGRAPHY

Ailsworth, K., Anderson, J., Atwood, L.A., Bailey, R.E., & Canavan, T. (2006). *ALSO: Advanced life support in obstetrics* (4th ed.). Leawood, KS: American Academy of Family Practice Physicians.

American College of Obstetricians and Gynecologists. (1998). *Obstetric aspects of trauma management* (ACOG Educational Bulletin 251). Washington, DC: Author.

Baldisseri, M. (2007). Amniotic fluid embolism. In B.D. Rose (Ed.), *UpToDate*. Wellesley, MA: UpToDate.

Bledsoe, B., Porter, R., & Cherry, R. (2003). *Essentials of paramedic care*. Upper Saddle River, NJ: Prentice Hall Health.

Bridges, E.J., Womble, S., Wallace, M., & McCartney, J. (2003). Hemodynamic monitoring in high-risk obstetrics patients I: Expected hemodynamic changes in pregnancy (Electronic version). *Critical Care Nurse, 23*(4), 53–62. Retrieved March 24, 2008, from http://ccn.aacnjournals.org/ cgi/content/full/23/4/53

Chamberlain, G., & Steer, P. (1999). ABC of labour care: Obstetric emergencies. *British Medical Journal, 318* (7194), 1342–1345.

Chang, A.K. (2006). *Pregnancy, trauma* (eMedicine, topic 484). Retrieved May 10, 2008, from http://www.emedicine.com/emerg/topic484.htm

Colburn, V. (1999) Trauma in pregnancy. *Journal of Perinatal & Neonatal Nursing*, 13 (3), 1–32.

Colwell, C. (2008). Management of shock in adult trauma. In B.D. Rose (Ed.), *UpToDate*. Wellesley, MA: UpToDate.

Curet, M., Schmer, C., Dermarest, G., Bieneic, E., & Curet, L. (2000). Predictors of outcome in trauma during pregnancy: Identification of patients who can be monitored for less than 6 hours. *Journal of Trauma: Injury, Infection, and Critical Care, 49* (1), 18–25.

Dobo S.M., & Johnson, V.S. (2000). Evaluation and care of the pregnant patient with minor trauma. *Clinics in Family Practice, 2*(3), 707–722.

Ernst, A. (2007). Critical illness during pregnancy and peripartum. In B.D. Rose (Ed.), *UpToDate*. Wellesley, MA: UpToDate.

Gabbe, S.G., Niebyl, J.R., & Simpson, J.L., Eds. (2007). *Obstetrics: Normal and problem pregnancies* (5th ed.). New York: Churchill Livingstone.

Gaieski, D., & Manaker, S. (2008). General evaluation and differential diagnosis of shock in adults. In B.D. Rose (Ed.), *UpToDate*. Wellesley, MA: UpToDate.

Gilbert, E.S. (2007). *Manual of high risk pregnancy and delivery* (4th ed.). St Louis: Mosby.

Gonik, B., & Leonardi, M.R. (2008). Treatment and outcome of septic shock in obstetrics and gynecology. In B.D. Rose (Ed.), *UpToDate*. Wellesley, MA: UpToDate.

Grossman, N.B. (2004). Blunt trauma in pregnancy. *American Family Physician, 70*(7), 1303–1310.

Gruenberg, Bonnie U. (2005). *Essentials of prehospital maternity care*. Upper Saddle River, NJ: Prentice Hall.

Howell, C., Grady, K., & Cox, C. (Eds.). (2007). *Managing obstetric emergencies and trauma: The MOET course manual* (2nd ed.) London: RCOG Press.

Jacobs, A.G., Bales, A.C, & Lang, R.M. (2007). Peripartum cardiomyopathy. In B.D. Rose (Ed.), *UpToDate*. Wellesley, MA: UpToDate.

Kilpatrick, S.J. (2007). Trauma in pregnancy. In B.D. Rose (Ed.), *UpToDate*. Wellesley, MA: UpToDate.

Krause, R.S. (2006). *Anaphylaxis* (eMedicine, topic 25). Retrieved March 14, 2008, from http://www.emedicine.com/emerg/topic25.htm

Leung, L.L.K. (2007). Clinical features, diagnosis, and treatment of disseminated intravascular coagulation in adults. In B.D. Rose (Ed.), *UpToDate*. Wellesley, MA: UpToDate.

Mattox, K., & Goetzl, L. (2005). Trauma in pregnancy. *Critical Care Medicine 33* (10 Suppl.), S385–S389.

Morris, S., & Stacey, M. (2003). Resuscitation in pregnancy. *British Medical Journal, 327* (7426), 1277–1279.

Neufeld, J.D.G. (2002). Trauma in pregnancy. In J.A. Marx, R.M. Walls, & R.S. Hockberger (Eds.), *Rosen's emergency medicine: Concepts and clinical practice* (5th ed.). St. Louis: Mosby.

Pearlman, M., Tintinalli, J., & Dyne, P. (2004). *Obstetric and gynecologic emergencies: Diagnosis and management*. New York: McGraw-Hill.

Podrid, P.J. (2007). Arrhythmias and conduction disturbances associated with pregnancy. In B.D. Rose (Ed.), *UpToDate*. Wellesley, MA: UpToDate.

Sharma, S. (2006b). *Shock and pregnancy* (eMedicine, topic 3285). Retrieved March 14, 2008, from http://www.emedicine.com/med/topic3285.htm

Siu, S.C., & Colman, J.M. (2001). Heart disease and pregnancy. *Heart, 85* (6), 710–715.

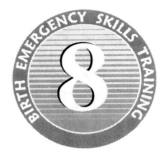

Preterm Labor

OBJECTIVES

▶ Describe the expected frequency and severity of neonatal complications resulting from preterm delivery. Describe the survival rates for preterm neonates based on age and weight.

▶ Discuss the indications for and complications of expectant management versus induction in preterm and term clients with PROM.

▶ Discuss how diagnosis is established for preterm rupture of the membranes.

▶ Identify risk factors and warning signs of preterm labor.

▶ Discuss the risks and benefits of interventions for preterm labor, including antibiotics, tocolytics, corticosteroids, cerclage, bed rest, alpha-hydroxyprogesterone, and serial cervical length evaluation.

AACT and ReACT
ALERT—Be alert ▶ Exercise hypervigilant attention
ANALYZE—Think about possible causes
CONSIDER—Use OLDCART ▶ Gather data
TREAT—Make first response ▶ Proceed to definitive care
ReACT | **ReAssess** ▶ **ReConsider** ▶ **Re-Treat**

✍ AACT—Alert and Analyze

Preterm Labor

Priority 2 or 1

Preterm labor is defined as the presence of uterine contractions with progressive effacement and dilation of the cervix before 37 completed weeks' gestation. The incidence of preterm delivery in the United States has actually increased by 27% in the last 20 years (Ross & Eden, 2007). Prematurity complicated 9.4% of births in 1981; but by 2001, the rate had increased to 11.9% (Ross & Eden). This increase may be partially attributed to more multiple births (caused by *in vitro* fertilization and other infertility treatments) and a greater willingness (encouraged by better neonatal intensive care) to deliver babies early when maternal complications occur.

In 2004, the United States infant mortality rate (6.8 per 1,000 live births) ranked 29th among selected countries, more than 3 times higher than Singapore's rate (2.0 per 1,000 live births) (March of Dimes, n.d.). Long-term consequences of prematurity can include learning disabilities, lung disease, blindness, hearing impairment, cerebral palsy, and developmental delay. The lower the birth weight, the more likely an infant is to die or suffer serious impairment.

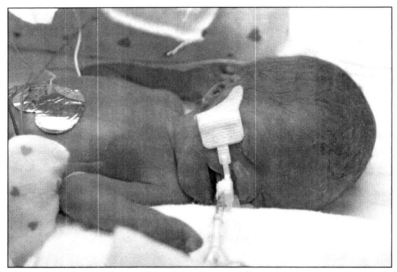

Figure 63. Facing challenges. This infant of 26 weeks' gestational age is at increased risk for learning disabilities, lung disease, blindness, hearing impairment, cerebral palsy, and developmental delay.

Certain pathogenic processes can result in preterm labor and delivery. The four primary processes are premature activation of the maternal or fetal hypothalamic-pituitary-adrenal axis (which triggers labor), inflammation or infection, decidual hemorrhage, or pathological uterine distention (Lockwood, 2007). Preterm delivery is often related to abruption, cervical incompetence, Müllerian duct abnormalities, fibroid uterus, infection, and uteroplacental insufficiency. Risk factors for preterm delivery include

▶ Previous preterm delivery—the more previous preterm deliveries, the higher the risk for this pregnancy.

▶ Uterine anomalies, cervical incompetence (tendency of the cervix to painlessly open in the second or third trimester), certain cervical surgeries such as Loop Electrosurgical Excision Procedure (LEEP) and cone biopsy.

▶ Excessive uterine enlargement, as in multiple pregnancy or polyhydramnios.

▶ Maternal infection—vaginal and urinary-tract infections increase the risk of preterm delivery.

▶ Low socioeconomic status, lack of adequate prenatal care, domestic violence.

▶ Tobacco, cocaine, or alcohol abuse.

▶ Short interval between pregnancies.

▶ Fetal anomalies.

▶ Chronic health problems such as hypertension, diabetes, or clotting disorders.

▶ Poor nutrition, poor weight gain, and being underweight or obese at the beginning of the pregnancy.

▶ Emotional stress.

▶ Physically strenuous work, long working hours, prolonged standing.

▶ Age less than 17 or greater than 35.

▶ African American ancestry.

▶ Uterine overdistention from multiple gestation or polyhydramnios.

▶ Frequent preterm contractions, vaginal bleeding.

▶ Abruption.

▶ History of multiple first-trimester elective abortions or one or more second-trimester elective abortions.

First Thought, Worst Thought

What is the most likely cause of cramping in the second half of pregnancy?

Dehydration or musculoskeletal pain.

What is the worst it could be?

Preterm labor and delivery can be one of the worst outcomes, especially if the fetus is pre-viable.

Preterm labor appears to be a long-term, multifactorial process rather than an acute condition. This condition is diagnosed when a woman has regular uterine contractions accompanied by dilation and thinning of the cervix and descent of the fetus.

The fetus plays a role in the initiation of labor, and appears to respond to adverse intrauterine conditions by initiating preterm labor. Relative contraindications to tocolytics include intrauterine growth restriction, oligohydramnios, nonreassuring fetal heart tracing, positive contraction stress test, cord

Doppler examination with absent or reversed diastolic, and abruption with significant bleeding.

Signs and symptoms of preterm labor may be vague. The woman may complain of contractions, generalized crampiness, pelvic pressure, rectal pressure, or back pain, but half of all women in preterm labor feel no pain at all. Diarrhea, intestinal cramping or a change in vaginal discharge can be associated with many unrelated conditions. Any amount of vaginal bleeding in the second or third trimester should be evaluated immediately, but some women spot benignly after intercourse. A gush of fluid may indicate rupture of membranes, but more often is related to normal vaginal discharge or bladder incontinence. Urinary-tract infections, appendicitis, and gastroenteritis can both cause and mimic preterm labor.

Women should be educated about the signs and symptoms of preterm labor, especially at and beyond the threshold of viability. Women who show symptoms of preterm labor are more likely to have an increase in symptoms during sexual activity (including breast stimulation and orgasm), long distance travel in cars, trains or buses, prolonged standing, or strenuous physical activity. The preterm delivery rate in heavy smokers (more than half a pack a day) is 20%, or more than twice the rate of nonsmokers (Ross & Eden, 2007).

Women in developing countries are at higher risk for preterm delivery, but most medical facilities in these regions are unable to care for premature infants.

Preterm labor cannot be identified on symptoms alone; 50% of clients hospitalized for PTL deliver at term, and many women have cramping throughout the second and third trimesters. Bacterial vaginosis increases the risk of preterm delivery, but so far no treatment regimen has improved outcomes. Uterine monitors are useful for following contractions to evaluate preterm labor, but cannot predict or prevent preterm birth. A short cervical length on transvaginal ultrasound (≤25 mm), particularly at 24–28 weeks' gestation, has been associated with a strikingly increased risk of preterm labor and delivery. Women at increased risk for preterm delivery should have serial cervical length measurements. The woman with both a short cervix and a positive fetal fibronectin test should be closely watched for preterm labor, and steroids should be considered.

Fetal fibronectin (FFN) is a protein that glues the amniotic membranes to the decidua. A swab in the vagina of a symptomatic woman between 24 and 34 weeks can determine the presence or absence of FFN. A negative FFN accurately identifies women who are unlikely to deliver within the next 1–2 weeks. A positive FFN has less predictive value.

✍ AACT—Consider and Treat

If a woman is complaining of cramping or is having contractions, investigate by performing a vaginal examination. Reassess and confirm her estimated delivery date. If she is between 24 and 34 weeks' gestation and has not had anything in the vagina in 24 hr (as in examinations or intercourse), consider performing a fetal fibronectin swab. The FFN sample must be collected first, because any jostling of the cervix as with a digital examination could cause a false positive result. Swabs for gonorrhea, chlamydia, group B strep and bacterial vaginosis/trichomonas can be collected at the same time. Antibiotics are given to the woman with PTL only for prophylaxis against group B beta-streptococcus, not as an adjunctive therapy.

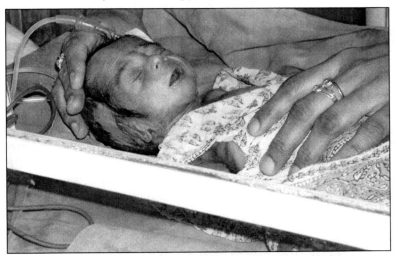

Figure 64. Infant of 28 weeks' gestation, at age 19 days, in NICU in Jaipur, India. Women in developing countries are at increased risk for preterm delivery, but most medical facilities in these regions are unable to care for premature infants.

Specific criteria for PTL include persistent uterine contractions (at least four every 20 min or eight every 60 min) with premature rupture of membranes or cervical change (transvaginal cervical length <2.5 cm, dilation of 1–3 cm, effacement exceeding 80% or fetal descent (Simhan & Caritis, 2008). If contractions continue without cervical change, the provider may opt for continued observation or therapeutic sleep (morphine sulfate 10–15 mg subcutaneous). If the FFN is negative, there is no cervical change, or the contractions cease, the client may be sent home with appropriate follow-up.

Glucocorticoids reduce the risk of neonatal death, respiratory distress syndrome, intraventricular hemorrhage, and necrotizing enterocolitis in premature neonates. Glucocorticoids also raise maternal blood sugar and increase the risk of infection. These steroids are given between 24 and 34 weeks when the risk of preterm delivery is high and there is no clinical infection. Betamethasone is given as two 12 mg IM doses 24 hr apart; dexamethasone is given as four IM doses of 6 mg each at 6-hour intervals. Repeated courses of glucocorticoids do not seem to benefit the fetus, except when steroids are given at 24–26 weeks and repeated after 28 weeks' gestation.

Tocolytic agents do not prevent preterm birth. These agents can stop contractions temporarily, but they do not affect the pathophysiology that set the process in motion. Between 24 and 33 weeks' gestation, the goal of treatment is to delay delivery for 48 hr to derive maximum benefit from glucocorticoids, but the fetus benefits if delivery is delayed by as few as 12 hr after steroid administration. Aggressive tocolytic therapy is generally not recommended beyond 34 weeks, because at that time risks outweigh benefits (Simhan & Caritis, 2008).

Tocolytics are contraindicated for any congenital anomaly incompatible with life and in chorioamnionitis. Other contraindications include intrauterine fetal demise, nonreassuring fetal status, severe IUGR, severe preeclampsia or eclampsia, and maternal hemodynamic instability.

Magnesium sulfate, indomethacin, and nifedipine are tocolytic agents commonly used to treat preterm labor. Although magnesium sulfate is associated with greater maternal toxicity, indomethacin is riskier for the fetus. A Cochrane review found no evidence of a clinically important tocolytic effect for magnesium sulfate. More studies are needed to determine efficacy (Simhan & Caritis, 2008). In 2008, however, the *New England Journal of Medicine* reported that fetal exposure to magnesium sulfate before anticipated early preterm delivery reduced the rate of cerebral palsy among survivors (Kaunitz, 2008). Terbutaline and ritodrine were once in common use; but these beta-mimetics have many side effects, such as tachycardia, hyperglycemia, palpitations, pulmonary edema, myocardial ischemia, and cardiac arrhythmia.

Tocolytics and Cerclage
Magnesium Sulfate
The usual loading dose for magnesium sulfate is 4–6 g IV over 20 min, followed by a maintenance dose of 1–4 g/hr depending on urine output and status of contractions. Common maternal side effects include flushing, nausea, headache, drowsiness, and blurred vision. Magnesium sulfate can cause neonatal respiratory and motor depression if given near the time of delivery. Extended magnesium sulfate therapy is not usually beneficial, except in the case of the fetus less than 28 weeks' gestation, who benefits from each additional day *in utero*. Another possible exception is when labor is triggered by self-limited conditions such as pyelonephritis or abdominal surgery.

Indomethacin
Indomethacin is prostaglandin synthetase inhibitor used as a first-line tocolytic for preterm labor <30 wks or preterm labor with polyhydramnios. Preterm labor before 30 weeks' gestation is more likely due to an inflammatory process, and indomethacin reduces prostaglandin synthesis. Indomethacin also works on the fetal kidneys and may decrease polyhydramnios.

Indomethacin is as effective as terbutaline but has fewer maternal side effects. It can cause oligohydramnios if used for more than 48 hr. Baseline CBC count and liver function tests (LFTs) should be ordered before starting therapy. The initial dose is usually 100 mg PR followed by 50 mg PO every 6 hr for 8 doses. If oligohydramnios occurs, the amniotic fluid index usually normalizes when the drug is discontinued, but fetal kidney damage and neonatal death have occurred. Use of indomethacin beyond 32 weeks' gestation and for longer than 72 hr increases risk for constriction or closure of the ductus arteriosus. Terbutaline is a better second-line agent in these circumstances. Avoid indomethacin in the woman with coagulopathy, liver or kidney disease, hypotension, gastrointestinal ulcers, concurrent use of beta-mimetics or magnesium sulfate, or hypersensitivity to aspirin.

Nifedipine

Nifedipine is a calcium-channel blocker that relaxes smooth muscle cells and is commonly used as an antihypertensive medication. It is used "off-label" as a very effective tocolytic, and appears to decrease neonatal morbidity. Initial dosage of nifedipine usually 20 mg orally, followed by 20 mg orally after 30 min. If contractions persist, therapy can be continued with 20 mg orally every 3–8 hr for 48–72 hr with a maximum dose of 160 mg/d. After 72 hr, if maintenance is still required, long-acting nifedipine 30–60 mg daily can be used. Contraindications include liver disease and transdermal nitrates or other antihypertensive medication. Nifedipine can cause maternal tachycardia, palpitations, flushing, headaches, dizziness, and nausea.

Tocolysis is unlikely to stop labor that has progressed beyond 3 cm. The mother should be transferred to a facility that can provide an appropriate level of neonatal care if she delivers preterm.

Because preterm labor is often overdiagnosed, inconsequential uterine irritability is often overtreated. Research shows that IV hydration, sedation, and bed rest do not reduce the rate of preterm delivery in symptomatic women. Tocolytic agents are generally safe, but can cause complications and should be used only if benefits outweigh risks. If the first tocolytic medication does not stop contractions, it should be discontinued and a second agent initiated. Simultaneous administration of multiple tocolytic drugs increases the risk of serious side effects and is not more effective than a single agent.

Beta-Mimetic Agents

Ritodrine and terbutaline relax the uterus by stimulating the beta2 receptors, resulting in relaxation of the uterine muscles and the smooth muscles of the lung with few effects on the beta1 cardiac receptors. The effect is similar to an adrenaline rush. Terbutaline is administered as 0.25 mg doses subcutaneously every 30 min initially, then every 4–6 hr. Oral terbutaline tablets, 2.5–5.0 mg, can be given every 4–6 hr; but while this regimen may suppress contractions, it does not appear effective in preventing preterm delivery. Ritodrine is given intravenously in an initial dose of 0.05–0.1 mg/min and increased at 15-min intervals to 0.35 mg/min. Tachycardia and palpitations are common side effects, and beta mimetics can also cause cardiac arrhythmias and hyperglycemia.

Cerclage

Cerclage is often placed between 13 and 17 weeks' gestation for a history of loss due to cervical incompetence. Sometimes a rescue cerclage is placed if the cervix is shortened, regardless of history. Inhibiting labor in the pre-viable pregnancy is controversial because tocolytics can only delay labor for a short time, and the infant is unlikely to survive if less than 23 weeks. Some authorities feel that etiology is more important than gestational age, and that inhibiting contractions after a self-limited event such as intra-abdominal surgery is reasonable.

Table 21. Recommendations from the National Guideline Clearinghouse

There are no clear "first-line" tocolytic drugs to manage preterm labor. Clinical circumstances and physician preferences should dictate treatment.

Antibiotics do not appear to prolong gestation and should be reserved for group B streptococcal prophylaxis in patients in whom delivery is imminent.

Neither maintenance treatment with tocolytic drugs nor repeated acute tocolysis improve perinatal outcome; neither should be undertaken as a general practice.

Tocolytic drugs may prolong pregnancy for 2 to 7 days, which may allow for administration of steroids to improve fetal lung maturity and the consideration of maternal transport to a tertiary care facility.

(ECRI Institute, 2004)

Preterm Premature Rupture of Membranes
Priority 2 or 1

First Thought, Worst Thought

What is the most likely cause of preterm leaking?
Urinary incontinence or vaginal discharge.
What is the worst it could be?
Preterm PROM, especially pre-viable or with chorioamnionitis.

✍ AACT—Alert

Premature rupture of the membranes, or amniorrhexis, is a complication of pregnancy responsible for about 30% of premature deliveries (Creasy & Resnik, 1999). The fetal membranes comprise a thin inner amnion and a thicker outer chorion, five distinct layers embedded in a collagenous matrix devoid of blood vessels or nerves (Gabbe, et al., 2007; Weitz, 2001). These membranes and the adjacent maternal decidua are metabolically active, transporting solutes and water to achieve homeostasis and secreting bioactive compounds such as peptides, growth factors, and cytokines. By the 26th week of gestation, the amnion is a single tough layer of cells, and the chorion is a mere four to six cells thick. But together these membranes can withstand great pressure and stress, especially when supported by a closed cervix.

✍ AACT—Analyze

The amniotic membrane protects the fetus from infection and trauma by encapsulating about 800 ml of amniotic fluid (Gabbe, et al., 2007). Beginning in the second trimester, the fetus largely determines fluid volume by balancing output of lung fluid and urine with swallowing and flow across the membranes. Near term, the fetus secretes 300–400 ml of lung fluid and 400–1,200 ml of urine into the amniotic cavity and swallows 200–500 ml (Gabbe, et al.). Far from being stagnant, amniotic fluid circulates with a total turnover time of one day (Creasy & Resnik, 1999). It equalizes pressure, makes umbilical cord compression less likely, allows for movement and musculoskeletal development, and promotes the development of healthy lungs and urinary tract. If fluid volume is inadequate for a long period, the fetus may suffer deformities and underdeveloped lungs.

Premature rupture of the membranes, or PROM, is usually defined as rupture of the chorioamniotic membranes before the onset of labor, but usage varies. Some sources define PPROM as *preterm* premature rupture of membranes (Star, Shannon, Lommel, & Gutierrez, 1999); others, as *prolonged* premature rupture of membranes (greater than 24 hr) (Creasy & Resnik, 1999). This text will use PPROM to mean preterm premature rupture of membranes.

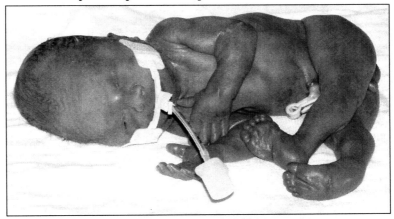

Figure 65. Compression deformities. This genetically normal infant remained in utero for about 9 weeks after spontaneous rupture of the membranes at 19 weeks. He was finally delivered via cesarean at about 28 weeks' gestation when the placenta abrupted. He survived, though he contended with many orthopedic and respiratory issues.

The latency period, or time between PROM and the onset of labor, is usually longer in preterm pregnancies. Women who rupture membranes at term go into labor within 24 hr in 80% of cases (Gabbe, et al., 2007). Seventy to 80% of women with PROM between 28 and 34 weeks' gestation deliver within 1 week. Half of these deliver within 4 days; 80–90%, within 1 week (Gabbe, et al.). Before 24 weeks, 50% start labor within a week of rupture (Creasy & Resnik,

 Risk factors for preterm premature rupture of membranes include PROM in a previous pregnancy; low socioeconomic status; cervical incompetence; DES exposure; placental pathology, such as placenta previa or marginal cord insertion; coitus; cocaine use; hypertension; diabetes; 2nd- and 3rd-trimester bleeding; Ehlers-Danlos syndrome; smoking; and nutritional deficiency of ascorbic acid, zinc, or copper.

1999). Regardless of management or clinical presentation, most cases of preterm PROM result in delivery within 1 week of membrane rupture (ACOG, 1998).

Studies suggest that preterm PROM is triggered by a flaw in membrane structure or an extrinsic cause of weakening, such as infective microorganisms, cerclage placement, or amniocentesis (Creasy & Resnik, 1999). Substances produced by adherent bacteria can weaken the membranes. Multiple gestation and polyhydramnios cause damage by excessive stretching, and certain cervical surgeries can weaken physical support.

Although infection appears to be a major cause of PROM, some women harbor suspicious microorganisms without suffering PROM or preterm labor. Clients who carry group B streptococci, *Gardnerella vaginalis*, gonococci, chlamydia, or trichomonas in early pregnancy are significantly more likely to suffer PROM; but studies differ on the risk level conferred by each microorganism (Creasy & Resnik, 1999). Bacterial vaginosis (BV) has been implicated in preterm delivery and seems to cause preterm PROM as well, but the largest cohort study to date shows no correlation between BV and rupture of membranes (Mercer, et al., 2002).

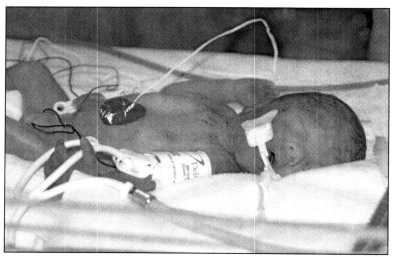

Figure 66. Compression deformities from prolonged ROM. This baby beat the odds. Preterm rupture of membranes occurred at 20 weeks, and he remained in utero until 28 weeks' gestation, when the placenta finally abrupted. His AFI remained at 3–4 for the 2 months of PPROM, but most of the fluid was pooled around his head, so his lungs developed adequately. His facial features and limbs do show signs of compression. At this writing, he is 1 year old and doing well.

Premature birth is one of the most significant risks of preterm PROM. Infection is both cause and sequela in preterm PROM. Bacteria ascend from the vagina and cause weakening and rupture of the membranes, then infection of the fetus, fluid, and placenta. Infection following PROM manifests as chorioamnionitis or endometritis in the mother and septicemia, pneumonia, urinary-tract infection, or localized infection in the fetus Chorioamnionitis occurs in 15–25% of preterm PROM cases, its likelihood increasing with younger gestational age to a rate of 40% with PROM before 24 weeks (Ross & Eden, 2007). More than half of chorioamnionitis cases develop within the first 7 days after rupture (McElrath, 2007). Ordinarily chorioamnionitis occurs before the fetus shows signs of infection, but in some cases the mother remains preclinical and only the fetus shows signs

Infection and preterm delivery are not the only risks to the fetus. Placental abruption occurs in 2–44% of clients with midtrimester PPROM, but in 0.4–1.3% of pregnant women overall (McElrath, 2007). Preterm fetuses frequently assume positions other than vertex with the presenting part high in the pelvis, increasing the likelihood of umbilical cord prolapse. Fetal distress from cord compression can occur without a protective cushion of fluid, especially during labor.

Oligohydramnios after preterm PROM can lead to growth restriction, malformations of face and limbs from compression, scoliosis, hip dislocation, limb reduction, and body-wall defects (Weitz, 2001). About 27% of fetuses born after prolonged PROM show skeletal deformities, though most resolve after 1 year (Gabbe, et al., 2007). Fetal breathing of amniotic fluid is necessary for proper lung formation. Pulmonary hypoplasia, a condition with high lethality, can result from insufficient fluid, especially when PROM occurs before 26 weeks (Gabbe, et al.).

Ruptured fetal membranes appear to reseal spontaneously in 7–14% of women with midtrimester PPROM. In this case, pregnancy outcomes are similar to those of women without a history of PPROM (Gabbe, et al., 2007). Other women continue to leak small amounts of fluid, but can reaccumulate a sizable pocket of fluid around the fetus.

✍ AACT—Consider

The client with preterm PROM should be managed by physicians, but midwives are often the first providers to assess for preterm PROM and frequently co-manage with physicians (Weitz, 2001). The client with preterm PROM will usually present with either a gush of fluid from the vagina followed by leakage or with persistent dampness (Gabbe, et al., 2007). Sometimes she may confuse either with involuntary urination or profuse, thin vaginal discharge. A woman with premature cervical dilation sometimes will have a watery discharge even with intact membranes (Creasy & Resnik, 1999). Sometimes the only diagnostic clue is bloody show, cramping, painless contractions, pelvic "heaviness," or symptoms of chorioamnionitis (Star, et al., 1999). It is important for the clinician to consider this diagnosis in the presence of oligohydramnios or complaints of persistent vaginal discharge.

Perform a sterile speculum examination to check for pooling of fluid; to observe the cervix for dilation, scars, or abnormalities; and to note membranes, umbilical cord, or fetal limbs protruding through the cervical os. If no fluid is seen, the clinician should ask the client to bear down (Valsalva maneuver) while watching for leakage through the os. During the speculum examination the clinician may also perform a Nitrazine test, take vaginal cultures, check for ferning, and make a wet mount.

The pH of amniotic fluid (7.1–7.3) is higher than that of the pregnant woman's vagina (4.5–6) and will turn Nitrazine paper dark blue. False positives, however, can occur in the presence of blood, semen, tap water, soap, cervical mucus, or infection (Weitz, 2001). A swab from the posterior fornix applied to a slide and allowed to dry shows a distinctive microscopic ferning pattern if it is amniotic fluid—but cervical mucus can also fern and confuse results.

If the initial sterile speculum examination is negative or inconclusive, the clinician should allow the woman to rest in a semi-Fowler's position for 30 min or more, then repeat the test, asking her to bear down while applying gentle fundal pressure. The clinician who suspects PROM must make every effort to avoid digital examinations. In PROM cases, serial digital cervical examinations more than 24 hr before delivery increase the risk of neonatal infection and mortality and shorten latency significantly. There is no change in infection rates or latency period when digital examinations are limited to two or fewer (Alexander, et al., 2000; Gabbe, et al., 2007).

A vaginal swab for fetal fibronectin, which is abundant in amniotic fluid, can help the clinician diagnose ROM (Gabbe, et al., 2007). AmniSure is a product that detects minuscule amounts of amniotic fluid in vaginal secretions without speculum examination, additional reagents or equipment. The result is evaluated visually at the bedside in 5–10 min with up to 99% accuracy (Park & Norwitz, 2005). A false positive result is likely in the presence of blood, and false negatives occur when the test is performed 12 hr or more after membrane rupture.

Ultrasonography usually reveals oligohydramnios following PROM. When results are ambiguous, a physician can inject dye via amniocentesis and observe its leakage through the cervical os or onto a tampon (Creasy & Resnik, 1999; Gabbe, et al., 2007).

✍ AACT—Treat

Immediate delivery is indicated in the case of chorioamnionitis, fetal distress, advanced active labor, or abruptio placentae (Creasy & Resnik, 1999). Infants delivered after chorioamnionitis develops, however, suffer a 2–4 times greater incidence of perinatal mortality, intraventricular hemorrhage, and neonatal sepsis than do gestational age-matched controls with noninfected mothers.

In other cases, accurate gestational age dating becomes the crucial factor in the management of preterm PROM, for the provider must weigh the complications of prematurity (respiratory distress syndrome, intraventricular hemorrhage, and necrotizing enterocolitis) against the consequences of expectant management (Creasy & Resnik, 1999). Before 30–32 weeks, the risks of prematurity usually outweigh the intrauterine risk of infection and oligohydramnios. The reverse is true after 34 or 35 weeks (Duff, 2007). Many providers allow the client to reach 36 or 37 weeks' gestation, but some prefer to induce when the fetal lungs are mature, regardless of gestational age (Creasy & Resnik).

Lung maturity is a significant consideration in managing the preterm PROM client after 32 weeks (Gabbe, et al., 2007). The provider can test pooled amniotic fluid for phosphatidylglycerol (PG), a good indicator of lung maturity in the fetus and the only accurate one in vaginal amniotic fluid. Many fetuses do have mature lungs when PG is absent; however, bacterial contaminants are reported to give false-positive results, and the lecithin/sphingomyelin ratio (L/S) verifies lung maturity at an earlier date. Therefore, when clinical management hinges on the status of lung maturity, it is prudent to follow with amniocentesis for L/S ratio if PG is absent from vaginal fluid (Creasy & Resnik, 1999).

Studies disagree about whether corticosteroids influence lung maturation in preterm PROM. PROM itself accelerates lung maturation: there is an observable decrease in the rate of respiratory distress syndrome with an increase in the duration of PROM up to 48 hr (Namavar Jahromi, Ardekany, & Poorarian, 2002). Corticosteroids slightly reduce rates of RDS and significantly reduce the incidence of intraventricular hemorrhage, necrotizing enterocolitis, and death in the immature neonate (Creasy & Resnik, 1999; Harding, Pang, Knight, & Liggins, 2001). Consequently, the National Institutes of Health deems antenatal corticosteroids appropriate for managing preterm PROM in the absence of chorioamnionitis before 32 weeks (Creasy & Resnik). Corticosteroids used with antibiotics reduce morbidity more than either medication used alone (Gabbe, et al., 2007).

Prophylactic antibiotics should be given to all women with preterm PROM (Gabbe, et al., 2007). Research shows that prophylactic amoxicillin and erythromycin reduce not only chorioamnionitis and endometritis, but also major neonatal morbidities (including sepsis, pneumonia, RDS, and necrotizing enterocolitis) and prolong the latency period by an average of 5–7 days (Creasy & Resnik, 1999). These benefits have greatest impact on preterm PROM clients with a gestational age less than 30–32 weeks. Prophylaxis for group B streptococci differs from that used for other pathogens, however, so the clinician must be sure to choose the proper antibiotic regime.

In most cases, the woman with preterm PROM will remain on bed rest for the duration of her pregnancy, ideally in a hospital with a NICU (Weitz, 2001). One clinical trial considered preterm PROM clients eligible for home discharge if after 72 hr they displayed negative cervical cultures, no signs of labor, no fetal distress, and no signs of infection. In the 18% of clients who were discharged, maternal and infant outcomes were comparable to those who had remained hospitalized (ACOG, 1998).

Pregnant clients on hospital bed rest show greater muscle atrophy, fatigue, indigestion, sleep disturbances, depression, weight loss, and risk of blood clots (Maloni & Kutil, 2000). Pulmonary embolism is a leading cause of maternal death in industrialized nations, and most cases arise from DVT in the legs (Kovacevich, et al., 2000).

Tocolytic therapy appears to do little to prolong pregnancy in women with preterm PROM. Short-term tocolysis may delay labor long enough to allow administration of corticosteroids and antibiotics. In most cases of PROM at or near viability, the woman will remain in the hospital until delivery. Occasionally the leak in the amnion seals, and the amniotic sac refills. In these cases, the woman can return home as if she had never suffered PROM.

Ultrasound evaluation should be performed on the woman with preterm PROM to assess gestational age, fetal reactivity, and amniotic fluid volume. The clinician should recognize that oligohydramnios can cause compression of the fetus and change measurements of biparietal diameter or abdominal circumference, giving a false estimation of maturity (Gabbe, et al., 2007). Ultrasound can also determine cervical length, placental location and grade, and fetal and pelvic abnormalities.

A biophysical profile is valuable for monitoring fetal wellbeing—a high score and reactive nonstress test correlate well with absence of infection in the fetus—but it says little about maternal infection (Lewis, et al., 1999). Daily biophysical profiles are indicated in pregnancies under 28 weeks until the fetus develops the neurological capacity for a reactive fetal heart tracing (Lewis, et al.).

If the woman's temperature is greater than 101°F and she shows uterine tenderness, leukocytosis greater than or equal to 20,000/mm (Gabbe, et al., 2007), a low biophysical profile score, persistent fetal tachycardia, or foul-smelling vaginal drainage, delivery must occur promptly regardless of gestational age (Gabbe, et al.). An intensive review of laboratory tests to detect intrauterine infection concluded that no single test is completely satisfactory, and the clearest clinical impression comes from looking at many different results.

In preterm PROM earlier than 25 weeks, only 25–40% of women will go on to deliver viable babies (Duff, 2007). Postponing delivery often results in serious complications, like abruption or severe infection, and neurologically damaged infants. Clients who rupture their membranes at very early gestational ages can occasionally be brought to viability with antibiotics and bed rest, but in most cases severe maternal infection ensues (Creasy & Resnik, 1999).

Some providers prefer to induce labor if the gestational age and estimated fetal weight are beyond a certain point (such as 32 weeks or 1,500–1,800 g). If the woman is not in labor and has no signs of infection or fetal distress, and there is no evidence of fetal lung maturity, the provider should opt for expectant management in the hospital.

The provider must remain vigilant for signs of infection in the fetus or mother, including elevated white blood cells, maternal or fetal tachycardia, uterine tenderness, fever, malaise, or foul-smelling vaginal discharge. The early presentation of chorioamnionitis is often subtle, and clues can be attributed to other causes. Amniocentesis can determine infection in a client with inconclusive signs (Creasy & Resnik, 1999).

Women with a history of preterm PROM, premature delivery, or cervical incompetence should be evaluated by a physician. A short cervical length (less than 2.5 cm) at 23–24 weeks' gestation consistently correlates with ROM at less than 35–37 weeks' gestation, so serial ultrasonographic assessments of the cervix for length and dilation should be performed in the at-risk woman (Odibo, Berghella, Reddy, Tolosa, & Wapner, 2001; Mercer, et al., 2002).

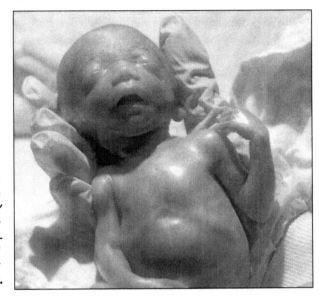

Figure 67. Too small to survive. This infant was almost 22 weeks' gestation when her mother presented unexpectedly in advanced labor. Sadly, she only lived about 5 min.

MANAGING THE PREMATURE INFANT

The premature infant born out of the hospital requires careful management. Babies born before the 37th week of gestation are considered premature, regardless of weight. The majority of premature babies under 35–36 weeks will need resuscitation or specialized supportive care following birth.

The scope of practice of the out-of-hospital midwife does not include planned preterm delivery, but preterm infants can be born with unexpected swiftness. Women in preterm labor often have vague or nonspecific symptoms until labor is advanced. The baby usually arrives shortly after the water breaks and is more likely to assume a nonvertex position for birth. Premature babies are extremely delicate, and the birth attendant can easily damage their delicate skin and organs. Allow the baby to deliver with as little assistance as possible. Position the mother on her side to reduce pressure on the fetal head.

The earlier the gestational age, the more the preterm baby will differ from the term baby. The extremely premature baby will need aggressive intervention if it is to have any chance of survival (see Neonatal Resuscitation in Chapter 11). Most infants weighing less than 1,500 g need resuscitation at birth, with the smaller infants needing the most intervention. Follow established resuscitation guidelines, making accommodations for prematurity. Babies born on the cusp of viability usually have severe, lifelong health problems, including cerebral palsy and blindness, if they survive. If a child is extremely premature, his organ systems may be insufficiently developed to sustain life.

The mother may report a reliable gestational age if she has had an early ultrasound scan or is sure of the conception or last menstrual date. Gestational dating is not always accurate, even if the woman has had prenatal care, and the infant may prove more or less mature than expected.

The 36-week infant will be very much like a small term baby, but may have initial breathing and feeding problems and more jaundice by day 4. The 32–34 week baby will be thin-skinned and gaunt because of minimal subcutaneous fat. Infants of this gestational age will often cry vigorously at birth, though they frequently need assistance to sustain adequate respirations.

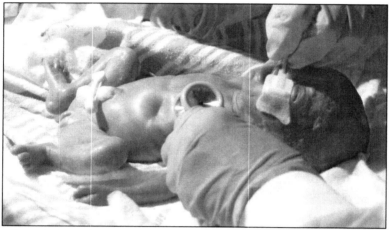

Figure 68. Amelia's birthday. Amelia was born at 26 weeks weighing 1 lb, 6 oz after her mother painlessly dilated and ruptured membranes.

The preterm infant is weak and not very active. Reflexes may be only partially developed, and sucking may be uncoordinated and ineffective. The preemie is easily overstimulated and may respond to noise or rough handling with apnea or bradycardia. Common complications include hypothermia, respiratory distress, patent ductus arteriosus, intracranial hemorrhage, hypoglycemia, necrotizing enterocolitis, infection, and retinopathy of prematurity. This risk increases with decreasing gestational age.

Premature infants require resuscitation more often than full-term infants. Other important considerations include

▶ **Warmth:** Small babies become chilled easily through conduction, convection, radiation, and evaporation. Premature infants have a relatively large body surface area and are unable to produce much heat. Hypothermia can start a spiral of complications ending in cardiovascular collapse. Temperature management is crucial.

▶ **Immature lungs:** The lungs of the very immature baby may be stiff and require more pressure when using a bag and mask. A lack of surfactant in the lungs may cause them to collapse after each breath.

- ▸ **Brain hemorrhage:** Delicate blood vessels in the brain may break during delivery and cause intracranial hemorrhage. Hypoxia, rapid changes in intravascular volume, and rough handling can also cause bleeding in the brain.
- ▸ **Blood sugar:** Preterm babies are more likely to develop hypoglycemia soon after delivery.

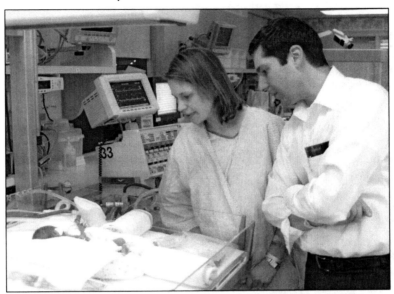

Figure 69. Bells and whistles. Amelia's parents are overwhelmed when they visit the NICU for the first time.

Neonatal ICUs are best suited for stabilizing and supporting any preterm infant. Ideally the baby should be directly transported to a hospital with a neonatal ICU if it does not greatly prolong transport to do so. Ideally, this transfer should take pace with the fetus still *in utero*, so that delivery can take place in a setting with optimal resources.

Intrauterine Growth Restriction

Low birth weight is the second leading cause of infant mortality, after congenital anomalies, but contributes disproportionately to the infant mortality rate. Growth failure can develop early in pregnancy, resulting in underdeveloped body organs, or later in pregnancy, resulting in normal organs that are smaller than usual. There is a higher risk of morbidity and mortality for both the fetus and the neonate when the weight falls below

 Low birth weight (LBW): <2,500 g
Very low birth weight (VLBW): <1,500 g
Extremely low birth weight (ELBW): <1,000 g

the 10th percentile. Common causes of IUGR include multiple gestation, maternal smoking, chronic maternal disease, high altitude, excessive exercise, abnormal placenta structure or placement, certain antepartal infections like rubella or syphilis, and fetal chromosomal abnormalities.

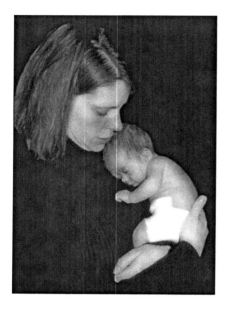

Figure 70. Amelia's discharge day. At discharge Amelia weighed almost 7 lb and appeared to have no deficits related to her preterm birth. Amelia is one of the lucky survivors. At the time of her birth, two other 26-week preemies were undergoing treatment in the same NICU. One has profound disabilities, and the other has a developmental delay and requires special care.

Symmetric IUGR results in chronic, prolonged restriction of the growth of organs, weight, length, and sometimes head circumference. Symmetric IUGR can be caused by any chronic maternal condition that diminishes blood flow or nutrients to the fetus, including longstanding hypertension, malnutrition, anemia, or tobacco use. Symmetric IUGR can also be associated with fetal genetic abnormalities. This condition can be diagnosed on ultrasound as early as early second trimester.

Asymmetric IUGR reflects an acute compromise in the blood flow to the placenta, such as with placental infarctions and pregnancy induced hypertension. The fetus with asymmetrical IUGR shows a normal head circumference and length, but decreased weight and abdominal circumference.

It is thought that the stressed fetus produces elevated levels of norepinephrine and epinephrine, which cause loss of fat stores, muscle mass, and glycogen stores and increase blood flow to the brain, heart and adrenal glands. The fetus retains a normal head circumference as it attempts to protect brain development, but suffers weight loss and poor growth elsewhere.

After delivery, the fetus with IUGR becomes an infant with limited reserves. He is at increased risk for hypoxia during labor and delivery and is more likely to need resuscitation at birth. He shows poor thermoregulation and is more likely to suffer hypoglycemia. Transfer to a facility capable of managing high-risk newborns.

Gestational Age in Weeks	Survival Rate	Neurologically Intact
24	40%	5%
25	70%	50%
26	75%	60%
27	80%	70%
28	90%	80%
29	92%	85%
30	93%	90%
31	94%	93%
32	95%	95%
33	96%	96%
34	97%	97%

Table 22. Gestational Age and Survival Rates

(Ross & Eden, 2007)

BIBLIOGRAPHY

Ailsworth, K., Anderson, J., Atwood, L.A., Bailey, R.E., & Canavan, T. (2006). *ALSO: Advanced life support in obstetrics* (4th ed.). Leawood, KS: American Academy of Family Practice Physicians.

Alexander J.M., Mercer, B.M., Miodovnik, M., Thurnau, G.R., Goldenberg, R.L., Das, A.F., et al. (2000). The impact of digital cervical examination on expectantly managed preterm rupture of membranes. *American Journal of Obstetrics and Gynecology, 183* (4), 1003–1007.

American College of Obstetricians and Gynecologists. (1998). *Obstetric aspects of trauma management* (Educational Bulletin 251). Washington, DC: Author.

Duff, P. (2007). Preterm premature rupture of membranes. In B.D. Rose (Ed.), *UpToDate*. Wellesley, MA: UpToDate.

ECRI Institute. (2004). *Management of Preterm Labor.* (National Guideline Clearinghouse Guideline 3130, Brief Summary.) Retrieved December 13, 2009, from http://www.guideline.gov/summary/summary. aspx?ss=15&doc_id=3993&nbr=3130

Foley, M.R. (2007). Maternal cardiovascular and hemodynamic adaptation to pregnancy. In B.D. Rose (Ed.), *UpToDate*. Wellesley, MA: UpToDate.

Freda, M.C., Patterson, E.T., & Wieczorek, R.R. (2004). *Preterm labor: Prevention and nursing management: Continuing education for registered nurses and certified nurse-midwives* (3rd ed.). White Plains, NY: Education & Health Promotion, March of Dimes.

Gabbe, S.G., Niebyl, J.R., & Simpson, J.L., Eds. (2007). *Obstetrics: Normal and problem pregnancies* (5th ed.). New York: Churchill Livingstone.

Gilbert, E.S. (2007). *Manual of high risk pregnancy and delivery* (4th ed.). St Louis: Mosby.

Gruenberg, Bonnie U. (2005). *Essentials of prehospital maternity care.* Upper Saddle River, NJ: Prentice Hall.

Heppard, M., & Garite, T. (2002). *Acute obstetrics: A practical guide* (3rd ed.). St. Louis: Mosby.

Iverson, Jr., R.E., DeCherney, A.H., & Laufer, M.R. (2007). Clinical manifestations and diagnosis of congenital anomalies of the uterus. In B.D. Rose (Ed.), *UpToDate*. Wellesley, MA: UpToDate.

Kaunitz, A.M. (2008, September 18). Does fetal exposure to magnesium sulfate prevent cerebral palsy in preterm infants? *Journal Watch Women's Health*. Retrieved December 13, 2009, from http://womens-health.jwatch.org/cgi/content/full/2008/918/4

Kovacevich, G.J., Gaich, S.A., Lavin, J.P., Hopkins, M.P., Crane, S.S., Stewart, J., et al. (2000). The prevalence of thromboembolic events among women with extended bed rest prescribed as part of the treatment for premature labor or preterm premature rupture of membranes. *American Journal of Obstetrics and Gynecology, 182* (5), 1089–1092.

Ladewig, P., London, M., Moberly, S., & Olds, S. (2002). *Contemporary maternal-newborn nursing care.* Upper Saddle River, NJ: Prentice Hall.

Lewis, D.F., Adair, C.D., Weeks, J.W., Barrilleaux, P.S., Edwards, M.S., & Garite, T.J. (1999). A randomized clinical trial of daily nonstress testing versus biophysical profile in the management of preterm premature rupture of membranes. *American Journal of Obstetrics and Gynecology, 181* (6), 1495–1499.

Lockwood, C.J. (2008). Pathogenesis of preterm birth. In B.D. Rose (Ed.), *UpToDate.* Wellesley, MA: UpToDate.

March of Dimes. (n.d.). International comparisons—infant mortality rates: 2004. Retrieved May 10, 2008, from http://www.marchofdimes.com/PeriStats/iim.aspx

McElrath, T. (2007). Midtrimester preterm premature rupture of membranes. In B.D. Rose (Ed.), *UpToDate.* Wellesley, MA: UpToDate.

Mercer, B.M., Goldenberg, R.L., Meis, P.J., Moawad, A.H., Shellhaas, C., Das, A., et al. (2002). The preterm prediction study: Prediction of preterm premature rupture of membranes through clinical findings and ancillary testing. The National Institute of Child Health and Human Development Maternal–Fetal Medicine Units Network. *American Journal of Obstetrics and Gynecology, 183* (3), 738–745.

Newton, E.R. (2007). Intraamniotic infection. In B.D. Rose (Ed.), *UpToDate.* Wellesley, MA: UpToDate.

Park, J.S., & Norwitz, E.R. (2005). Technical innovations in clinical obstetrics [Electronic version]. *Contemporary OB/GYN, 50*(9), 6–20. Retrieved May 5, 2008, from http://www.modernmedicine.com/modernmedicine/article/ articleDetail. jsp?ts=1209993749394&id=364759

Pearlman, M., Tintinalli, J., & Dyne, P. (2004). *Obstetric and gynecologic emergencies: Diagnosis and management.* New York: McGraw-Hill.

Queenan, J., Hobbins, J., & Spong, C. (Eds.). (2005). *Protocols for high-risk pregnancies* (4th ed). Hoboken, NJ: Wiley-Blackwell.

Roberts, D.J. (2007c). Placental infections. In B.D. Rose (Ed.), *UpToDate.* Wellesley, MA: UpToDate.

Ross, M.G., & Eden, R.D. (2007). *Preterm labor* (eMedicine, topic 3245). Retrieved March 15, 2008, from http://www.emedicine.com/ med/topic3245.htm

Scorza, W.E. (2007). Management of premature rupture of the fetal membranes at term. In B.D. Rose (Ed.), *UpToDate.* Wellesley, MA: UpToDate.

Sherman, M., & Otsuki, K. (2006). *Maternal chorioamnionitis* (eMedicine, topic 89). Retrieved March 4, 2008, from http://www.emedicine.com/ped/topic89.htm

Simhan, H., & Caritis, S. (2008). Inhibition of acute preterm labor. In B.D. Rose (Ed.), *UpToDate.* Wellesley, MA: UpToDate.

Sinclair, C. (2004). *A midwife's handbook.* St. Louis: Saunders.

Star, W.L., Shannon, M.T., Lommel, L.L., & Gutierrez, Y. (1999). *Ambulatory obstetrics: Protocols for nurse practitioners-nurse midwives* (3rd ed.). San Francisco: UCSF Nursing Press.

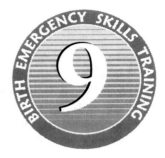

Multiple Gestation

OBJECTIVES

- ▶ List four intrapartum complications that may occur with vaginal delivery of multiple gestation.
- ▶ Compare risks and benefits of vaginal birth and cesarean section for multiple gestation.
- ▶ Formulate a plan of management for the delivery of undiagnosed twins.

AACT and ReACT
ALERT—Be alert ▶ **Exercise hypervigilant attention**
ANALYZE—Think about possible causes
CONSIDER—Use OLDCART ▶ **Gather data**
TREAT—Make first response ▶ **Proceed to definitive care**
ReACT | ReAssess ▶ ReConsider ▶ Re-Treat

✍ AACT—Alert and Analyze

Fertility treatments and a rising average maternal age at childbirth have increased the incidence of multiple gestation in the developed world.

Twins

Priority 1, 2, or 3

The rate of occurrence for identical twins remains fairly stable at about 1 in 225 births, unaffected by variables such as race and parity. The tendency to bear fraternal twins is hereditary, and these births occur naturally at a rate of about 1 set of twins per 86 births. Twins increased to 3.15% of live births in 2003 in the United States (ACOG, 2004b). Since 1980, assisted reproductive technology has doubled the rate of twins and escalated the rate of triplets and high order births by 500% (ACOG, 2004b). Women between the ages of 35 and 40 are more likely to conceive twins, as are overweight and tall women.

There is significant variation between races between in the incidence of dizygotic twins, from fewer than 1 in 100 births in Japan to 1 in 30 births in Nigeria (Chasen & Chervenak, 2007a). The advent of ultrasonography has allowed us to observe pregnancies from soon after conception, and it has revealed that twin conceptions occur far more frequently than previously suspected. Loss of one twin while the second is carried to term is not an uncommon occurrence.

Twin conceptions occur through one of two mechanisms. Identical, or monozygotic, twins (31%) arise when a single fertilized ovum divides into two separate clusters of cells that give rise to two separate individuals that share identical genes (Cunningham, et al., 2005). They are always of the same sex, except for the rare case of a divided trisomy. Fraternal, or dizygotic, twins (69%) originate from separate ova and sperm that happen to be fertilized about the same time (Cunningham, et al.). Genetically, they are as closely related as any other siblings. They can be of different sexes, they can even have different fathers, and they may be conceived more than a week apart. "Vanishing twins" are common; spontaneous death of one fetus will occur in about 36% of twins diagnosed prior to seven weeks of gestation (Chasen & Chervenak, 2007a).

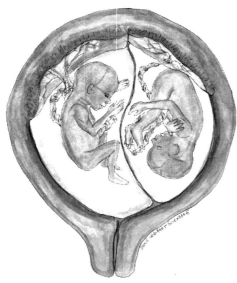

Figure 71. Twelve-week twins. Twins with separate amnions and chorions (diamniotic, dichorionic placentation) arise when division takes place before the morula stage (within 3 days after fertilization).

Twins with separate amnions and chorions (diamniotic, dichorionic placentation) arise when division takes place before the morula stage (within 3 days after fertilization). All dizygotic and one third of monozygotic twins are diamniotic, dichorionic.

Twins with two amnions, one chorion (diamniotic, monochorionic placentation) follows division between days 4 and 8 post fertilization. All monochorionic twins are monozygotic.

Two twins within the same sac, sharing both a chorion and an amnion (monoamniotic, monochorionic placentation) occurs with division between days 8 and 12 after fertilization. All are monozygotic and may be mirror image twins (one twin is left-handed and the other is right-handed, opposite hair whorl directions). Perinatal mortality is 30–70%, usually from cord entanglement (Roqué & Lockwood, 2008). If division takes place at or after day 13, conjoined twins occur.

Higher-order pregnancies tax both mother and babies, and carry a higher incidence of complications. Fifty-four percent of twins and 93% of all triplets and higher order multiples are delivered preterm (Jones, 2007). Over 90% of triplets have birth weights less than 2500 g and 40% are less than 1500 g (Jones, 2007). Preeclampsia, maternal anemia, gestational diabetes, placental abnormalities, hyperemesis, fetal growth restriction, malpresentations, abruption, cord prolapse, fetal death and maternal hemorrhage are all more likely with multiple gestations. The risk of congenital anomalies and developmental defects are doubled for each twin, and more than doubled for monozygotic twins and higher-order multiples (Chasen & Chervenak, 2007a). Cerebral palsy is 4 times more common in twin pregnancies and 17 times more common in triplet pregnancies (ACOG, 2004b). Velamentous insertion of the umbilical cord is common in triplet gestations.

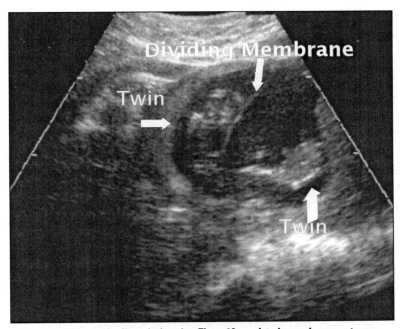

Figure 72. Dichorionic, diamniotic twins. These 13-week twins are in separate sacs, but it is unclear whether they are identical or fraternal.

Potential intrapartum complications include malpresentations (especially breech), cord prolapse, abruption, dysfunctional labor, and postpartum hemorrhage. More than half of multiple births involve at least one breech, conveying all the usual problems associated with breech delivery. Sometimes the breech first twin locks heads with the vertex twin during delivery, making vaginal birth impossible.

Identical twins can grow in separate amniotic sacs or, more rarely, share a sac. The latter situation is riskier to the twins because of the likelihood of cord entanglement. Identical twins who share placental blood vessels can suffer growth discordance (twin-to-twin transfusion syndrome). One twin is engorged with a superabundance of blood to the point of congestive heart failure; the other is wasted and anemic from insufficient circulation. Untreated cases have a poor prognosis, mortality of 70–100%, and severe damage to survivors (Roqué & Lockwood, 2008).

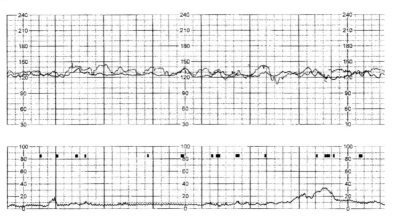

Figure 73. Twins on external fetal monitor tracing. It can be difficult to determine which heart rate belongs to which twin if intermittent auscultation is used in multiple gestation. Rates may be similar, and the movements of one baby stimulate the other.

At delivery, the majority (43%) of twins present with both babies vertex, which is also the presentation most favorable for vaginal delivery (Chasen & Chervenak, 2007). In the hospital, many obstetricians choose vaginal delivery over cesarean section when both twins are vertex. Even in the most favorable circumstances, vaginal twin delivery can be complicated by abruption of the second placenta after delivery of the first twin; cord prolapse; and hemorrhage before, during, or after the delivery of the second twin.

The twin with the presenting part closest to the cervix is termed twin A. Thirty-eight percent present with twin A vertex and twin B nonvertex; 19% present with twin A nonvertex and twin B either vertex or nonvertex (Chasen & Chervenak, 2007a).

The biggest risk to the twin fetus is spontaneous preterm birth. Fifty-seven percent of twins are born before 37 weeks' gestation, 19% before 33 weeks, and 2% before 28 weeks (Chasen & Chervenak, 2007a). A cervix shorter than 25 mm at 24 weeks by transvaginal ultrasound is one of the most reliable indicators that the babies will deliver prematurely, but a cervical length of 3.5 cm or greater is reassuring (Gabbe, et al., 2007). Contrary to conventional wisdom, low birth weight babies from a multiple gestation do not have better outcomes than equivalent babies from a singleton gestation; twins, in fact, may have more morbidity due to IUGR (ACOG, 2004b).

Discordant fetal growth occurs when one fetus is 15–25% smaller than the other. It is associated with structural malformations, stillbirth, IUGR, preterm delivery, acidosis, and neonatal death in the first week of life (ACOG, 2004b).

Twin-to-twin transfusion syndrome occurs when fetuses (usually monozygotic) share blood vessels. One twin becomes engorged with excessive blood and develops polyhydramnios, while the other twin becomes severely anemic with oligohydramnios. In this situation, either or both twins can suffer heart failure and die. One therapy is to remove excess fluid from the sac of the engorged twin through amniocentesis. By reducing the pressure within the sac, the release of pressure on placental vessels normalizes blood flow to both twins. In certain very early, severe cases, laser coagulation can be used to seal the vascular connection between the twins. If twin-to-twin transfusion is suspected, the babies are usually delivered as soon as they are likely to survive.

The average length of pregnancy for singletons, twins, and triplets is 39, 35, and 34 weeks, respectively (Jones, 2007). Modified bed rest is often prescribed to prevent preterm birth, but studies have failed to prove that activity restriction prolongs pregnancy. Likewise, prophylactic cerclage does not seem to increase gestation, nor do 17 alpha-hydroxyprogesterone caproate injections (Chasen & Chervenak, 2007a). Routine antenatal testing of twins has not been shown to improve outcomes unless there are complications such as discordant growth or IUGR.

In the absence of a clear maternal or fetal indication for delivery, perinatal mortality in twin gestations is the lowest if delivery occurs at 37–39 weeks' gestation. The lowest rate for singletons is 39–41 weeks (Chasen & Chervenak, 2007b). If elective delivery is considered before 38 weeks, fetal lung maturity should first be determined via amniocentesis if there is no pressing medical reason to deliver. ACOG recommends delivering all twin pregnancies by 40 weeks' gestation. Antepartum fetal demise cannot be prevented in monoamniotic twins, and the provider must weigh the risks of prematurity with the risks of continuing the pregnancy. The optimal gestational age for intervention in this situation is still undetermined, but many institutions employ close fetal surveillance from the time of viability and deliver by 32 weeks.

Multiple gestations are at increased risk of intrapartum complications. Providers differ in comfort level and experience. Some providers deliver twins routinely by cesarean. ACOG and SOGC agree that twins may be delivered vaginally if cesarean section is immediately available, with anesthetic, obstetrical, and neonatal staff present in the hospital at the time of birth (ACOG, 2004b) (Barrett & Bocking, 2000).

Continuous electronic fetal monitoring and real-time ultrasound should be employed to ensure that each twin is monitored individually. ACOG (2004b) states that retrospective case series validate vaginal delivery as a potential mode of birth for triplets, though most providers opt for cesarean to reduce risks. The mode of delivery is controversial if twin A is vertex and twin B is breech or transverse. Studies disagree on whether vaginal delivery increases risk to the babies.

Cesarean delivery is the method of choice if the first twin is nonvertex or if the twins are monoamniotic. Cesarean is also safer than vaginal delivery if the presenting twin is not vertex. Besides the risk of head entrapment, cord prolapse, and other problems inherent with breech delivery if the twins are face-to-face and twin B is vertex, the chins can lock and obstruct delivery. Cesarean delivery improves outcomes if one of the twins is less than 1500 g (Gabbe, et al., 2007). Six percent to 25% of second twins will require cesarean delivery (Chasen & Chervenak, 2007b).

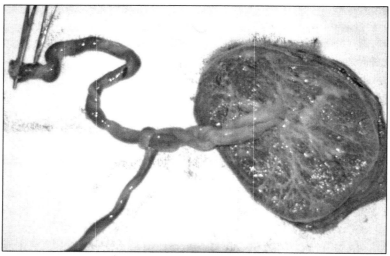

Figure 74. Mono-mono twins are extremely vulnerable. This placenta graphically demonstrates the cord entanglement common with monoamniotic-monochorionic twins. These twins died suddenly at 30 weeks' gestation.

First Thought, Worst Thought

What could cause a large fundal height and irregularly shaped abdomen?

Fibroids, Müllerian abnormality, obesity, polyhydramnios, or malpresentation.

What is the worst it could be?

Multiple gestation with cord prolapse, malpresentation, entrapped head, hemorrhage, or depressed or stillborn infants.

Some authorities have suggested that neonatal outcomes could be improved through routine cesarean delivery for all twin pregnancies, but this policy would necessitate a large number of unnecessary cesareans to save one baby (Chasen & Chervenak, 2007a).

Both ACOG and the SOGC state that it is reasonable to attempt vaginal delivery if twin A is vertex and twin B is breech, as long as usual criteria for breech delivery are met and twin B is between 2000 and 3500 g (ACOG, 2004b). Often twin B will start as vertex and flip to breech or transverse lie after twin A vacates the uterus. Breech extraction carries an increased risk of uterine rupture and fetal trauma. The breech with an extended head is at high risk of sustaining spinal cord injury during the birth process.

Contraindications to breech extraction include

▶ Estimated fetal weight of the second twin (B) is ≥20% more than that of the first twin (A)

▶ Prolonged second stage or marked molding of the head during the delivery of twin A

▶ Gestational age less than 32 weeks

Some authorities recommend converting the second twin to vertex after the first twin is delivered. These procedures should be performed by an experienced provider in a hospital setting.

Triplets
Priority 1 out of hospital, priority 1 or 2 in hospital

Multiple gestation is risky. In 2002, infant mortality rates for quadruplets were 160/1000, for triplets 60/1000, for twins 30/1000 and for singletons 6/1000—mostly due to the increased rate of preterm delivery (Jones, 2007).

Triplets most commonly present vertex-breech-breech (18%), vertex-vertex-breech (16%), vertex-vertex-vertex (15%), and breech-breech-breech (13%) (Jones, 2007).

Many providers elect to deliver all triplets by Cesarean section. Others may consider trial of labor if the presenting triplet is vertex, all three triplets are continuously monitored, the babies are at least 34 weeks of gestation; delivery should be performed in a room equipped to perform a cesarean delivery (Jones, 2007). Vaginal triplet birth should occur in a hospital setting, attended by an experienced provider who is skilled with intrapartum ultrasonography, intrauterine manipulation, and operative delivery. Epidural anesthesia is beneficial should intrauterine manipulation or emergency cesarean section be required. Ten percent to 35% of women will hemorrhage after delivering triplets (Jones, 2007).

✍ AACT—Consider and Treat

Considerations for Twin Delivery

Of all pregnancy variations, multiple gestation presents the greatest range of potential complications, including malpresentations, locking of twins, cord prolapse, abruption, fetal distress, dysfunctional labor, and postpartum hemorrhage (Ailsworth, et al., 2006). While maternal and fetal safety is significantly improved if delivery occurs in a hospital setting with physician backup, out-of-hospital midwives may find themselves surprised by twins or triplet gestations. In women who have not had a routine first- or second-trimester ultrasound, 38% of twin pregnancies remain unrecognized until after 26 weeks of gestation, and 13% of twins are not diagnosed until delivery (Chasen & Chervenak, 2007a).

Although ultrasound is the only safe and reliable method of diagnosis, discrepancies between uterine size and menstrual dates and elevations in maternal serum alpha-fetoprotein (MSAFP) may raise the provider's suspicion of multiple gestation. Twins and triplet pregnancies are more likely to involve hyperemesis, hypertension, and impaired glucose tolerance. The abdominal contour may feel unusually lumpy, and the midwife may have trouble palpating the fetal outline. The midwife's intuition may suggest that something is not quite normal.

Table 23. OOH Management of Undiagnosed Twins

(Order of steps may vary)

Call EMS, initiate transfer protocol

Explain situation to the client and her family

Avoid clamping and cutting nuchal cord of first baby

Deliver first twin as usual

Monitor heart rate of twin B continuously

Palpate abdomen carefully to determine position of twin B

Perform external version to longitudinal lie, if necessary

Perform vaginal exam for presentation and to check for cord prolapse

Expect 20–30 min delay before delivery of twin B. There is no need to hurry the birth if fetus and mother are stable.

Avoid rupture of membranes if the presenting part is not in the pelvis.

Start intravenous line, draw blood, and bolus with 1000 cc lactated Ringer's or normal saline

Expedite delivery for twin B if

    Fetal heart tones are nonreassuring

    Mother is hemorrhaging

    Mother resumes heavy labor

Clamp the cord of twin B with 2 clamps

Prepare for postpartum hemorrhage and neonatal resuscitation

As many as three ambulances may be necessary if both infants and the mother are in need of resuscitation.

Deliver twins as you would individual infants, being especially gentle with delicate premature babies. Usually the second twin will deliver within 15–20 minutes of the first. You will need an infant resuscitation kit for each baby, including cord clamps, baby hats, endotracheal tubes, suction catheters, oxygen delivery equipment, neonatal resuscitation bags, blankets, and the like.

The heart rates of twins are often synchronous, and the provider must watch carefully to ensure that both babies are monitored. If there is any question, the rates can be checked via ultrasound. If separate monitors are used, the internal clocks must be synchronized, paper speeds must be identical, and contractions must be displayed on both tracings. Intermittent auscultation is impractical and riskier because it can be difficult to distinguish one twin from the other (Chasen & Chervenak, 2007b).

The most critical time follows the delivery of twin A, when the second is still *in utero*. Once his sibling has vacated the uterus, twin B is at significant risk for cord prolapse, placental abruption, or maneuvering into an undeliverable malpresentation such as transverse lie. If twin B is larger than twin A, the cervix may not be sufficiently dilated to accommodate twin B after the birth of twin A. In some cases the cervix recloses after the birth of the first twin.

Use caution when cutting the cord. There have been instances in which the cord of the second twin was wrapped tightly several times around the neck of the first twin, and in cutting it to free twin A, the birth attendant cut off circulation to the twin still *in utero*. Be sure to clamp the cord twice before cutting—if the twins share placental circulation, allowing the cord to drain after cutting might exsanguinate the twin still *in utero*.

Both babies may need resuscitation, and the mother may hemorrhage. If the infants are obviously not the same size, both are extremely likely to develop respiratory distress, intracranial hemorrhage, seizures, or other complications.

Mark the umbilical cords' progressive numbers of clamps—one clamp on twin A's cord, two on twin B's. Twin A on ultrasound may not be first born. After delivery of the first twin, evaluate the position and heart rate of the second. Second-born twins have a higher incidence of morbidity and mortality. If the heart rate is reassuring, there is no rush to deliver the second twin. Perform amniotomy after the presenting part is engaged.

After the delivery of the first twin, the uterus may stop contracting and the cervix may start to close, making rapid delivery of the second twin difficult or impossible. Meanwhile, the cord may prolapse or the placenta may abrupt. Although some second twins may require rapid delivery, research has shown good outcomes for fetuses with reassuring heart rates born more than 2 hr after the first twin (Gabbe, et al., 2007).

A facility with the capability of immediate cesarean should be readily available in case of prolapsed umbilical cord, nonreassuring fetal heart rate, or failed breech extraction. In the United States, 10–30% of planned vaginal twin births result in emergency cesareans (Chasen & Chervenak, 2007b).

BIBLIOGRAPHY

Ailsworth, K., Anderson, J., Atwood, L.A., Bailey, R.E., & Canavan, T. (2006). *ALSO: Advanced life support in obstetrics* (4th ed.). Leawood, KS: American Academy of Family Practice Physicians.

American College of Obstetricians and Gynecologists. (2004b). *Multiple gestation: Complicated twin, triplet, and high order multifetal pregnancy. Clinical management guidelines for OB-GYN* (Practice Bulletin 56). Washington, DC: Author.

Barrett I, Bocking A. (2000) *Management of twin pregnancies* (part 2). Society of Obstetricians and Gynaecologists of Canada (SOGC) Consensus Statement. J SOGC.91:5–15.

Chasen, S.T., & Chervenak, F.A. (2004). Intrapartum management of twin gestations. In B.D. Rose (Ed.), *UpToDate*. Wellesley, MA: UpToDate.

Chasen, S.T., & Chervenak, F.A. (2007a). Antepartum assessment of twin gestations. In B.D. Rose (Ed.), *UpToDate*. Wellesley, MA: UpToDate.

Chasen, S.T., & Chervenak, F.A. (2007b). Delivery of twin gestations. In B.D. Rose (Ed.), *UpToDate*. Wellesley, MA: UpToDate.

Cruikshank, D.P. (2007). Intrapartum management of twin gestations. *Obstetrics & Gynecology, 109*(5), 1167–1176.

Cunningham, F., Grant, N., Leveno, K., Gilstrap, L., Hauth, J., & Wenstrom, K. (2005). *Williams's obstetrics* (22nd ed.). New York: McGraw-Hill.

Hofmeyr, G.J. (2007). Approach to breech presentation. In B.D. Rose (Ed.), *UpToDate*. Wellesley, MA: UpToDate.

Howell, C., Grady, K., & Cox, C. (Eds.). (2007). *Managing obstetric emergencies and trauma: The MOET course manual* (2nd ed.) London: RCOG Press.

Jones, D.C. (2007). Triplet pregnancy: Mid and late pregnancy complications and management. In B.D. Rose (Ed.), *UpToDate*. Wellesley, MA: UpToDate.

Queenan, J., Hobbins, J., & Spong, C. (Eds.). (2005). *Protocols for high-risk pregnancies* (4th ed). Hoboken, NJ: Wiley-Blackwell.

Roqué, H., & Lockwood, C.J. (2008). Monoamniotic twin pregnancy. In B.D. Rose (Ed.), *UpToDate*. Wellesley, MA: UpToDate.

Simpson, K.R., & Creehan, P.A. (2007). *AWHONN's perinatal nursing* (3rd ed.). Hagerstown, MD: Lippincott Williams & Wilkins.

Sinclair, C. (2004). *A midwife's handbook*. St. Louis: Saunders.

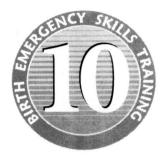

Malpresentations and Shoulder Dystocia

OBJECTIVES

▶ Discuss the management of umbilical-cord prolapse.
▶ Describe maternal and fetal conditions associated with a higher incidence of breech presentation.
▶ Explain the risks of vaginal breech delivery.
▶ Discuss risks, benefits, and efficacy of techniques for resolving shoulder dystocia.

MALPRESENTATIONS

Mechanism of Normal Delivery

Most commonly, the fetus will traverse the pelvis in an occiput anterior (OA) position—head down, back toward the mother's abdomen, chin flexed to chest, presenting the smaller suboccipitobregmatic diameter (averaging 9.5 cm) to the pelvic passage. After the cervix is fully dilated, the fetus must rotate while negotiating a maze of bony maternal projections and stretching the musculature of the pelvic floor. Vertex delivery occurs through predictable alterations in fetal position:

Engagement: The widest part of the head enters the pelvic inlet, the first bony obstacle to be negotiated.

Descent: The head enters the pelvis in a transverse position to conform to the shape of the pelvic inlet.

Flexion: As the fetal head descends, it encounters resistance from the muscles of the pelvic floor, which increases flexion. Flexion allows the smallest diameter of the head to move through the pelvis. (If the head is not flexed, a wider portion of fetal skull must negotiate the pelvic passage.)

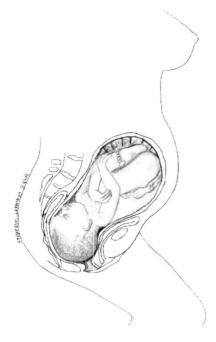

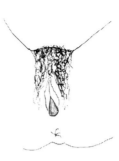

Figure 75. Internal rotation. The fetal head faces the maternal sacrum. The birth attendant may see gaping of the vagina and a dark hollow within.

Internal rotation: The midpelvis is widest from front to back, so the fetus rotates to face his mother's sacrum. Only the head makes this turn—the shoulders remain oblique (diagonally positioned).

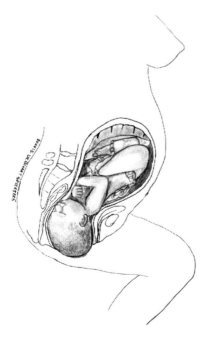

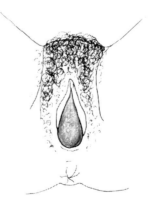

Figure 76. Extension. The fetal head reaches the pelvic floor and begins to extend. The birth attendant can glimpse the fetal scalp with each push, but it recedes between pushing efforts.

Extension: The back of the head reaches the pubic bone and pivots beneath it. Then the fetus extends his head to follow the curve of Carus. At this point, the birth attendant observes perineal bulging, crowning, and then the birth of the head, facing the mother's anus.

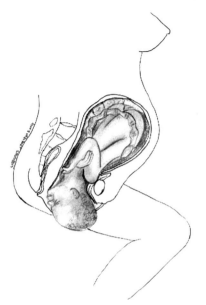

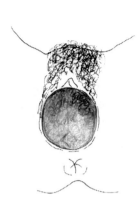

Figure 77. Full crowning. The vagina encircles the widest part of the fetal head. Birth is imminent.

Restitution: When the baby's head is born, it faces the anus while his shoulders remain positioned diagonally inside the pelvis. As soon as the head is free, the baby's neck turns to the right or the left to realign with the shoulders.

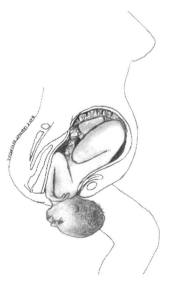

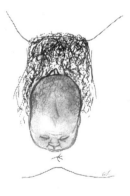

Figure 78. The head emerges.

External rotation: Now the head turns farther to the side as the shoulders rotate internally to the anteroposterior diameter.

Expulsion: The anterior shoulder slides under the pubic bone and is born by lateral flexion. The posterior shoulder is born next, and the body should follow quickly.

Presentation is defined by the fetal part that leads into the birth canal: face, brow, occiput (vertex), shoulder, or breech (frank, footling, double footling, complete). Approximately 96% of fetuses present vertex—head down with chin flexed to the chest. This posture efficiently introduces the smallest diameter of the baby's head to the pelvis, simplifying the birth process. Premature infants are more likely to adopt unusual birth positions, because they are small in relation to amniotic fluid volume and can easily change position.

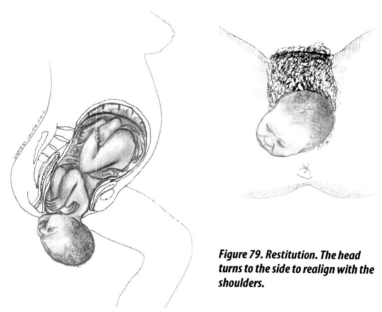

Figure 79. Restitution. The head turns to the side to realign with the shoulders.

The "Four P's"

Successful delivery involves interplay among the "four P's" of childbirth: the Passage, the Passenger, the Powers, and the Psyche.

Passage

The woman's birth passage comprises the bony pelvis and the overlying soft tissues. The female pelvis is designed for childbearing, and the unique internal dimensions determine whether a baby of a particular size and orientation will fit. The resistance of the cervix and pelvic-floor muscles can also affect the progress of labor, and maternal position can affect the ability of the pelvis to expand.

Passenger

The size and position of the fetus are crucial to the success of labor and delivery. Fetal position is a result not only of uterine shape and available space, but also of the mother's position and movements and the fetus's own activities. The fetus is not a passive passenger—fetal position is voluntary to some extent, and even a last-minute alteration like a tilted or deflexed head can obstruct progress. A stillborn infant, in contrast, is utterly passive and is more likely to deliver as a brow or face presentation because of his lack of tone and tactile responsiveness.

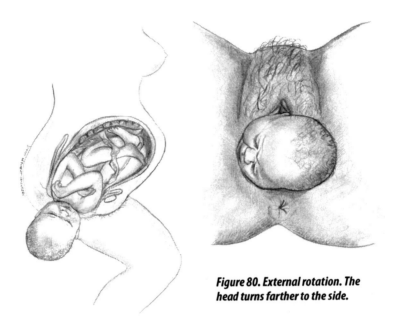

Figure 80. External rotation. The head turns farther to the side.

Powers

This refers to the power generated by uterine contractions. Strong, long, frequent, well-coordinated contractions hasten delivery. If the uterus does not contract hard enough or frequently enough, vaginal birth will not occur. Maternal position influences the powers of labor. Supine positioning decreases the strength of contractions but increases frequency; left lateral increases strength and decreases frequency. Ambulation can increase the intensity and frequency of contractions.

Psyche

The expectant mother's psychological state—self-concept, attitude, confidence, level of preparation, experience of pain, coping ability, and social support—can all affect the course of her labor and her reaction to circumstances.

Cephalic Malpresentations

For birth to occur, the fetus must pass through his mother's pelvis. The fetus finds the best fit in the intrauterine space by arranging his buttocks and flexed legs in the broad fundal cavity and his head in the narrower lower segment of the uterus. The fetus who presents head-down, but with head extended to some degree or tilted to the side instead of in alignment with the shoulders (asynclitism) faces a more difficult birth because he presents a wider diameter of his head to the pelvis. Abdominal palpation can be highly inaccurate in determining fetal head position; fetus head position is aligned neutrally with the spine only 48% of the time (Peregrine, O'Brien, & Jauniaux, 2007).

Face Presentation

Priority 2 or 3

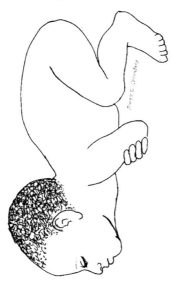

Figure 81. Face presentation. The face presentation is the most extreme example of deflexion.

The face presentation is the most extreme example of deflexion. The fetal neck is hyperextended, and the face from forehead to chin is first fetal part to enter the pelvis. More than half of fetuses that assume a face position have a deformity such as anencephaly, microcephaly, multiple nuchal cord loops, or tumors of the neck. Face presentation is also associated with macrosomia, contracted pelvis, and platypelloid pelvis. The multiparous woman may have a lax abdominal wall, which allows the fetal trunk to shift anterior and the neck to extend. Face presentation occurs in 1 of every 250–690 live births, somewhat more frequently in the case of fetal demise.

Many fetuses with face presentation begin labor in the brow position. While descending, pressure of contractions and resistance from the maternal pelvis causes the fetal head to either flex or extend. If it extension occurs, with engagement the increased pressure causes the fetal neck to hyperextend until the occiput touches the back. Internal rotation occurs between the level of the ischial spines and ischial tuberosities, so that the chin (mentum) is the actual presenting part. As the face descends onto the perineum, the fetal chin passes under the maternal symphysis pubis, the head is born by flexion and externally rotates, and the shoulders move into the usual position for delivery. The rest of the delivery proceeds as usual. The fetus may suddenly adopt a face presentation just before delivery, surprising the birth attendant by the crowning of the mouth, nose, and eyes.

The newborn born in face presentation may have facial swelling and bruising that interferes with his airway. This usually resolves within the first 24–48 hr of life. Difficulty in ventilation during resuscitation has been attributed to tracheal and laryngeal trauma and edema. Therefore, equipment and personnel to perform endotracheal intubation should be readily available at the time of delivery

A persistent face presentation can be identified by Leopold maneuvers. The cephalic prominence can be palpated on the same side as the fetal back with an indentation between them. Upon vaginal examination during labor, the mouth, nose, orbital ridges, and malar bones are palpable. Take the time to identify all presenting structures. Because the mouth may be mistaken for the anus, and the malar bones or orbital ridges may feel like fetal ischial tuberosities it is easy for even an experienced provider to misidentify the face presentation as a frank breech. The mouth and orbital ridges of the face presentation form a triangle, whereas the greater trochanters and anus form a straight line on the breech—and fetal genitalia may be palpable.

Most face presentations are mentum anterior position (60%). Less frequent are mentum transverse (15%) and mentum posterior (26%) (Julien & Galerneau, 2007). Many of these will spontaneously convert to mentum anterior for delivery. Severe variable and late decelerations are more common with face presentation during labor. Some authorities recommend internal monitoring by carefully placing the electrode on the fetal chin.

Cephalopelvic disproportion is more likely with a face presentation. Attempts at manual conversion of the mentum posterior face to a vertex or mentum anterior position can result in uterine rupture, cord prolapse, and fetal cervical spine trauma. If the face presentation is mentum anterior or transverse, labor may be allowed to progress with close monitoring. Cesarean delivery is necessary for 12–20% of fetuses with face presentation (Julien & Galerneau, 2007). The mentum posterior face presentation cannot deliver vaginally unless rotation occurs or the fetus is very small. Commonly, the baby will continue to hold the hyperextended posture for days after birth.

Brow Presentation

Priority 2 or 3

Brow presentation involves extension of the fetal head midway between full flexion (vertex) and hyperextension (face) in a cephalic longitudinal lie. The presenting part of the head is the brow area between the orbital ridge and the anterior fontanel. The frontal bones are the point of designation; when the sagittal suture is transverse and the anterior fontanel is on the right maternal side, the fetus would be in the right frontotransverse position (RFT).

Brow presentation is uncommon, and diagnosis is often made late in labor. When the abdomen is examined, a prominent occipital prominence is felt along the fetal back. The examiner can palpate the fetal orbital ridge, eyes, nose, frontal sutures, and anterior fontanel on vaginal examination, but not the mouth or chin. Most brow presentations are frontum anterior—frontum transverse and frontum posterior positions are more likely to necessitate cesarean delivery.

Spontaneous labor is usually allowed to progress. If internal rotation does not occur, the mentoparietal diameter (the largest diameter of the fetal head) presents at the pelvic inlet and must pass through it. Oftentimes, this is not physically possible, and the fetus may spontaneously convert to a face (30%) or vertex (20%) presentation (Julien & Galerneau, 2007). Delivery in brow position can be accomplished only if the pelvis is roomy, the infant is small, or the infant is a macerated stillborn. Persistent brow presentation with obstructed labor is an indication for cesarean section.

Compound Presentation

A compound presentation refers to the fetus with a combination of fetal parts presenting. One or more extremities may present with the vertex, face, or breech, or multiple small fetal parts will present simultaneously. The most common scenario is a hand or arm alongside the vertex. Compound presentations are associated with premature rupture of membranes, preterm labor, pelvic masses displacing the fetus, or with inductions with a high presenting part. Usually, a hand or arm prolapses, but sometimes a foot can present with the vertex, especially if premature.

A hand beside the head does not usually obstruct labor, but it may suffer circulatory compromise and become bruised and traumatized during the birth process. Many providers will move to cesarean delivery if a hand or arm has prolapsed beyond the presenting part or if labor is not progressing normally.

The fetus often spontaneously retracts the arm and may withdraw the hand if the fingers are pinched between contractions. Gentle pressure on the extremity may be used to replace it above the head. Excessive force applied to the extremity can cause injury, or may disengage the head and cause a cord prolapse.

A foot may be harder to retract, and its presence is more likely to obstruct labor. Compound presentation with breech birth is less common. Compound presentations can cause extensive maternal lacerations.

No intervention is necessary for the vertex fetus with an arm or hand presenting as long as labor progresses normally. A dysfunctional labor pattern may be followed by tetanic contractions leading to uterine rupture, and cesarean should be performed before this occurs.

Occiput Posterior

Priority 3 or 4

The most common fetal malpresentation is occipitoposterior position (OP), occurring in 10–20% of labors at onset (Ratcliffe, et al., 2008). The occiput posterior fetus lies with his occiput at the maternal sacrum and the fetal face toward maternal symphysis pubis, often in a deflexed attitude. The head is born by flexion first, then extension. The head externally rotates as the shoulders move into the usual anterior-posterior position.

Previously, OP fetuses were thought to enter labor in an unfavorable position and then fail to rotate. Recent research demonstrates that fetal position changes are common during labor, and the position at onset is not a strong predictor of position at delivery. Fewer than 10% of fetuses who are OP at labor onset remain OP at delivery, and two thirds of babies who are OP at delivery begin labor in a more favorable position and rotate to OP (Peregrine, et al., 2007). About 8% of neonates deliver in occiput posterior position, increasing the risk of 5-minute Apgar score less than 7, acidemia, meconium-stained amniotic fluid, birth trauma, and admission to the neonatal intensive care nursery (Ponkey, Cohen, Heffner, & Lieberman, 2003).

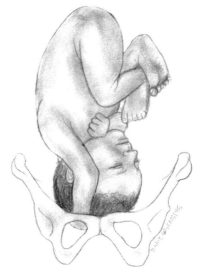

Figure 82. Compound presentation. The most common scenario for compound presentation is a hand or arm alongside the vertex.

The hospital-based research of Peregrine, O'Brien, and Jauniaux (2007) shows that occiput posterior presentation increases the risk of cesarean section due to failure to progress or relative cephalopelvic dysproportion (CPD), but one may speculate that the likelihood of spontaneous delivery would increase in the home or birth-center setting, aided by increased mobility and lack of interventions such as epidural anesthesia. Most vertex babies begin descent through the pelvis in occipitotransverse position. Resistance from the pelvic contours, cervix, and maternal musculature increases flexion and encourages rotation towards either an anterior or posterior presentation. A well-flexed fetus of average size propelled by adequate contractions will usually rotate to anterior on the pelvic floor. In other cases, the occiput anterior fetus may rotate to OP during labor.

A fetal occiput posterior position at delivery is more likely among women who are given epidural analgesia during labor, a situation which contributes to the higher rate of cesareans associated with epidurals. It was theorized that because women with occiput posterior fetuses have longer and more painful labors, they are more likely to request epidural analgesia. Research indicates that the fetus tends to move into the occiput posterior position *after* the epidural.

Occipitoposterior positioning creates a setting of relative cephalopelvic disproportion. The occiput drops into the hollow of the sacrum and deflexes the head, presenting a much larger "military" diameter to the pelvis. The head is less effective as a dilating wedge, which leads to slow progress and less effective contractions. At the end of the first stage, the anterior cervix tends to become compressed between the fetal head and the pubis, causing a persistent anterior lip or cervical edema.

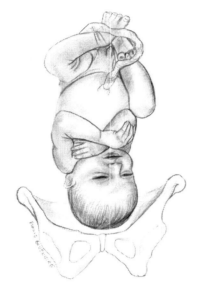

Figure 83. Occiput posterior. The occiput posterior fetus lies with his occiput at the maternal sacrum and the fetal face toward maternal symphysis pubis.

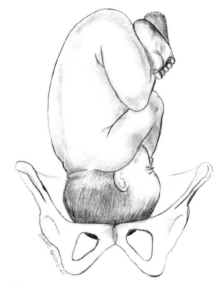

Figure 84. Occiput anterior. The occiput anterior fetus is in the optimal position to move efficiently through the pelvis.

Perineal and periurethral lacerations are more common as the large diameters of the deflexed head push through the tissues of the pelvic floor. The neonate born in the OP position is more likely to have a 5-min Apgar score less than 7, acidemia, meconium-stained fluid, birth trauma, and require admission to the NICU.

Occipitoposterior position is diagnosed by Leopold's maneuvers and observation of the abdominal shape (many small parts in front and central concavity to abdominal contour). Eighty-five percent of OP positions are right occiputoposterior (ROP), with the fetal small parts directed toward the left side of the maternal abdomen. Fetal heart tones are more easily auscultated towards the flank, usually the right. On cervical examination, the provider may observe asymmetric cervical dilation or persistent anterior lip. The fetal anterior fontanel may be prominent in the anterior pelvis. The woman complains of back pain as the contractions press the fetal skull against the sacrum. In the hospital or clinic, a transabdominal ultrasound scan may reveal eye sockets gazing up towards the maternal abdomen.

If the fetus is occiput posterior, the provider should take steps to encourage fetal rotation to anterior. In many cases, it is advantageous to leave the membranes intact as long as possible. Intact membranes give the fetus a pocket of slippery fluid in which to rotate, while rupture of membranes may wedge the fetus against the pelvic bones. Conversely, if contractions have been weak and irregular, rupture of membranes may produce stronger contractions that can facilitate rotation of the fetus.

Table 24. Technique for Rotating Occiput Posterior Fetus

After complete dilation:

Flex the fetal head

Place hand in posterior pelvis behind occiput

Wedge head into flexion

Rotate head during contraction while woman pushes

OP: Provider pronates dominant hand on examination

ROP: Provider pronates left hand clockwise

LOP: Provider pronates right hand counterclockwise

Maternal positions such as knee-chest, lunging, hands-and-knees, kneeling, squatting, pelvic rocking, side-lying or exaggerated Sims, or asymmetrical sitting have been utilized to correct persistent occipitoposterior or asynclitic fetal positions. The double hip squeeze involves applying pressure to the anterior iliac crests. Another strategy is the abdominal lift. The woman hugs her abdomen and lifts, allowing the long axis of the fetus to align with the pelvic inlet, relieving back pain, and possibly facilitating fetal rotation. Anecdotally, these methods seem to achieve fetal rotation to occiput anterior, but research has not yet confirmed the efficacy of these techniques.

Manual rotation is a technique that significantly increases the likelihood of spontaneous vaginal delivery. It is a clinical skill that requires training and practice. After full dilation, ensure the maternal bladder is empty. Place your hand palm-upward behind the fetal head, to serve as a wedge to cause the head to flex. With a contraction, the mother pushes while the fingers exert pressure to rotate the occiput to the anterior.

Another method of manual rotation is to grasp the head with the fingers over one ear and the thumb over the other, rotating with a contraction. The provider should first find the posterior fetal ear to confirm presentation. Sometimes the baby will spontaneously rotate after the ear is palpated.

Android and anthropoid pelvises encourage the fetus to rotate to the OP position, because the wider diameters of the fetal head fit more easily into the roomy posterior dimensions. OP is more common after 40 weeks, probably because the deflexed head of the OP baby applies less pressure to the cervix, causing a delay in the commencement of labor. Though many exercises and positional variations have been proposed to reduce the incidence of OP positioning, research has yet to validate the efficacy of any of them.

Noncephalic Malpresentations
Transverse Lie

Transverse lie occurs when the longitudinal axis of the fetus is perpendicular to the long axis of the uterus. The fetal spine may be oriented "back-up" or dorsosuperior, where fetal small parts present at the cervix, or "back-down" or dorsoinferior, where the fetal shoulder presents at the cervix. Transverse and oblique lies are unusual at term, occurring in about one in 300 deliveries (Bowes, 2008).

Most transverse lies are associated with premature delivery, multiple gestations, placenta previa, contracted pelvis, uterine anomalies or tumors, polyhydramnios, fetal anomalies, and grand multiparity. Transverse lie will sometimes present as a prolapsed arm or cord, which is a life-threatening situation for the fetus. Maternal and perinatal mortality/morbidity with this complication is high in developing countries with limited resources, usually secondary to uterine rupture.

Many authorities believe that gravity and fetal comfort are primary influences on fetal position. Noncephalic presentations are common early in pregnancy when the fetus has a large pool of fluid in which to maneuver. By later pregnancy, the fetal pole with the greatest mass—the buttocks with flexed thighs—seems more comfortably accommodated in the uterine fundus unless placenta previa, uterine abnormalities, or uterine distention change internal dimensions. A longitudinal lie aligns the body axis posture with the line of gravity and presents less restriction to fetal movement.

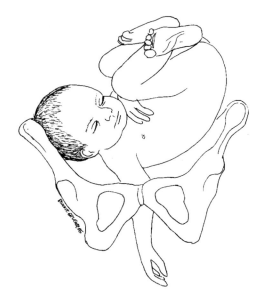

Figure 85. Transverse lie. Transverse lie will sometimes present as a prolapsed arm or cord, which is a life-threatening situation for the fetus.

Leopold's maneuvers will reveal the fetal head bulging at the maternal flank and the absence of a presenting part above the symphysis pubis. It can be more difficult to distinguish whether the fetal back is up or down. Fundal height may measure less than expected for gestational age. Because the fetus will sometimes assume this position if the placenta is across the cervix, do not perform a vaginal examination until placenta previa has been excluded. Ultrasound scan will clarify the exact fetal position and may reveal maternal and fetal anatomical deviations that may have precipitated the malpresentation.

If placenta previa is present, cesarean is necessary. If the fetus is pre-viable or has died, vaginal delivery may be possible due to a tendency for the macerated fetal body to collapse. Occasionally, the experienced obstetrician may perform an internal podalic version, a delicate procedure that carries a high risk of uterine rupture and fetal trauma.

The fetus in the transverse position may be turned to either a cephalic or breech presentation via external version under tocolysis, or delivered by cesarean section. After successful version many fetuses will spontaneously revert to transverse or breech.

If transverse lie is diagnosed before labor begins beyond 37 weeks' gestation, some providers will perform external version to cephalic presentation, then rupture the membranes and induce.

During the cesarean procedure, the dorsosuperior (back up) transverse lie may be delivered as a footling breech through a low transverse incision. The dorsoinferior (back down) position is harder for the obstetrician to grasp through transverse incision; vertical incision in the uterus is usually necessary.

AACT and ReACT

ALERT—Be alert ▶ Exercise hypervigilant attention
ANALYZE—Think about possible causes
CONSIDER—Use OLDCART ▶ Gather data
TREAT—Make first response ▶ Proceed to definitive care

ReACT | ReAssess ▶ ReConsider ▶ Re-Treat

✍ AACT—Alert and Analyze

Breech Presentation

Priority 1, 2, or 3

Breech presentation (buttocks or feet at the cervix) is the most common of the noncephalic malpresentations. Breech presentation is considered normal until late in gestation and only becomes a concern during labor and delivery. About 16% of fetuses are breech at 32 weeks, but the incidence of breech presentation at term is about 3–4% (Hofmeyr, 2007b).

Twenty-five percent of fetuses who are breech at 36 weeks will turn to cephalic presentation before delivery (Hofmeyr, 2007b).

Breech presentation may occur as a random incident, or may arise as a consequence of maternal, fetal, or placental conditions. Contributing factors involve conditions that alter the shape of either the uterus or the fetus: grand multiparity, polyhydramnios or oligohydramnios, placenta previa, uterine abnormalities or fibroid tumors, contracted maternal pelvis, multiple gestation, certain fetal anomalies (anencephaly, hydrocephaly, sacrococcygeal teratoma), neurological impairment, short umbilical cord, fetal death, or a fetus who becomes wedged in place with extended legs. Other risk factors include preterm delivery, nulliparity, and previous breech presentation.

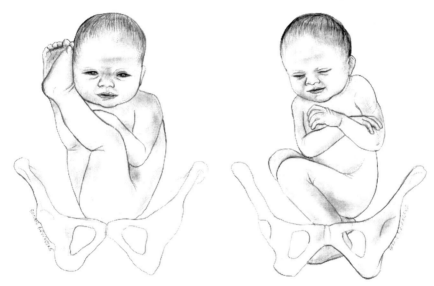

Figure 86. Frank breech.   **Figure 87. Footling breech.**

Frank Breech (50–70%)

The fetal buttocks enter the pelvis; hips are flexed, legs extended, and the feet by the baby's head. The extended legs make it difficult for the baby to somersault to vertex, and often he remains lodged in the frank breech position. Frank breech accounts for about half of all breech presentations and is most favorable for a vaginal delivery.

Complete Breech (5–10%)

With complete breech, the fetus is squatting or sitting cross-legged on the cervix.

Footling Breech (10–30%)

One or both hips and knees are extended and one or both feet are presenting. A variation of this is the kneeling breech.

Complications of Breech Presentation

Breech babies have more neurological deficits than non-breech babies, whether delivery occurs vaginally or by cesarean, suggesting that poor perinatal outcome may stem from the underlying causality that gave rise to the breech presentation as much as from injury during delivery. Perhaps the fetus that does not assume a cephalic presentation has failed to achieve its first developmental milestone.

Vertex delivery places the largest part of the baby first and allows the head to mold for hours, presenting the smallest possible diameter to the pelvis and conforming to its shape. In a breech delivery, the body is born first, followed by the larger shoulders, and then the largest and most solid part, the head, without the benefit of molding. If the head is unable to fit the pelvis, this fact may not become apparent until the body is born. The head of the preterm fetus is proportionately larger than that of a mature baby, and is more and is more likely to become entrapped if the body descends before the cervix is fully dilated.

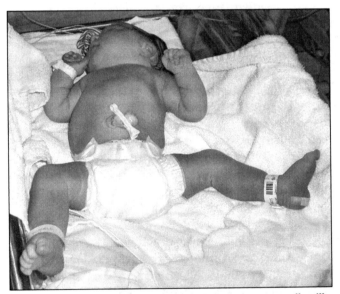

Figure 88. Babies who remain frank breech for months antenatally will maintain the position after birth. Developmental dysplasia of the hip occurs in 25% of breech babies.

Cord prolapse is a significant risk with breech presentation. In an engaged cephalic presentation, the fetal head effectively corks the cervix. With breech presentation, the irregular shape of the presenting part or parts creates gaps where the cord might fall through. This poor fit also means that severe hypoxia from cord compression is less likely to occur than in other cases of cord prolapse. Overall likelihood of cord prolapse is influenced by whether the fetus is frank breech (0–2%), complete breech

(5–10%), or footling breech (10–25%) (Belogolovkin, Bush, & Eddleman, 2008). Breech-associated cord prolapse is more likely with multiparas (6%) than with primigravidas (3%) (Belogolovkin, et al.).

The child may suffer birth trauma, especially if the birth attendant tugs on the body in an effort to free the baby. Sometimes the partially empty uterus will contract and release the placenta, causing hemorrhage and cutting off the baby's oxygen supply before it is completely born. When the fetal head is hyperextended before labor, vaginal breech delivery can cause serious cervical spinal cord lesions in up to 21% of cases (Gabbe, et al., 2007).

Mode of Delivery

The management of breech presentation in term pregnancy is highly controversial. Providers often choose the mode of delivery based on personal experience, local standard of care, or fear of litigation. Vaginal breech deliveries carry a risk of perinatal death 3–5 times that of cephalic deliveries—but these statistics include breech deaths due to anomalies or prematurity, and so the figures are misleading. The Farm Midwifery Center boasts safety statistics drastically above the national average, and those statistics include breech and twin deliveries (Gaskin, n.d.). Cesarean delivery for breech presentation, which might benefit the infant, has been shown to increase both short- and long-term maternal morbidity, and often necessitates future cesareans.

Hannah, et al. (2000), upended the obstetrical community with a term breech trial suggesting that planned cesarean results in superior neonatal outcomes for the breech fetus. This large, multicenter randomized clinical trial involved 2,088 term fetuses in frank or complete breech presentations at 121 institutions in 26 countries. The study concluded cesarean delivery for term breech presentation significantly decreases perinatal/neonatal mortality and neonatal morbidity, possibly decreases long-term morbidity and slightly increases maternal morbidity.

This study has design flaws that bring clinical relevance into question. Investigators failed to eliminate cases where adverse outcomes were unrelated to birth route, and defined serious neonatal morbidity imprecisely. Complications and contraindications such as twin pregnancy, antepartum fetal demise, footling breech and hyperextended neck were included in the study. Inexperienced practitioners delivered a significant number of the babies with poor outcomes. When the corrected numbers are compared, the difference between groups appears no longer significant.

A follow-up study by the authors of the term breech trial involving children who were part of the initial study found no differences between planned cesarean delivery and planned vaginal breech delivery in infant death rates or neurodevelopmental delay by age 2 years (Hannah, et al., 2004). Subsequent research has demonstrated that with experienced providers, careful client selection, and appropriate intrapartum management protocols, vaginal breech delivery can be as safe for the infant as spontaneous cephalic birth.

Based on the term breech trial, ACOG published a Committee Opinion in 2001 stating that "planned vaginal delivery of a singleton term breech may no longer be appropriate" unless the woman presents in advanced labor or the breech in question is a second twin. Before this recommendation was made, about 50% of women with breech fetuses were candidates for vaginal delivery (Fischer, 2006). Of these candidates, 60–82% had successful vaginal deliveries (Fischer). The World Health Organization recommends vaginal birth if the fetus is frank breech with a flexed head, the maternal pelvis is adequate for fetal size, and the woman has not undergone prior cesarean section for cephalopelvic disproportion, but maintains that *every breech delivery should ideally occur in a hospital with surgical capability.* The obstetrical community remains polarized on this issue.

The ideal candidate for vaginal breech delivery is at least 36 weeks' gestation and has a normal labor pattern and no contraindications to vaginal birth. Estimated fetal weight should be about 2,000–4,000 g, the head must be flexed, and the fetus should have no anomalies that may obstruct delivery (Hofmeyr, 2007). The birth attendant should be skilled in breech delivery, and emergency cesarean should be readily available if necessary.

Frank or complete breech presentations are more favorable for vaginal delivery; if the body and thighs come easily, cephalopelvic disproportion is unlikely to occur. Footling or kneeling presentations are riskier, because an increasingly larger circumference must pass sequentially through the pelvis, potentially risking entrapment of the aftercoming head.

Version

Exercises may encourage the breech fetus to turn, although studies disagree on the efficacy of this intervention. Instruct the woman to assume a knee-chest position for 20 min three times a day, at times when the fetus is usually active (Ratcliffe, et al., 2008). This posture tends to move the baby out of the pelvis, providing there is more room to turn. Hypnosis and moxibustion have been validated by studies as effective methods of turning breech fetuses.

External cephalic version (ECV) is the transabdominal manual rotation of the fetus into a cephalic presentation. It was popular in the 1960s, but fell out of favor when fetuses reportedly died after the procedure. Today, version is back in vogue, and it is about 58% successful in converting a fetus to a cephalic presentation (Ailsworth, et al., 2006).

Complications resulting from ECV are unusual, but may include fractured fetal bones, rupture of membranes, placental abruption, fetomaternal hemorrhage (0–5%), and cord entanglement (Fischer, 2006). Transient bradycardia may occur in as many as 40% of versions, presumably a vagal response to head compression that does not increase risk to the fetus (Fischer). Women with active labor, uterine scarring, polyhydramnios, oligohydramnios, fetal growth restriction, uterine malformation, or fetal anomaly are not good candidates for ECV.

ECV is typically offered only to women with no contraindications who have reassuring nonstress tests before and after ECV. Rh immune globulin is given to Rh-negative women to prevent isoimmunization. Version is typically performed in or near a delivery suite in case of fetal compromise. Some providers induce labor following version, because some babies will revert to breech, but labor is more likely to be successful if the provider waits for spontaneous labor with an engaged head. If ECV is unsuccessful, the client may be sent home in hopes of spontaneous version, or the provider may proceed with a cesarean. The rate of cesarean delivery ranges from 0–31% after successful ECV (Fischer, 2006).

✎ AACT—Analyze

Assessing the Breech

Even experienced providers miss breech presentations on occasion. On vaginal examination, the solid sacrum of a frank breech can feel like a skull, and in early labor a high station may confuse diagnosis. An edematous face presentation feels similar to the breech on cervical examination until the provider carefully assesses landmarks—the greater trochanters and anus form a straight line, whereas the malar bones and mouth form a triangle. With the breech, fetal genitalia may be palpable, and meconium may be present on the examiner's finger. If a limb is felt alongside the presenting part, determine whether it is a foot or a hand. Sometimes ultrasound confirmation is necessary.

Assessment of fetal lie and presentation is part of a routine prenatal examination toward the end of pregnancy. With Leopold's maneuvers, a breech in the lower uterine segment is not as rigid as a fetal skull, and the groove that divides head from shoulders is absent. A fetal head can be balloted (bounced between the examiner's thumb and fingers) in the fundus. Ballottement of the breech moves the baby's body and is accompanied by more resistance. Breech presentation often causes maternal rib pain and lower abdominal cramping from the fetal feet kicking the bladder.

If the lie is unstable near term or the provider is uncertain about presentation after 34–36 weeks, the client should be referred for ultrasound examination.

✎ AACT—Treat

Managing the Breech Delivery

It is impossible to know whether a breech delivery will proceed easily or become obstructed. In breech labor the bitrochanteric diameter (about 9.25 cm) enters the pelvis in the transverse orientation, rotating in midpelvis and arriving at the pelvic outlet in the anterior-posterior position. After the buttocks deliver, the body rotates, usually with the back anterior, and the shoulders descend in the same way. The anterior shoulder delivers as the flexed head enters the pelvis in the transverse diameter. The baby rotates internally so that the chin appears at the perineum, then the face, followed by the rest of the head, which delivers by flexion.

Adequate descent is determined if the breech is at the level of the ischial spines when the cervix is 6 cm dilated, and reaches the pelvic floor at full dilatation. If the breech does not descend further with pushing efforts, cesarean delivery is usually necessary. Nulliparas usually deliver within 1 hr of active pushing, multiparas in about half the time.

Assist the woman to an upright, supported squat, or semi-Fowler's at the edge of a bed. The woman may have a strong urge to push, but it is crucial that she refrain from pushing until she is fully dilated. Even when fully dilated, passive descent of the fetus or open glottis pushing may be safer than vigorous Valsalva pushing until the breech is on the perineum. Episiotomy, if required, is not performed until the fetal anus has appeared at the introitus.

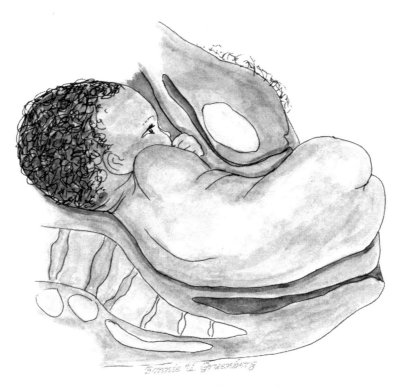

Figure 89. Breech delivery. A hands-off approach encourages the fetus to maintain a position of flexion during birth, simplifying delivery.

A hands-off approach encourages the fetus to maintain a position of flexion during the birth, simplifying delivery. The sensation of being grasped can startle the emerging baby, causing his hands and arms to extend in a Moro "startle" reflex and potentially causing shoulder dystocia. This can extend the neck and present larger diameters of the head to the pelvis or even wedge an arm up alongside the head. Allow the breech to hang and keep your hands off the baby. Interference can cause serious injury to the infant, including organ damage and limb fractures. Breech extraction is associated with a birth injury rate of 25% and a mortality rate of approximately 10%, and should only be performed by obstetricians in the management of breech second twin (Fischer, 2006).

The frank breech usually delivers with one hip toward the pubic bone and the other toward the mother's sacrum, his back to either the right or left. First the anterior hip delivers, then the posterior hip with lateral flexion, the body emerging to the umbilicus. Encourage the mother to push with contractions. External rotation should occur until the baby's back faces up, and you should gently guide the infant to a back-up position if he does not naturally achieve that on his own. There is no evidence that pulling a loop of cord down to create slack is of any benefit, and in fact may cause spasm of the cord vessels (Howell, et al., 2007).

This is the crucial point of the delivery. At this stage, the head has entered the pelvis, and the cord is probably compressed between the pelvic bones and the baby's head. To reduce the risk of anoxia, the head should be born within 4 minutes.

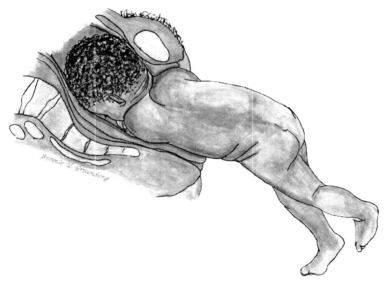

Figure 90. Dorsum anterior. The baby should spontaneously achieve a back-up position. If not, encourage his back to rotate anteriorly.

Eventually, the feet should spring free as the body descends. When the legs are extended, the attendant may need to flex each knee individually (Pinard maneuver), pushing it to the side of the baby so that the foot can be delivered. The birth attendant may wrap the emerging infant in a warm towel or blanket. Cool air may cause hypothermia, and can stimulate breathing efforts with the head still unborn.

If the arms are extended, slide a finger along the baby's scapula over the shoulder and into the antecubital fossa to deliver the elbow between the body and the side of the vagina.

If the arms are behind the fetal neck, the midwife may place both hands on the bony fetal pelvis, with thumbs on the sacroiliac regions and fingers on the iliac crests (Lovset's maneuver). Apply *gentle* downward traction while lifting the body slightly towards the symphysis. Rotate the baby gently through 180 degrees, bringing the posterior arm under the symphysis, and flex the elbow with your fingers to deliver the arm. Without changing your grip, rotate the baby back through 180 degrees and repeat for the opposite arm (Howell, et al., 2007). You are relieving an obstruction, not pulling the baby out.

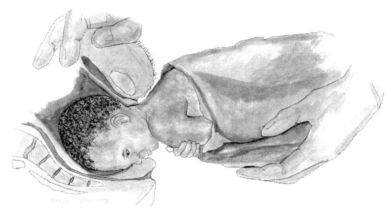

Figure 91. The birth attendant may wrap the emerging infant in a warm towel or blanket.

With maternal pushing, the shoulders present in (or are turned to) the anterior-posterior plane and emerge sequentially.

Table 25. Delivering the Footling Breech

If you are faced with the need to deliver a footling breech, ensure the woman's bladder is empty.

Do not pull on the feet

If fetal heart rate is stable and there is no evidence of cord prolapse, use expectant management to allow the cervix to completely dilate around the breech.

Proceed as with delivery of frank breech

Consider increased risk of cord prolapse (17%) and head entrapment, especially if preterm.

(Fischer, 2006)

For the head to appear, the occiput must be low enough in the pelvis to hinge around the back of the symphysis. Support the body at this point—allowing the baby to hang may cause the head to extend rather than flex (Howell, et al., 2007). Allow the head to descend through the pelvis.

When the hairline appears, gently lift the fetal body upwards. Hyperextension of the neck or excessive pressure on the cervical spine will occlude the vertebral arteries and can lead to necrosis of the cervical cord. An assistant can apply pressure directly behind the maternal pubic bone (not fundal pressure) to keep the fetal head flexed and aid delivery. In most cases, the head will spontaneously deliver.

Typically, the fetal chin is posterior. The Mauriceau-Smellie-Veit maneuver is performed by draping the baby's body over one arm and placing a finger on each side of the baby's nose, on the fetal maxilla. Place one or two fingers of your other hand on the fetal occiput. Flex the head with pressure from both hands. Avoid compressing the neck or inserting fingers in the mouth.

The midwife may insert two fingers and check for an anterior lip of cervix, which sometimes descends with the occiput and can obstruct delivery. Reducing the cervix also encourages the fetal head to flex optimally.

Breech Delivery? Remember "BHIND":
BRING the woman into position that facilitates pelvic expansion.
HANDS OFF until delivered past the umbilicus, then gently ensure that the back rotates to anterior.
INSERT fingers to splint humerus and sweep the forearm across the chest and out.
NESTLE emerging body in blanket and support baby's weight as it emerges.
DELIVER after-coming head by elevating baby and applying suprapubic pressure.

If the head does not deliver, rapid transport is critical. Immediately insert your hand into the vagina and make an airway for the baby by keeping the maternal tissue away from his face. Thread oxygen tubing into the space you have created and supply blowby oxygen at a rate of 6–8 L/min. If the umbilical cord is still pulsing, keep it warm and moist and avoid handling it. If the circulation between mother and fetus remains intact, the child has a vastly improved chance for survival. Ensure the fetal body remains wrapped in dry, warm towels or blankets to preserve heat. Establish IV access in the mother with a large bore catheter and a crystalloid solution, and put her on high-flow oxygen. Have the mother continue to push hard with contractions, while you lift the fetal body parallel to the floor and have an assistant apply suprapubic pressure.

Nuchal Arms

When a baby delivers breech, one or both arms may be wrapped around the back of the neck. One of four of these babies will suffer brachial plexus injuries or other trauma. Nuchal arms are managed by gently rotating the baby to reduce the tension so that first one then the other shoulder delivers under the symphysis pubis, always keeping the back upwards. Hold the baby by the thighs and wrap him in a towel for traction.

Head Entrapment

Head entrapment can be lethal for the baby. The head of the vertex baby molds over time, gradually decreasing circumference for a better fit. The head of the breech fetus has no opportunity to mold, and must negotiate the pelvis with its original diameters. Fetal head entrapment is most likely if the fetus is earlier than 32 weeks' gestation, due to the proportionately larger head. An incompletely dilated cervix can also trap the head and prevent delivery.

Table 26. OOH Management of Undiagnosed Breech

Call EMS and initiate transfer protocol

Explain the situation to the client and her family

Empty the bladder with a catheter

Assist the woman into a position that allows the breech to dangle

When the presenting part is seen at the vaginal opening, encourage strong pushing

Allow the baby to deliver unassisted—hands off the breech

After baby delivers to umbilicus, ensure that delivery occurs within 4 minutes of this point

Assist delivery of the legs if necessary

If there is progress, keep hands off

Wrap the baby's emerging body in a towel and gently provide support

Assist birth of the arms as necessary

Encourage the back to rotate anteriorly

When the baby's hairline is seen, position his body on your forearm and place fingers on the fetal maxilla

Place your opposite hand over the baby's back with two fingers over his shoulders and middle finger pressing on the occiput

Lift the baby to the horizontal plane to deliver the face with flexion from your fingers

Prepare for postpartum hemorrhage and neonatal resuscitation

Piper or Wrigley's forceps are used by obstetricians and can effectively achieve delivery of the head. Dührssen incisions are sometimes made at the 2 o'clock or 10-o'clock position to facilitate delivery of a fetal head trapped by an incompletely dilated cervix. Extension into the lower uterine segment can occur and cause severe bleeding. The Zavanelli maneuver can be used to replace the fetus into the uterus to be delivered by cesarean, but this technique carries a high risk of uterine rupture and fetal injury or death (Hofmeyr, 2007a). In low resource settings, symphysiotomy is sometimes performed.

Head entrapment can even occur during cesarean delivery, especially with preterm breeches, and low transverse uterine incision. Many physicians opt for vertical uterine incisions for preterm breeches prior to 32 weeks' gestation to avoid head entrapment and subsequent neonatal trauma.

Be on guard for maternal hemorrhage. After the fetal body delivers, the uterus might clamp down and attempt to expel the placenta. With the head and placenta still retained in the mother's body, the uterus might not be able to control its own bleeding, and hemorrhage may ensue. If she begins to bleed heavily, IV fluid bolus is indicated, along with the high-flow oxygen and rapid transport that should already be underway.

Vaginal breech delivery has declined in recent years, but still occurs in the case of mother's preference for vaginal birth, precipitate delivery, out-of-hospital delivery, severe fetal anomaly or stillbirth. The optimal way to gain expertise in breech deliver is hands-on clinical experience. Educational tools such as videos and mannequins are also helpful.

Umbilical Cord Prolapse

Priority 1

✍ AACT—Alert and Analyze

Umbilical cord prolapse occurs when the cord slips down alongside or ahead of the fetal presenting part. This is most likely to occur when the fetal presenting part is unengaged, or with multiple gestation, with preterm premature rupture of membranes, polyhydramnios, or fetal presentation other than vertex. If the cord becomes compressed or if the cord vessels begin to spasm, the fetus becomes hypoxic or anoxic.

Overt prolapse is the descent of the cord in advance of the fetal presenting part, usually through the cervix and into or through the vagina. The amniotic membranes are ruptured and the cord can be seen or felt on examination. Occult prolapse occurs when the cord slips down alongside, but not beyond, the presenting part. Membranes may or may not be ruptured.

✍ AACT—Consider and Treat

Cord prolapse often causes a sudden, protracted fetal heart-rate deceleration or moderate to severe variable decelerations after a previously normal tracing. Other conditions that present similarly include maternal hypotension, placental abruption, uterine rupture, and vasa previa. The cord may be palpable on vaginal examination or felt by the client if the prolapse is overt, but occult prolapse may not be diagnosed until a cesarean delivery is performed, if at all. Prolapse can occur at any cervical dilation from minimal to complete, but is most common at 5–6 cm and –1 to –2 station.

Vaginal delivery is seldom possible, except in the case of a fully dilated multiparous client that can be delivered within 4 minutes of cord prolapse. To manage cord prolapse, the first step is to place the mother in a knee-chest position immediately or lay her on her back with several pillows elevating her hips. Knee-chest is probably better for sustaining a good fetal heart rate, but may be hard to maintain in a moving ambulance. Immediately don sterile gloves and insert your entire hand into the woman's vagina. Find the presenting part of the fetus and push it upward, off the cord.

Have someone call EMS, and if possible inform the obstetrical unit at the receiving hospital that a cord prolapse is en route and will need immediate cesarean delivery. The cervix might be only partially dilated, so displacing the fetal presenting part is not always easy to manage. Uterine contractions force the baby toward you at regular intervals, but your task is to hold the fetus back and prevent compression of the cord.

Once your hand is in the vagina, it will remain there until the baby is delivered by cesarean section at the hospital. You will probably remain under the drapes between her legs during the surgery until the baby is delivered.

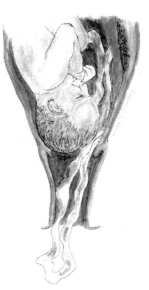

Figure 92. Cord prolapse.
Overt prolapse occurs when the cord drops down ahead of the presenting part, into or through the vagina.

Another technique is to insert a Foley catheter and rapidly fill the maternal bladder with 500–700 ml of normal saline with the client in steep Trendelenberg. The distended bladder raises the presenting part and alleviates cord compression. Tocolytic therapy with ritodrine or terbutaline increases the efficacy of this technique and has not been associated with postpartum hemorrhage.

Table 27. OOH Management of Cord Prolapse

(Order of steps may vary)

Call EMS and initiate transfer protocol

Explain the situation to the client and her family

Place woman into knee-chest or Trendelenberg

Elevate the fetal head using manual pressure, bladder distention, or both

Wrap cord loosely in warm saline compresses if it protrudes from vagina

Avoid handing or moving the cord

Supply high-flow oxygen

Continuously monitor fetal heart rate

If fetal heart rate is not reassuring, try changing maternal position *without* discontinuing head displacement

Obtain intravenous access with blood draw and bolus 1000 cc of lactated Ringer's or normal saline

Consider vaginal delivery only if the client is multiparous, complete, and pushing and delivery can be accomplished in less than 4 minutes

If the baby delivers, prepare for resuscitation and postpartum hemorrhage

A pulsing cord is reassuring if you feel it against your hand, but do not compress the cord to check the pulse. Cold can cause the cord vessels to spasm. If part of the cord protrudes outside of the vagina, keep it moist and warm with saline and plastic wrap.

Immediate transport is crucial. The woman should be placed on high-flow oxygen by mask, and IV access should be achieved, but ideally this should all be accomplished *en route*. The fetus might only have minutes of adequate blood supply remaining, and his best chance for survival lies in immediate rapid transport and immediate cesarean section upon arrival at the hospital.

The longer the interval between cord prolapse and delivery, the greater the risk of anoxia, but other factors come into play such as the degree of cord compression. One of the largest studies to date demonstrated that if cesarean delivery takes place within 30 min of diagnosis, neonatal outcomes are usually good.

SHOULDER DYSTOCIA

Priority 2 (1 If not resolved by McRobert's maneuver and initial fetal repositioning)

✍ AACT—Alert and Analyze

Shoulder dystocia is most accurately defined as failure of the shoulders to spontaneously negotiate the pelvis after delivery of the fetal head, requiring additional obstetric maneuvers beyond gentle downward traction to achieve delivery (ACOG, 2002). The provider must extricate the fetus rapidly to minimize damage to mother and baby.

Although most cases of shoulder dystocia resolve without injury, the condition carries a fairly high incidence of postpartum hemorrhage and injuries to the infant such as hypoxic brain injury, clavicular and humeral fracture, nerve damage, and death—even with appropriate management. This complication can occur without warning, so the attendant must anticipate and recognize the problem, and then rapidly extricate the baby using a systematic series of maneuvers.

Normally, the fetal biacromial diameter (the measurement between the most distal portions of the fetal shoulders) enters the pelvis obliquely, leading with the posterior shoulder. The pelvis is narrower front to back than in the oblique dimension, and the fetus gravitates towards the roomier dimension. The fetus rotates to the anterior-posterior position at the pelvic outlet when the head externally rotates, allowing the anterior shoulder to slide beneath the symphysis pubis and deliver. If the shoulders enter the pelvis in an anteroposterior orientation rather than obliquely, or come through the pelvic inlet simultaneously rather than sequentially, the anterior shoulder can lodge behind the symphysis pubis. The posterior shoulder can also become wedged on the sacral promontory.

If the baby's head continues to descend, the brachial plexus nerves, which supply motor function to the arm, may stretch or tear, sustaining irreversible damage. (The birth attendant can also cause brachial plexus injury by pulling or twisting the head, by lateral traction, or by applying pressure to the baby's anterior axilla.) Infants who survive are at risk for asphyxia, fractures of the clavicle or humerus, and brachial plexus nerve damage. It is often difficult to determine whether shoulder dystocia-related injuries originate as a prenatal insult, trauma from the impaction of the shoulder through the natural process of labor, acidemia from cord compression or other intrauterine events, or from the provider's attempts at extrication.

Some authorities have attempted to standardize the designation of shoulder dystocia by measuring a "normal" time from delivery of the head until delivery of the body, but this definition is problematic. Some argue that the head normally delivers with one contraction and the shoulders with the next. Medical texts advocate delivering the shoulders immediately after the birth of the head.

Fetal macrosomia (weight over 4,500 g) is a major risk factor for shoulder dystocia. Shoulder dystocia occurs with less than 1% of deliveries involving fetuses weighing less than 4,000 g, and 5–7% of deliveries with fetuses weighing more than 4,000 g (Rodis, 2007a). Infants born to mothers with diabetes are two to six times more likely to suffer shoulder dystocia, not only because diabetes is associated with macrosomia, but also because these fetuses have proportionately wider shoulders. Male infants are more likely to suffer shoulder dystocia, presumably because they are at greater risk for macrosomia.

Identification of a truly macrosomic fetus can be difficult. Sonography is only 22–69% accurate in identifying fetuses over 4,500 g, about as accurate as Leopold's maneuvers. Macrosomia tends to recur in subsequent pregnancies, as does shoulder dystocia, which carries a recurrence risk of about 14% (Rodis, 2007a). The risk of birth trauma increases with subsequent shoulder dystocias.

Risk increases with greater maternal weight gain, labor abnormalities such as precipitous delivery or prolonged second stage, fetal congenital anomalies and tumors, fetus heavier than previous fetuses, postdate pregnancies, maternal pelvic deformities, and short maternal stature. Women with epidural anesthesia may experience impaired rotation due to relaxed muscle tone and inability to push effectively. A combination of risk factors may be more meaningful—one small study showed that in women with macrosomic infants and a history of shoulder dystocia, the recurrence rate was above 50% (Rodis, 2007a).

The provider creates some shoulder dystocias. When vacuum or forceps are applied, the shoulders often abduct to a wider diameter that is more likely to impact. One study showed that the combination of macrosomia, prolonged second stage, and mid-pelvic operative delivery resulted in a 21% incidence of shoulder dystocia (Rodis, 2007a). There is also a relationship between oxytocin augmentation and shoulder dystocia.

Shoulder dystocia can be prevented by cesarean delivery, but physicians would have to perform 3,695 prophylactic cesareans to prevent just one brachial plexus injury among nondiabetic clients with fetal macrosomia (Rodis,

2007a). One study of 110 infants with birth weights over 5,750 g (12.5 lb) showed that 60% emerged without shoulder dystocia (Rodis, 2007a). Cesarean delivery harms the mother's future reproductive capabilities, and the pain of recovering from major surgery complicates the postpartum period. Inducing early to avoid macrosomia results in an increased cesarean rate and does not improve outcomes.

Most authorities discourage routine prophylactic cesarean delivery or induction of labor for suspected macrosomia unless the client is otherwise at very high risk of shoulder dystocia. Elective cesarean delivery is recommended for the woman with a history of prior shoulder dystocia with a brachial plexus injury.

There are several physical clues that shoulder dystocia is developing. Whereas babies often birth quickly after being born to the eyebrows, the baby with shoulder dystocia is often very slow to emerge from brows to neck. The birth attendant may have to press back the perineum to aid the birth of the face. The head then retracts tightly against the perineum—"turtle sign." Whereas most babies spontaneously restitute to the right or left, the baby with shoulder dystocia usually remains with the face oriented posteriorly, looking toward the mother's anus. The head begins to darken as it congests with blood secondary to impaired venous return, a condition that can result in brain hemorrhage.

Often the umbilical cord is compressed, and the fetus rapidly becomes hypoxic. If the baby has been well oxygenated before the shoulder impacts, it will take about 7 minutes of cord compression for the fetal pH to decline from the normal 7.25 to the damaging 6.97 (Rodis, 2007b). If the fetus suffers cord compression or other compromise *before* the shoulder impacts, the brain's maximal damage-free interval shortens accordingly.

✎ AACT—Consider and Treat

Shoulder dystocia cannot be resolved by traction on the baby. Attempts to pull or pry the baby out, twisting the head, or pressing on the fundus can stretch and injure the brachial plexus, rupture the uterus, or worsen the obstruction. Extrication maneuvers attempt to dislodge the anterior shoulder from behind the symphysis pubis by changing the orientation of the fetus or maternal pelvis. These interventions should be attempted with a sense of urgency. After about 7 min of entrapment, the infant risks brain damage, so all interventions should be tried in rapid sequence and immediate transport initiated if they fail.

First, stay calm and remember that most shoulder dystocias resolve with maternal position changes and strong pushing if the birth attendant is prepared and moves quickly. Get assistance. Enlist as many hands as possible—your birth assistant, the father of the baby, the birth photographer—to help with maneuvers. Anticipate the need for neonatal resuscitation and the likelihood of postpartum hemorrhage, and call for backup as needed.

Position the woman with buttocks at the edge of the bed to provide optimal access for maneuvers to effect delivery. If her bladder has not been recently emptied, drain it with a catheter. Many experts advocate a large episiotomy; but shoulder dystocia is a bony obstruction and not affected by soft tissue, so by itself episiotomy does not help to free the baby (Rodis, 2007b). In some cases episiotomy is needed so the birth attendant can insert her hands deeply enough to maneuver the fetus. Episiotomy in this situation also risks extension into a 3rd- or 4th-degree laceration.

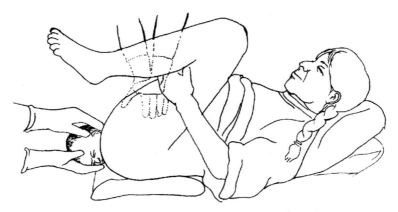

Figure 93. McRobert's maneuver with suprapubic pressure. McRobert's maneuver by itself can resolve almost half of all shoulder dystocias.

Shoulder dystocia management is best practiced in a progression from simple to complex, less invasive to more invasive. You will learn these steps in a linear fashion, but in the context of an actual emergency situation, you should vary application as the circumstances demand. Because no single maneuver has been shown to be more effective than any other, it is acceptable to rearrange the steps in your own practice as indicated. The goal of management is to free the baby without asphyxia or permanent Erb's palsy without causing undue injury to the infant.

McRobert's Maneuver

McRobert's maneuver is a technique to expand pelvic diameters by flexing the maternal thighs onto the abdomen, which mimics a deep squatting position. McRobert's maneuver works better if there are two assistants helping the woman to get her legs back, and if the woman herself grasps the underside of her thighs and retracts her legs. This posture causes ventral rotation of the symphysis pubis, brings the pelvic inlet into alignment with the maximum expulsive force, increases pushing efficiency, flattens the sacral promontory, straightens the lumbosacral lordosis, and increases the available space in the posterior pelvis. McRobert's also increases intrauterine pressure, amplitude of uterine contractions, and expulsive force. McRobert's maneuver by itself can resolve almost half of all shoulder dystocias. A word of caution: although the activity must be focused on extricating the baby, overzealous application of McRobert's can occasionally cause injury to the mother, including symphyseal separation, sacroiliac joint dislocation, and transient dysfunction of the femoral nerve.

Suprapubic Pressure

An assistant to the midwife (preferably the strongest person available) should then stand on the side of the fetal back and apply moderately deep lateral suprapubic pressure with a fist and with locked elbows. This maneuver adducts the fetal shoulder toward the fetal chest or shifts it into an oblique orientation, to help it to move beneath the symphysis. Pressure should be applied into the soft tissue above the pubic bone, not over the bone itself. Sometimes you will have more success if you apply suprapubic pressure first, and then bring the woman into McRobert's position while the pressure is applied. Fundal pressure is always contraindicated because it may rupture the uterus or worsen the impaction.

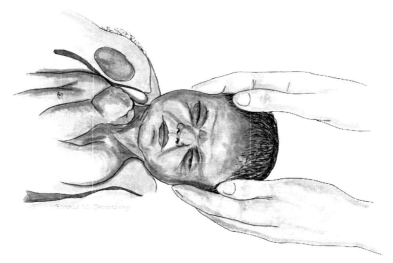

Figure 94. Guiding the head. Gently guide the head downwards with the goal of helping the posterior shoulder to slip into the hollow of the sacrum.

Reattempt Delivery

With the woman in McRobert's position, and the assistant applying suprapubic pressure, the midwife should grasp the fetal head between two hands and ask the mother for her strongest pushing effort. Gently guide the head downwards, toward the mother's anus, with the goal of helping the posterior shoulder to slip into the hollow of the sacrum, making room for the anterior shoulder to move beneath the pubis. Only careful, gentle, symmetric pressure should be used—the mother's expulsive efforts are the force that delivers the baby. Meanwhile, maintain McRobert's position with suprapubic pressure.

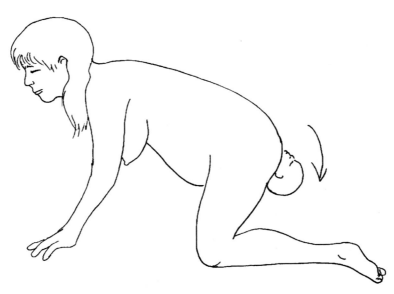

Figure 95. Gaskin's maneuver. Gaskin's maneuver may be the most appropriate choice for initial management, and may be chosen in preference to the McRobert's maneuver as the first intervention.

In most cases, this combination will free the fetus. Outward traction or excessive pressure can cause permanent damage to the infant.

Gaskin's Maneuver

Ina May Gaskin, CPM, introduced the Gaskin Maneuver to mainstream medicine. To perform the Gaskin maneuver, turn the mother to hands and knees—NOT knee-chest. The act of changing position to hands and knees and the effects of gravity are often enough to bring the anterior shoulder forward and make room for the posterior shoulder (now uppermost) to move through the hollow of the sacrum and deliver first. The midwife should apply gentle downward traction to deliver the uppermost, posterior shoulder first, then upward traction on the anterior shoulder (which rests against the symphysis pubis). Although medical texts often list this maneuver near the bottom of possible interventions for shoulder dystocia, for the mobile, unanesthetized woman delivering out of the hospital, Gaskin's maneuver may be the most appropriate choice for initial management. The midwife may choose to employ this technique in preference to McRobert's maneuver as the first intervention.

Scope It Out

Insert your hand into the vagina and reach back to the anterior shoulder. Feel the shoulders and note how they fit into the pelvis. Is the anterior shoulder difficult to reach because it is lodged above the pelvic brim? Are the shoulders transverse and jammed sideways? If so, suprapubic pressure will not be useful.

Is there a fetal hand blocking progress, or an abducted arm? Is a tight nuchal cord impeding birth?

Modified Rubin's Maneuver

The modified Rubin's maneuver, employed with the woman in McRobert's position, involves adducting the fetal shoulder and orienting it obliquely in the pelvis. This action creates more space for delivery and allows the posterior arm to enter the pelvis. Rubin's maneuver requires less traction force than McRobert's and involves significantly lower brachial plexus extension (Gurewitsch, et al., 2005). Place your hand in the vagina behind the posterior fetal shoulder and then rotate it toward the fetal chest. If the fetal spine lies to the left, use your right hand; if it lies to the right, use your left. This maneuver may be difficult and painful for the unanesthetized client, and it may be difficult to get your hand into the vagina of a primipara without cutting an episiotomy. A study involving a laboratory birthing simulator demonstrated that the modified Rubin's maneuver puts less force on the fetus and may cause less brachial plexus stretching than McRobert's maneuver. A variation of this technique is the Rubin II maneuver, which involves displacing the anterior fetal shoulder toward the fetal chest and beyond the midline of the maternal symphysis, from the 12 o'clock position to either 11 o'clock or 1 o'clock.

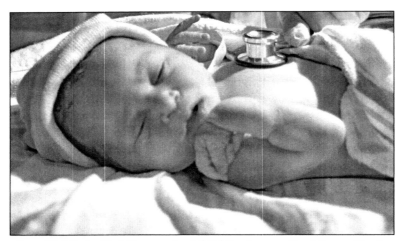

Figure 96. Infant with right arm motor deficit following operative delivery without shoulder dystocia. This infant (5 lb, 8 oz) was born to a primigravida after a long first stage and hours of pushing through a pelvis that appeared adequate. When the vacuum popped off her head twice, the obstetrician delivered her with forceps. Upon delivery, the baby had abnormal rotation and movement of her right arm. She was right occiput anterior, and her left shoulder was uppermost at delivery. Upon closer look, her right arm was hypoplastic, and there was an indentation across her right forearm. Her right arm had been restrained by an amniotic band that interfered with growth and mobility restricted descent in labor. The band had not been identified on ultrasound. The baby is responding well to physical therapy and is likely to have normal use of her arm.

Reattempt Delivery
Woods Screw

Woods compared shoulder dystocia to the "crossed thread" of a bolt in a nut. A bolt cannot be forced into a nut, but advances when turned repeatedly. The Woods screw maneuver turns the baby through the pelvis like a bolt through a nut until the anterior shoulder advances from behind the pubic symphysis. The midwife rotates the fetus by exerting pressure on the clavicular surface of the posterior shoulder. Do not twist the fetal head and neck. Like the Rubin's, it can be difficult in the unanesthetized or primiparous client.

Reattempt Delivery
Posterior Arm

The delivery of the posterior arm is an extremely effective method for extricating the baby. This can be difficult to accomplish in the primiparous client without an episiotomy, and painful for the unanesthetized woman. The midwife inserts an entire hand into the vagina. If the fetal abdomen faces the maternal right, use your left hand (your right hand if the fetus faces the maternal left). Find the posterior arm and follow it to the elbow. Flex the elbow across the fetal chest by applying pressure in the antecubital fossa, then grasp the forearm or hand, and guide the arm gently across the fetal chest and out of the vagina. Delivery of the posterior arm brings the posterior shoulder into the pelvis. If the anterior shoulder is still wedged, rotate the baby and deliver the other arm. A major risk of this maneuver is inadvertent fracture of the baby's humerus. If the arm is trapped behind the fetus, you must maneuver the arm gently to the front of the fetus, then sweep it across the chest and out of the vagina.

Other Measures
Clavicular Fracture

If the baby is still impacted and time is running out, the midwife can intentionally fracture the baby's clavicle to narrow the shoulder width. This can be very difficult to accomplish, and it carries the risk of injury to the fetal lungs and vasculature.

Zavanelli Maneuver

As a last resort, the Zavanelli maneuver is undertaken only at the hospital where immediate cesarean delivery is possible. This technique was first described in the delivery of a 6 ft, 300 pound woman, G18P17, giving birth to a 6,824 gm fetus (Gurewitsch, et al., 2005). The provider administers terbutaline or another tocolytic to stop contractions, rotates the head back to the occiput anterior position, flexes the head, and pushes it back into the vagina as far as possible with the palm of the hand. Cesarean delivery is performed immediately thereafter. Zavanelli maneuver has a 91% success rate when used with anesthesia to relax the musculature and undertaken soon after shoulder dystocia is recognized.

Symphysiotomy

Symphysiotomy, or bisecting the symphysis pubis, effectively frees the baby, but can create lifelong pain and ambulation difficulties for the mother. This technique requires minimal equipment and is frequently used in developing countries. It poses little risk to the fetus and is effective when performed early (Menticoglou, 1990). Under local anesthesia, the provider displaces the urethra and cuts through the cartilage that unites the two bony halves of the symphysis. This technique is not recommended, and it is employed only if all other maneuvers fail and cesarean delivery is not possible (Rodis, 2007b).

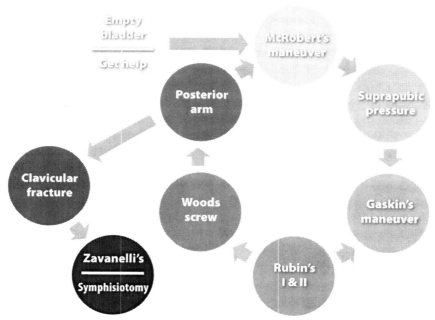

Although disimpaction maneuvers need not be performed in a specific order, it is helpful to memorize a sequence of interventions and modify them as the situation dictates.

Rapid Transport

If initial attempts to dislodge the baby fail, rapid transport is essential. You may transport the mother either on hands and knees or in McRobert's position, and you should continue to repeat the above maneuvers en route. In most areas, transport by an advanced life support EMS squad is preferable to use of a private car if response times are rapid. Paramedics carry life-saving medications and equipment for IV infusions and resuscitation, and they are trained to handle medical emergencies. The mother should receive high-flow oxygen by mask and should have at least one large-bore IV line of crystalloid solution. The mother is likely to hemorrhage after delivery, and hemorrhage can lead to shock and even death.

Shoulder Dystocia? Remember "FUDGE" (as in "Oh, Fudge! A shoulder dystocia!"):

FLEX maternal legs to abdomen in McRobert's position.

USE suprapubic pressure to disimpact shoulder

DISIMPACT anterior shoulder with Woods Screw or Rubin's II

GASKIN'S maneuver—flip mother to hands and knees, reattempt delivery with downward pressure and maternal pushing

EXPEDITE transport if no delivery, repeating above steps *en route*, and
EXPECT maternal hemorrhage and the need for neonatal resuscitation

If delivery is accomplished, the baby who has suffered a significant shoulder dystocia will often require resuscitation. Clavicular and humeral fractures are fairly common following a shoulder dystocia, but usually heal well with no long-term damage. Transient brachial plexus palsy occurs with only 15% of all shoulder dystocia cases, and less than 2% of brachial plexus palsies are permanent (Rodis, 2007b). Many cases of infant injury following shoulder dystocia cannot be attributed to the birth attendant; a significant number of infants with or without shoulder dystocia sustain these fractures or nerve injuries secondary to the forces of labor, position, and maternal pushing efforts, and even cesarean delivery cannot prevent them. Half of all babies with brachial plexus injuries are delivered spontaneously without shoulder dystocia. In fact, brachial-plexus injury has been documented in babies delivered by Cesarean section (Gherman, Ouzounian, & Goodwin, 1999).

Because every delivery carries the potential for shoulder dystocia, mothers should be instructed prenatally that strong pushing efforts may be necessary to accomplish delivery. This is especially true for women who have learned Hypnobirthing and other childbirth courses that encourage the natural descent of the infant and discourage Valsalva pushing. Although open-glottis pushing is beneficial in many cases, shoulder dystocia requires strong pushing efforts.

Table 28. Documentation for Shoulder Dystocia

Should Include

Demonstration of thought processes through delivery of the fetal head

Times of delivery of head and trunk

Need (or lack of need) for episiotomy

Force, direction, and duration of traction

Sequence, description, and duration of maneuvers used

Personnel involved and their roles

Tight Shoulders and Slow Descent

Actual shoulder dystocia is comparatively rare, but many babies will have tight-fitting shoulders at delivery. In this situation, the birth attendant will notice that the head is slow to restitute after delivery and that it is difficult to reach the neck when checking for a nuchal cord. Tight shoulders can be aggravated by maternal position, fetal position, full bladder, or excessive adipose tissue that interferes with the birth. "Bed dystocia" occurs when delivery is attempted on a soft mattress with the woman supine, limiting the capacity of the pelvis to expand and the ability of the birth attendant to guide the head downward. Tight shoulders differ from true shoulder dystocia in that the baby will usually deliver easily with maternal position change or emptying of the bladder.

Other impediments to birth can mimic shoulder dystocia. The body may not deliver spontaneously in the event of a short cord, a tight cord wrapped around the neck or body, an amniotic band, a fetal hand or foot wedged awkwardly and preventing birth, Bandell's ring, uterine rupture, certain fetal deformities, maternal pelvic tumors, or entanglement with a twin still *in utero*.

BIBLIOGRAPHY

American College of Obstetricians and Gynecologists. (2002c). *Shoulder dystocia* (Practice Bulletin 40). Washington, DC: Author.

Ailsworth, K., Anderson, J., Atwood, L.A., Bailey, R.E., & Canavan, T. (2006). *ALSO: Advanced life support in obstetrics* (4th ed.). Leawood, KS: American Academy of Family Practice Physicians.

Alarab, M., Regan, C., O'Connell, M.P., Keane, D.P., O'Herlihy, C., & Foley, M.E. (2004). Singleton vaginal breech delivery at term: Still a safe option. *Obstetrics & Gynecology, 103* (3), 407–412.

Belogolovkin, V., Bush, M., & Eddleman, K. (2008). Umbilical cord prolapse. In B.D. Rose (Ed.), *UpToDate*. Wellesley, MA: UpToDate.

Bowes, Jr., W.A. (2008). Management of the fetus in transverse lie. In B.D. Rose (Ed.), *UpToDate*. Wellesley, MA: UpToDate.

Cheng, Y.W., Shaffer, B.L., & Caughey, A.B. (2006). The association between persistent occiput posterior position and neonatal outcomes. *Obstetrics & Gynecology, 107* (4), 837–844.

Cunningham, F., Grant, N., Leveno, K., Gilstrap, L., Hauth, J., & Wenstrom, K. (2005). *Williams obstetrics* (22nd ed.). New York: McGraw-Hill.

Fischer, R. (2006). *Breech presentation* (eMedicine, topic 3272). Retrieved May 10, 2008, from http://www.emedicine.com/med/topic3272.htm

Gabbe, S.G., Niebyl, J.R., & Simpson, J.L., Eds. (2007). *Obstetrics: Normal and problem pregnancies* (5th ed.). New York: Churchill Livingstone.

Gaskin, I.M. (n.d.). The Farm Midwifery Center: Outcomes of 2,028 pregnancies: 1970–2000. Retrieved May 10, 2008, from http://inamay.com/archive/ statistics.php

Gherman R.B., Ouzounian, J.G., & Goodwin T.M. (1999). Brachial plexus palsy: An in utero injury? *American Journal of Obstetrics and Gynecology, 180* (5), 1303–1307.

Gruenberg, Bonnie U. (2005). *Essentials of prehospital maternity care.* Upper Saddle River, NJ: Prentice Hall.

Gurewitsch, E.D., Kim, E.J., Yang, J.H., Outland, K.E., McDonald, M.K., & Allen, R.H. (2005). Comparing McRoberts' and Rubin's maneuvers for initial management of shoulder dystocia: An objective evaluation. *American Journal of Obstetrics and Gynecology, 192* (1), 153–160.

Hannah, M.E., Hannah, W.J., Hewson, S.A., Hodnett, E.D., Saigal, S., & Willan, A.R. (2000). Planned caesarean section versus planned vaginal birth for breech presentation at term: A randomized multi-centre trial. *Lancet, 356* (9239), 1375–1383.

Hannah, M.E., Whyte, H., Hannah, W.J., Hewson, S., Amankwah, K., Cheng, M., et al. (2004). Maternal outcomes at 2 years after planned cesarean section versus planned vaginal birth for breech presentation at term: The international randomized term breech trial. *American Journal of Obstetrics and Gynecology, 191* (3), 917–927.

Hart, J., & Walker, A. (2007). Management of occiput posterior position. *Journal of Midwifery & Women's Health, 52* (5): 508–513.

Heppard, M., & Garite, T. (2002). *Acute obstetrics: A practical guide* (3rd ed.). St. Louis: Mosby.

Hofmeyr, G.J. (2007a). Delivery of the fetus in breech presentation. In B.D. Rose (Ed.), *UpToDate*. Wellesley, MA: UpToDate.

Hofmeyr, G.J. (2007b). Breech presentation: Incidence and management. In B.D. Rose (Ed.), *UpToDate*. Wellesley, MA: UpToDate.

Julien, S., & Galerneau, F. (2007). Face, brow, and compound presentations in labor. In B.D. Rose (Ed.), *UpToDate*. Wellesley, MA: UpToDate.

Lockwood, C.J., & Russo-Stieglitz, K. (2008b). Vasa previa and velamentous umbilical cord. In B.D. Rose (Ed.), *UpToDate*. Wellesley, MA: UpToDate.

Menticoglou, S.M. (1990). Symphysiotomy for the trapped aftercoming parts of the breech: A review of the literature and a plea for its use. *Australian & New Zealand Journal of Obstetrics & Gynaecology, 30* (1), 1–9.

Oxorn, H. (1986). *Oxorn-Foote human labor and birth* (5th ed.). New York: McGraw-Hill.

Peregrine, E., O'Brien, P., & Jauniaux, E. (2007). Impact on delivery outcome of ultrasonographic fetal head position prior to induction of labor. *Obstetrics & Gynecology, 109* (3), 618–625.

Ponkey, S.E., Cohen, A.P., Heffner, L.J., & Lieberman, E. (2003). Persistent fetal occiput posterior position: Obstetric outcomes. *Obstetrics & Gynecology, 101*(5, pt. 1), 915–920.

Ratcliffe, S.D., Baxley, E.G., Cline, M.K., & Sakornbut, E.L. (2008). *Family medicine obstetrics* (3rd ed.). Philadelphia: Mosby Elsevier.

Rodis, J.F. (2007a). Diagnosis and management of pregnancies at risk for shoulder dystocia. In B.D. Rose (Ed.), *UpToDate*. Wellesley, MA: UpToDate.

Rodis, J.F. (2007b). Intrapartum management of shoulder dystocia. In Rose, B.D. (Ed.), *UpToDate*. Wellesley, MA: UpToDate.

Sandberg, E.C. (1999). The Zavanelli maneuver: 12 years of recorded experience. *Obstetrics and Gynecology, 93* (2), 312–317.

Satin, A.J. (2007). Abnormal labor: Protraction and arrest disorders. In B.D. Rose (Ed.), *UpToDate*. Wellesley, MA: UpToDate.

Simkin, P., & Ancheta, R. (2000). *The labor progress handbook*. Oxford: Blackwell Science.

Simpson, K.R., & Creehan, P.A. (2007). *AWHONN's perinatal nursing* (3rd ed.). Hagerstown, MD: Lippincott Williams & Wilkins.

Sinclair, C. (2004). *A midwife's handbook*. St. Louis: Saunders.

Varney, H. (2004). *Varney's midwifery* (4th ed.). Sudbury, MA: Jones & Bartlett.

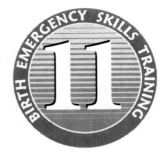

Fetal Heart Monitoring and Neonatal Resuscitation

OBJECTIVES

▶ Describe the possible causes and clinical significance of fetal heart-rate patterns:
  - ▶ Accelerations
  - ▶ Bradycardia
  - ▶ Tachycardia
  - ▶ Increased variability
  - ▶ Decreased/absent variability
  - ▶ Early decelerations
  - ▶ Variable decelerations
  - ▶ Late decelerations

▶ Describe how to perform basic newborn resuscitation using a self-inflating bag and mask.

▶ Discuss how to manage the infant with meconium-stained fluid.

▶ Explain the difference between primary and secondary apnea.

▶ Describe how to perform intrauterine resuscitation for the fetus in distress.

AACT and ReACT
ALERT—Be alert ▶ Exercise hypervigilant attention
ANALYZE—Think about possible causes
CONSIDER—Use OLDCART ▶ Gather data
TREAT—Make first response ▶ Proceed to definitive care
ReACT | ReAssess ▶ ReConsider ▶ Re-Treat

FETAL HEART-RATE INTERPRETATION

▶ **Reassuring pattern**—Baseline is normal, variability moderate, accelerations present, no decelerations present

▶ **Nonreassuring/ominous pattern**—Profound bradycardia, recurrent late and variable decelerations, absent variability.

Interpretation of fetal heart patterns is a fundamental skill of midwifery. The principles underlying fetal heart monitoring are similar whether the provider uses an electronic fetal monitor, a Doppler, or a fetoscope. Characteristics of the fetal heart rate can provide insight into whether the fetus is well-oxygenated or hypoxic, stressed or compensating. The same patterns represented visually by a fetal monitor tracing can be recognized audibly through intermittent auscultation. This chapter will provide an overview of fetal heart-rate interpretation. The reader is encouraged to pursue a more comprehensive program of study to develop expertise.

Although about 30% of neonatal encephalopathy cases are due to events during labor, the majority stem from a causative event before the onset of labor (ACOG, 2003). Epilepsy, autism, mental retardation, and attention deficit disorder are not caused by birth asphyxia (Sorem & Druzin, 2004).

If the laboring woman is low-risk, ACOG considers intermittent auscultation of the fetal heart rate acceptable. SOGC *prefers* this method of fetal surveillance, because evidence shows lower intervention rates with intermittent auscultation, and equivalent neonatal outcomes (Liston, Sawchuck, & Young, 2007). Both agencies recommend electronic fetal monitoring for high-risk pregnancies.

 When the outcome is known, it is easy to correlate features of the EFM tracing with acidosis, even if no such relationship exists. This bias could be eliminated if the expert witness were presented with several tracings, all nonreassuring. One tracing is associated with the case in question, the others with healthy babies. The EFM tracing would only carry weight in the courtroom if the expert witness could correctly identify the fetal heart tracing of the injured baby.

In active labor, the midwife should auscultate heart tones at least every 15–30 min, listening immediately after a contraction for 15–60 seconds. As contractions become longer, stronger, and closer, the midwife should assess the heart rate more often. In second-stage labor, auscultation should occur every 5 min or after every contraction.

Electronic fetal monitoring does not reduce the incidence of cerebral palsy or infant morbidity and mortality. In spite of this, many obstetric liability cases hinge on the interpretation of electronic fetal-monitoring strips.

Observers often differ in interpretation. It is difficult to correlate FHR patterns and neonatal outcome. Indicators of fetal distress are much easier to find if the examiner knows that the baby suffered damage. Abnormal heart-rate patterns sometimes do indicate intrapartum asphyxia, but most abnormal FHR patterns result in healthy babies with normal outcomes.

✍ AACT—Analyze

FHR Patterns

The atrial pacemaker sets the baseline FHR, and the beat-to-beat variations in the heart rate are influenced by interplay between the sympathetic and parasympathetic branches of the autonomic nervous system. The fetal vagus nerve inhibits the heart rate while the sympathetic nervous system stimulates, resulting in constant adjustments in response to changes in the fetal environment. Vagal influence becomes progressively dominant as the fetus matures, causing the baseline FHR to gradually decrease with advancing gestational age.

Table 29. Analyzing the Fetal Heart Monitor Tracing

Is the strip adequate for interpretation?

What is the baseline?

Is there variability? Short term or long term?

Are there accelerations?

Are there decelerations?

What is the contraction pattern? Consider regularity, rate, intensity, duration, and baseline tone.

What is the relationship between the accelerations/decelerations and the contractions?

Is the tracing reassuring, nonreassuring or ominous?

Are there trends evolving over time?

The normal baseline fetal heart rate in the third trimester is 120–160 bpm. Fetal activity stimulates the peripheral nerves and causes the heart rate to accelerate. Hypoxia, excess carbon dioxide, and acidosis can cause fetal tachycardia and hypertension. Prematurity, maternal anxiety and maternal fever may elevate the baseline rate, while increasing fetal maturity decreases the baseline.

A tracing is recorded on standard scaled paper, where one small square equals 10 seconds and one large square equals 60 seconds. The baseline fetal heart rate is the heart-rate range that occurs between contractions. The heart rate should be rounded to the nearest 5 bpm increment, excluding any marked FHR variability, periodic or episodic changes.

Table 30. Nonreassuring and Ominous FHR Patterns	
Nonreassuring Patterns	**Ominous Patterns**
Fetal tachycardia	Persistent late decelerations with minimal variability
Bradycardia 80–100 bpm	Nonreassuring variable decelerations associated with minimal variability
Saltatory pattern	Bradycardia <80 for greater than 3 minutes
Variable decelerations with slow return to baseline	Sinusoidal pattern
Late decelerations with normal variability	"Flat" tracing with minimal variability.

Fetal Tachycardia

Fetal tachycardia is defined as a baseline heart rate greater than 160 bpm and is considered a nonreassuring pattern. Tachycardia is further classified as mild (160–180 bpm) or severe (greater than 180 bpm). Continued tachycardia greater than 180 bpm suggests chorioamnionitis, especially when the mother is febrile. Rates above 200 bpm usually indicate a fetal tachyarrhythmia or congenital anomalies rather than hypoxia alone. Fetal tachycardia may result from administration of medications such as ritodrine or terbutaline or may be an early sign of hypoxia. Fetal tachycardia lasting more than 10 min may indicate increased fetal stress, but does not usually signify severe fetal distress unless decreased variability or another aberration is present.

Fetal Bradycardia

Fetal bradycardia is defined as a baseline heart rate less than 120 bpm for greater than 10 min. Mild bradycardia between 100 and 120 bpm with normal variability is not associated with fetal acidosis and is often seen in post-dates pregnancies with occiput posterior or transverse presentations. Bradycardia <100 bpm indicates a congenital heart anomaly or heart block, which may be related to maternal collagen vascular disease. Moderate bradycardia of 80–100 bpm is a nonreassuring pattern, and prolonged bradycardia <80 bpm that persists for three minutes or longer may indicate severe hypoxia.

Fetal hypoxia, maternal hypotension, congenital heart block, maternal hypothermia., uterine contractions, fetal head compression, certain medications, and possibly fetal Valsalva can cause bradycardia. Prolapse or compression of the umbilical cord stimulates a vagal response, causing bradycardia.

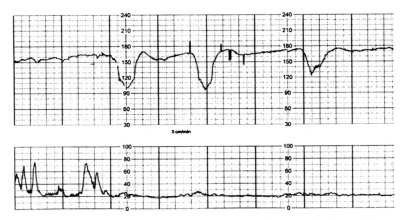

Figure 97. Fetal tachycardia with variables and loss of variability. This fetus has been experiencing variable deceleration and is beginning to decompensate. Tachycardia was the first sign of increasing distress, followed by loss of variability. The combination of late or severe variable decelerations with decreasing variability is associated with poor perinatal outcomes.

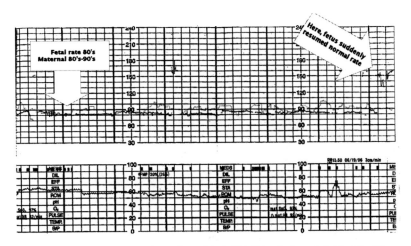

Figure 98. Fetal bradycardia due to heart block. This fetus had a rate in the 70s–80s for hours or days at a time from 27 to 34 weeks' gestation. Delivery was not indicated because the low rate was not related to hypoxia, and prematurity was a greater risk than the arrhythmia. Fetuses with heart blocks tend to compensate for the slow rate by increasing contractile force and are often able to maintain acceptable cardiac output despite the alarmingly slow rate. This baby was born healthy at term and with no evidence of cardiac problems.

Variability

The push and pull between sympathetic and parasympathetic influences in the healthy fetus causes a variable baseline. This variability is indicative of a well-oxygenated fetus and a healthy nervous system, chemoreceptors, baroreceptors, and cardiac responsiveness. Graphed out on a fetal monitor tracing, this variability is a jagged irregular line. When auscultating, count the fetal heartbeat in 6-second intervals, and multiply by 10 to get the heart rate. If normal variability is present, the 6-second counts will vary (for example, 14, 15, 15, 14, 16, 14, 14, 15), rather than maintaining a constant rate.

At about 28 weeks, the nervous system begins to mature, and by 32 weeks all healthy fetuses should show variability. Decreased variability may be related to fetal hypoxia and acidosis, congenital heart defects, and fetal tachycardia.

Beat-to-beat or short-term variability is the 5–10 bpm fluctuation of the FHR around the baseline. It is described as either present or absent and is most accurately measured with an internal spiral electrode. Long-term variability is a somewhat slower rise and fall of the fetal heart rate over 1 min, with a frequency of 3–10 cycles/min and an amplitude of 10–25 bpm. Loss of beat-to-beat variability is more worrisome than loss of long-term variability and may indicate hypoxia.

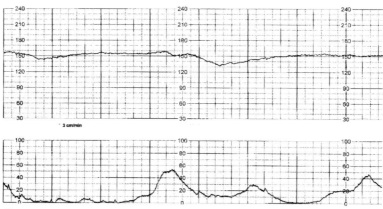

Figure 99. Minimal variability with late decelerations. Notice that the heart rate stays between 150 and 160 bpm except when decelerating.

A normal, healthy fetus should display average to moderate variability, decreasing benignly with fetal sleep cycles and with the administration of certain medications. Medications that decrease variability include morphine, diazepam (Valium), magnesium sulfate, atropine, hydroxyzine (Atarax), and methyldopa (Aldomet).

A saltatory ("jumping") pattern is one of exaggerated variability, swinging erratically between acceleration and deceleration, with oscillations greater

 Long-Term Variability (LTV) is described as
Absent = 0–2 bpm
Minimal = 3–5 bpm
Average = 6–10 bpm
Moderate = 10–25 bpm
Marked = > 25 bpm

than 25 bpm. It usually indicates cord compression or sudden hypoxia. The saltatory pattern is a nonreassuring pattern, but the fetus will often recover with hydration, position change, and/or oxygen.

Sinusoidal Pattern

A sinusoidal pattern is a regularly undulating pattern typical of a sine wave, persisting at least 10 min with 3–5 cycles/min and an amplitude range of 5–15 bpm. There are no accelerations and no short-term variability. When oscillation is greater than 25 bpm, mortality is much greater. The sinusoidal pattern is rare but usually indicates severe distress from isoimmunization, severe fetal anemia, and sometimes asphyxiation.

The "pseudosinusoidal" pattern can resemble the sinusoidal but the waveforms are less regular in shape and amplitude, and beat-to-beat variability is present, Pseudosinusoidal patterns are benign and transient and commonly follow the administration of narcotic medications.

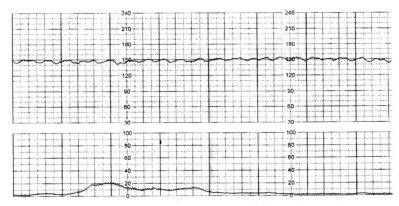

Figure 100. Pseudosinusoidal pattern. This pseudosinusoidal pattern developed after the mother was given 15 mg of morphine sulfate with 12.5 mg of Phenergan for therapeutic rest after a 60-hr labor prodrome. She woke up in effective labor and delivered quickly.

Accelerations

Accelerations are transient escalations in FHR precipitated by movement, vaginal examinations, uterine contractions, fetal scalp stimulation or external acoustic stimulation. Accelerations, including those that precede or follow a variable deceleration (shoulders), occur only in well-oxygenated fetuses. If the fetus is very active, accelerations can coalesce into a pattern that may be difficult to distinguish from fetal tachycardia. An elevated rate for longer than 10 min is considered a baseline change.

The nonstress test (NST) establishes fetal wellbeing by documenting at least two accelerations in 20 min, each lasting 15 seconds or more and rising to 15 bpm above baseline. The tracing that meets these criteria is termed "reactive."

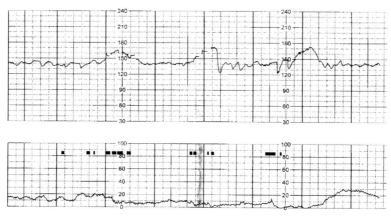

Figure 101. Reactive tracing. This reassuring fetal heart tracing shows long term variability and accelerations.

Late Decelerations

Late decelerations indicate decrease in uterine blood flow or placental dysfunction during a contraction. Precipitating factors may include maternal hypotension, uterine hyperstimulation, and calcified placenta from a variety of conditions. Uteroplacental insufficiency may be secondary to pregnancy-induced cardiovascular or renal disease, chorioamnionitis, hypertension, diabetes, smoking, or postmaturity.

A late deceleration is a gradual decrease in fetal heart rate, beginning at or following the peak of the uterine contraction and returning to baseline after the contraction has ended. Onset to nadir is greater than or equal to 30 seconds. The descent and return form a symmetric, gradual depression. The depth of the deceleration is irrelevant—a subtle late deceleration is just as worrisome as a deeper one. Decreased short-term variability in the setting of persistent late decelerations is an ominous sign. Late or variable decelerations in the setting of normal variability, while considered nonreassuring, indicates that the fetal stress is of minor degree or of recent origin.

Early Decelerations

Early decelerations are a decrease of the heart rate in response to vagal stimulation, usually caused by fetal head compression during uterine contraction. "Earlies" have a uniform shape, with a gradual onset at the start of the contraction and a gradual resolution coinciding with the end of the contraction. On a fetal heart tracing, the deceleration appears to be the mirror image of the contraction. Early decelerations are not associated with fetal distress.

Variable Decelerations

Variable decelerations are variable in duration, intensity and timing. They are shaped like the letters "U," "V" or "W," and may or may not be associated with contractions. Variable decelerations are caused by umbilical cord compression. Initially, cord pressure occludes the more compressible umbilical vein, which triggers an acceleration (the shoulder of the deceleration), a reassuring response. As pressure increases, the more resilient umbilical arteries compress, causing the steep down slope. They are especially common with ruptured membranes, oligohydramnios, and tight nuchal cord. As the compression resolves, the heart rate sharply returns to baseline and may show another shoulder acceleration, indicating adequate oxygenation.

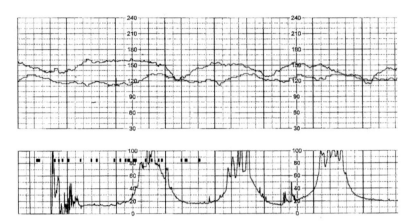

Figure 102. Late decelerations in second stage. The depth of the late deceleration is irrelevant—a subtle late deceleration is just as worrisome as a deeper one. The fetal heart rate only begins to decrease after the contraction peaks.

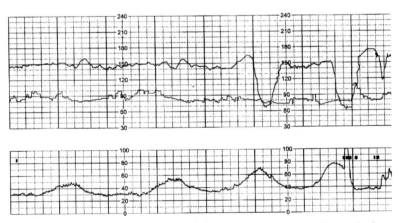

Figure 103. Variable decelerations. These variable decelerations were the result of a thin, tight nuchal cord. The baby was otherwise well-oxygenated, as evidenced by the shoulders on the variables and the good variability. Apgars were 8/9. The lighter line represents the maternal heart rate via pulse oximetry.

Unlike late decelerations, variables are more concerning when they are deep or prolonged. A mild variable deceleration is no deeper than 80 bpm and is no more than 30 seconds in duration. A moderate variable reaches a nadir of 70–80 bpm, and lasts for 30–60 seconds, while severe variables drop below 70 bpm and last longer than 60 seconds. The fetus with variable decelerations often has a good outcome, but persistent variables can lead to hypoxia and fetal distress. Variable decelerations in the setting of decreased or absent beat-to-beat variability may indicate fetal acidosis.

⟁ AACT—Consider and Treat

It is difficult to determine how long a pattern of ominous FHT can persist before the fetus suffers irreversible damage. A fetus sinking into acidosis will gradually show decreased variability, loss of accelerations, and/or persistent episodic or periodic deceleration.

Fetal heart-rate patterns are termed reassuring, nonreassuring, or ominous. A reassuring FHR pattern indicates a healthy, well oxygenated fetus with good reserves. A nonreassuring pattern requires further assessment and intervention to differentiate between acidotic and well-compensated fetuses. A nonreassuring fetal heart tracing (FHT) may be associated with maternal dehydration or hypotension, prolonged labor, medications such as narcotics or magnesium, intrauterine infection, abruption, fetal anomaly, fetal anemia, cord compression, or decreased placental perfusion.

The fetal and maternal heart rates may be indistinguishable during labor. Fetal bradycardia can result in a rate in the maternal ranges, while pain, stress or fever can drive the maternal pulse into the 140s or higher. Periodically compare the fetal heart rate with the maternal pulse to distinguish between mother and fetus, or apply a pulse oximeter (if available) to display the maternal pulse. An internal fetal electrode is not definitive because in some cases of demise the dead fetus will conduct the maternal rate.

When a nonreassuring or ominous FHT pattern arises, act quickly. Shift the mother's position from one side to the other, knee-chest, Trendelenberg, or knee-elbow. Position changes may dislodge an occult cord prolapse or otherwise relieve cord compression. Avoid the supine position, which carries the risk of vena caval compression.

Bolus her intravenously with 1,000 ml normal saline or lactated Ringer's unless her condition puts her at risk for volume overload. Hydration can improve placental perfusion if she is hypovolemic. Perform a digital examination to check for umbilical cord prolapse or rapid cervical dilatation and fetal descent. Give oxygen by mask (10 L/min) to maximize fetal oxygenation. There is no evidence that giving oxygen benefits the fetus in any way, but most authorities recommend the practice. If the uterus is hyperstimulated, consider tocolysis with subcutaneous terbutaline 0.25 mg (Acker, 2007).

In the hospital setting, the provider would turn off the oxytocin infusion, if present. Amnioinfusion may be considered to alleviate persistent variables.

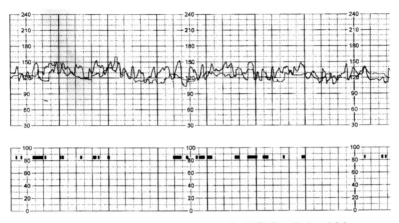

Figure 104. Maternal or fetal rate? At times it can be difficult to distinguish between maternal and fetal rates. The FHT (darker line) shows marked variability as it interweaves with the tachycardic maternal rate (lighter line) during second-stage labor.

Table 31. OOH Management of Nonreassuring Fetal Heart Rate

(Order of steps may vary)

Explain concerns to the woman and her family

Change maternal position to whichever posture yields the greatest improvement in fetal heart rate

Monitor fetal heart tones as continuously as possible

Assess the contraction pattern

Give 100% oxygen via mask

Perform a vaginal exam—evaluate for bleeding, cervical dilatation and cord prolapse; give scalp stimulation

Call for EMS and implement emergency transport plan

Obtain intravenous access with a large-bore catheter and administer fluid bolus (lactated Ringer's solution)

Assess maternal blood pressure, temperature, pulse, and respirations

Consider tocolysis for uterine tetany or hyperstimulation

After the deceleration, monitor the baseline rate and variability. Moderate variability is the most important hallmark of fetal wellbeing, indicating that the fetal brain is well oxygenated despite bradycardia or tachycardia or decelerations. If the baseline is within the normal range with moderate variability and accelerations, the fetus is unlikely to be acidotic. Significant acidemia is much more likely in fetuses with minimal/absent variability (10–30%) or minimal/absent variability and persistent bradycardia (80%) (Acker, 2007).

Fetal heart-rate acceleration with scalp stimulation suggests fetal pH greater than 7.20, but lack of such acceleration does not necessarily mean the fetus is in trouble. In a hospital setting, fetal scalp pH measurement or sonographic biophysical profile may be used to determine fetal well being.

✍ AACT—Alert
The Transition from Fetus to Neonate

The first breath of air taken at delivery marks a major anatomical and physiological transformation. Before birth, the lungs receive just enough blood supply to allow them to grow and develop. A hole between the atria of the heart (foramen ovale) and a shunt between the pulmonary artery and the aorta (ductus arteriosus) divert blood from the fetal lungs. To ready them for the task of breathing and to encourage lung expansion, the fetus breathes amniotic fluid in the absence of air.

At birth, the infant suddenly must obtain his own oxygen, and his lungs become vital to life-support. The changes in pressure and temperature stimulate him to draw his first breath, which distends the alveoli with air. The pressures of birth squeeze much of the fluid and mucus from his respiratory tract, and then as the baby draws a breath the lungs absorb any retained amniotic fluid. Oxygen from the air begins to diffuse into the newborn's bloodstream in much greater quantities than he was able to absorb from his mother *in utero.*

The distention of the alveoli and the abundant oxygen cause the network of tiny blood vessels in the lungs to relax, creating a dramatic increase in blood flow through the lungs. The baby breathes deeply or cries to bring air into the lungs and expand more and more alveoli. The climbing levels of blood oxygen have a relaxing effect on pulmonary vessels and cause the ductus arteriosus to constrict, sending blood flow from the heart to the lungs as in adult circulation. These pressure changes also close the foramen ovale. Abundant oxygen causes the infant's skin to quickly turn pink.

The first breath requires more effort than the breaths that follow. In the term infant, a surfactant within the alveoli reduces surface tension and prevents these small air sacs from collapsing with each exhalation, thus decreasing the work of breathing.

Blood pressure also increases in the minutes following birth. Recall that the blood in the placenta and umbilical cord is fetal in origin and is circulated by the fetal heart. The placenta is typically one sixth the size of the infant and holds a substantial amount of blood. When the umbilical vessels spasm and the cord is cut, the newborn is freed from the vast network of placental vessels and needs only to perfuse his own body. Consequently, his blood pressure rises.

If the baby is compromised at birth, this normal transitional process is disrupted. If the baby does not breathe deeply at birth, the lung vessels remain constricted and the blood continues to course through the ductus arteriosus, largely bypassing the lungs. Small arteries in the intestines, kidneys, muscles, and skin then constrict to maintain adequate blood flow to the heart and brain. If the newborn does not begin breathing, compensatory mechanisms begin to fail, leading to organ damage and death. Apnea in a newborn is classed as primary or secondary, and it can begin before, during, or after delivery. When a baby suffers a hypoxic episode, either *in utero* or after birth, heart rate and tone decrease, and the baby either gasps ineffectively or shows no respiratory effort. This is primary apnea. In the neonate, primary apnea can be corrected with oxygen and stimulation. Resumption of oxygen delivery to the fetus will correct primary apnea *in utero*. Often the prehospital provider will be unaware that there is a problem with the unborn baby. But if a bradycardic fetal rhythm is identified, maternal position change, oxygen administration, and an IV fluid bolus will often correct the problem.

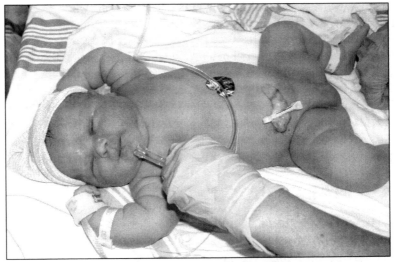

Figure 105. Macrosomia. This 12-lb girl, 37 weeks' gestation, is the child of a woman with uncontrolled diabetes and limited prenatal care. Her risk for complications such as congenital heart defects and persistent hypoglycemia are high.

Secondary apnea can occur if hypoxia is persistent or if the baby is not resuscitated. The heart rate and blood pressure decrease further, and the baby shows no respiratory effort. Aggressive resuscitation is necessary to reverse this condition.

A fetus can pass through primary apnea *in utero* and be in secondary apnea at delivery. No amount of stimulation and oxygen will initiate spontaneous breathing in the baby with secondary apnea. Therefore, if an infant does not respond immediately to back rubs and brisk toweling, the responder should immediately initiate more aggressive resuscitation efforts.

Ellis-van Creveld (EvC) Syndrome is a type of dwarfism that is seen in as many as 1 in 200 births among the Old Order Amish of Pennsylvania, but is rare in the population at large. Heart defects occur in 50–60% of babies with EvC (usually atrial septal defects or lack of an atrial septum), and many of these children also have pulmonary hypoplasia as well (Chen & Laufer-Cahana, 2007). Half of these babies will die in early infancy due to cardiorespiratory problems (Chen & Laufer-Cahana, 2007). Many of these babies are born at home with no prior suspicion of a problem. Children with EvC who have a normal heart, lungs, and chest have a normal life expectancy. There are always six fingers on each hand and sometimes six toes on each foot, along with short limbs and a normal torso that seems disproportionately long. The midwife who attends births with Amish women should stand ready to resuscitate babies that have these characteristics and arrange to transfer the infant as appropriate. If a couple has a child with EvC, odds are 1 in 4 that they will have another.

NEONATAL RESUSCITATION

About 10% of newborns require some assistance to begin breathing at delivery, and 1% need extensive resuscitation ("2005 American Heart Association Guidelines," 2006). Neonatal resuscitation can be stressful for the most seasoned provider. The provider who memorizes the steps of resuscitation and mentally rehearses them on the way to a delivery is likely to find that the events flow smoothly and are more likely to have a successful outcome.

Immediately after birth, assess the infant:

▶ Is the baby clear of meconium? (If meconium is present, skip to section on meconium, below.)

▶ Breathing or crying?

▶ Good tone? Color pink or cyanosis confined to hands and feet?

▶ Is baby full-term?

▶ No obvious anomalies?

The infant who passes this assessment does not need resuscitation and should be placed on the mother's abdomen, dried, and covered with blankets for warmth. The birth attendant should unobtrusively monitor breathing, activity, and color as bonding ensues.

The infant who requires resuscitation receives support at one or more of the following levels of care:

- ▶ Basic management, including warming, positioning, stimulation, and repositioning.
- ▶ Oxygen or assisted respirations
- ▶ Chest compressions
- ▶ Medications or fluid administration

If the first level of care does not stabilize the infant within 30 seconds, the provider moves to the next level of care. If the infant begins to improve, the provider withdraws intervention level by level until the baby is stable with warmth and positioning.

The vast majority of babies make a smooth, spontaneous transition to extrauterine life. At least one attendant at every birth should be trained in neonatal resuscitation (including positive-pressure ventilation and chest compressions) whose primary responsibility is managing the newborn. A person with intubation skills and capable of administering medication should be either present at the birth or readily available.

Table 31. The ABCs of Neonatal Resuscitation

As with adult patients, neonatal resuscitation follows the ABCs.

Airway, Warm and Stimulate—Open and clear the airway. Dry and stimulate the baby and provide warmth, position the head in a "sniffing" position to open the airway. Give oxygen if indicated by cyanosis. Flick or rub his feet and rub his back. These steps should be accomplished in the first 30 seconds following birth.

After 30 seconds, simultaneously assess respirations, heart rate, and color. After the first few breaths, the infant should maintain a heart rate >100 bpm and pink mucous membranes without oxygen administration.

Breathing—If breathing is ineffective and gasping or not spontaneous, or if the heart rate is under 100, assist respirations with a bag and mask connected to 100% oxygen for the next 30 seconds. Oxygen ideally should be warmed and humidified.

After 30 seconds of ventilation have passed (1 min after delivery), reassess.

Circulation—If pulse is less than 60 after 30 seconds of positive-pressure ventilation, begin chest compressions while continuing positive-pressure ventilation.

Reassess. If heart rate remains below 60 after 30 seconds of compressions, continue compressions and positive-pressure ventilations, and administer epinephrine.

Steps of Resuscitation

- ▶ 1. **Warm, dry, suction, and stimulate** the infant for the first 30 seconds after birth while he rests on his mother's abdomen.

▶ **2. Open and clear the airway** by positioning the baby and suctioning the mouth, then nose, as indicated, —or use a DeLee suction trap or mechanical suction set at 80–100 mmHg. Use an 8 or 10 French catheter. Do not suction for more than 5 seconds. Suctioning may cause vagal stimulation resulting in bradycardia.

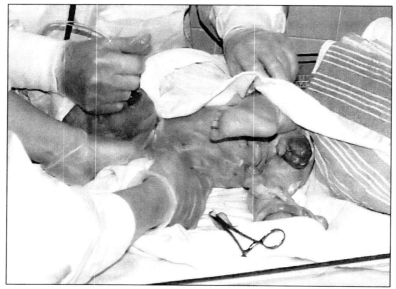

Figure 106. Initial steps after delivery. Warm, dry, suction, and stimulate the infant and replace wet linen to reduce heat loss.

▶ **3. Replace the wet linen beneath the baby with dry to reduce heat loss.** Reposition to open the airway, placing him on his back with his head slightly lower than his body and his neck slightly extended.

If the baby is not on the mother's abdomen, place a 1-inch thickness of folded blanket beneath his shoulders, especially if the baby is large and has a molded or edematous occiput. While accomplishing these steps, determine the baby's heart rate by palpating the cord, and note color, tone, and respiratory efforts. All this should be accomplished within the first 30 seconds after delivery.

If the baby is not vigorous, preserve several inches of umbilical cord when clamping and cutting, to provide access for umbilical catheter placement if necessary.

▶ *Reassess 30 seconds after delivery.*

▶ **4. Start positive-pressure ventilations if the baby is gasping or not breathing,** has persistent central cyanosis despite free-flow oxygen, or if the pulse is below 100 bpm. Ventilate with 100% oxygen (5–10 L/min) and a bag and mask.

Select a mask that fits the baby's face properly without air leakage, and then extend the neck slightly to the "sniffing" position. Suction the airway to clear any mucus. This is best accomplished with the baby placed on a firm surface (while taking care to avoid chilling). With light downward hand pressure, the mask should seal evenly on the infant's face without air leakage. A correctly sized mask covers the tips of the chin, mouth and nose without putting pressure on the eyes. Hold the mask so that your little, ring, and middle fingers extend over the mandible like the letter E, and the thumb and index fingers form a C-shape over the mask. Lift the chin forward with your ring and fifth fingers to maintain an airtight seal.

Effective ventilation can be achieved with a flow-inflating bag, a self-inflating bag, or with a T-piece.

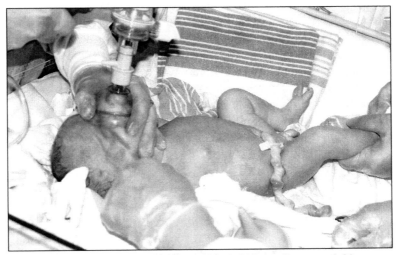

Figure 107. Positive-pressure ventilations. If the baby is gasping or apneic 30 seconds after delivery, shows persistent cyanosis despite free-flow oxygen, or has a pulse below 100 bpm, begin positive-pressure ventilations.

The flow-inflating bag, or anesthesia bag, is filled by gas flowing from a compressed source. This bag requires a tight face-mask seal, but it gives a better feel for lung compliance. A pressure manometer must be used to reduce risk of over-inflating the lungs.

The self-inflating bag reinflates when released, and does not require a compressed gas source. It is useful in resource-limited areas and when the provider chooses to resuscitate with room air. Without a reservoir, it only delivers up to 40%, but with a reservoir, it can deliver up to 100% oxygen.

A T-piece is similar to the flow-inflating bag, but has an adjustable flow-control valve that optimizes inflation pressure and inspiratory time. It requires a compressed-gas source.

Bags used for newborns should have a volume of 200–750 cc (optimal is 450 cc). Remember that the infant's tidal volume is only 20–30 cc. Larger bags increase the risk of lung overinflation. The bag should also have a pop-off valve set to 30–45 cm H_2O to release pressure if the bag is squeezed too vigorously. The pressure required for the initial breath may be as high as 60 cm H_2O), so for the first few breaths it may be necessary to deactivate the pop-off.

The addition of an oxygen reservoir allows the rescuer to deliver nearly 100% oxygen to the baby. Self–inflating bags cannot be used to deliver free-flow oxygen; so if the patient is breathing, use a mask or blowby to ensure oxygen delivery.

Compress the bag until the chest rises, taking care not to overinflate the lungs. The first breath requires more pressure than the breaths that follow, and premature infants may have more lung resistance. If the chest does not rise, check mask size and positioning for air leaks and equipment for proper functioning. Ventilate 40–60 times per minute. You are likely to maintain the correct rate if you repeat to yourself "BREATHE . . . two . . . three . . . BREATHE. . . . two . . . three . . . " as you ventilate, compressing the bag every time you say "BREATHE," then allowing the baby to exhale while you finish the count.

If you must provide positive-pressure ventilations for more than a few minutes, or the stomach appears distended, insert an orogastric or nasogastric tube.

▶ *Reassess after 30 seconds of positive-pressure ventilation.*
  ▶ If the heart rate increases to more than 100 bpm and the baby begins breathing effectively on his own, you may discontinue ventilations.
  ▶ Continue to provide supplemental oxygen until the baby's trunk and face are pink.
  ▶ If the heart rate exceeds 100 bpm, but the baby is still not breathing effectively, continue ventilation.

▶ **5. Begin chest compressions if the heart rate is ≤60 bpm** despite adequate ventilation with supplementary oxygen for 30 seconds.

Chest compressions press the heart against the spine, increasing intrathoracic pressure and helping to perfuse vital organs. Newborns are more likely to be revived by ventilations than by chest compressions, however, so ensure that the compressions do not disrupt effective ventilation. One person should compress the chest while another ventilates.

Two hand positions are acceptable, either encircling the baby's chest with the thumbs over the sternum below the nipple line and above the xyphoid, or with two fingers of one hand positioned over the same location. The baby should be on a firm surface and protected against heat loss. The down stroke of each compression should be quicker than the release. Keep your fingers or thumbs on the sternum at all times while performing compressions. Compressions should be approximately one-third the depth of the chest.

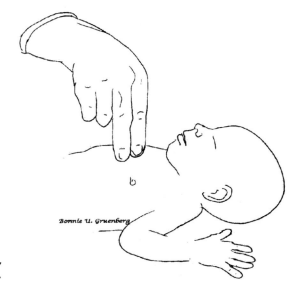

Figure 108. Chest compressions. If the heart rate is ≤60 bpm despite adequate ventilation with supplementary oxygen for 30 seconds, begin chest compressions.

Babies must be ventilated when chest compression is deemed necessary, and ventilations must be timed to avoid simultaneous delivery of compressions and ventilations. Blood flow seems to improve when the relaxation phase is slightly longer than the compression phase. Allow the chest to recoil after compression, but the provider's thumbs should not leave the baby's chest. The ventilation should be administered after every third compression, yielding a total of 30 breaths and 90 compressions every minute. It helps if the person giving compression repeats the words "One-and-Two-and-Three-and-BREATHE-and-One-and. . . ." with the bag squeezed for a breath on the cue "BREATHE-and," with compressions suspended to allow for the breath.

▶ *Reassess after 30 seconds of chest compressions with positive-pressure ventilation.*
  ▶ If ventilation is adequate, in most cases the heart rate will quickly improve—if not, confirm chest rise.
  ▶ If the heart rate is above 80, you may discontinue compressions, but continue to breathe for the baby at 40–60 breaths per minute.
  ▶ Once the heart rate surpasses 100 bpm, gradually stop ventilation and provide oxygen until the baby remains centrally pink.

- ▶ Reassess respirations, heart rate, and color every 30 seconds, and continue cardiopulmonary respiration until the spontaneous heart rate is ≥60 bpm.
- ▶ If the baby does not improve, reassess the effectiveness of CPR techniques.
- ▶ Check to be sure that 100% oxygen is being delivered to the infant—did the tubing disconnect from the oxygen source or has the tank run out?

Table 33. Criteria To Establish Acute Hypoxic-Ischemic Insult

Arterial cord blood at delivery with pH <7.0 or base excess ≥ 12 mmol/L, demonstrating metabolic acidosis present at birth

Early onset of moderate or severe neonatal encephalopathy in infants ≥ 34 weeks' gestation at birth

Spastic quadriplegic or dyskinetic cerebral palsy

Exclusion of other identifiable causes

Criteria Suggestive of Intrapartum Origin of Insult

Sentinel hypoxic event occurring immediately before or during labor

Sudden sustained fetal bradycardia or absent variability with persistent late or variable decelerations

Apgar score of less than 3 at 5 min

Onset of multisystem pathology within 72 hr of delivery

Early imaging studies demonstrate acute nonfocal abnormality.

(ACOG, 2003)

- ▶ **6. Consider intubation if positive-pressure ventilation with bag and mask is ineffective, if ventilation is likely to continue for a prolonged period, if endotracheal administration of medications is required, if birth weight is extremely low (<1,000 g), or if diaphragmatic hernia is suspected.**

  Intubation maintains an open airway but eliminates PEEP—the physiologic positive end-expiratory pressure created when the baby cries or coughs, necessitating the addition of a PEEP valve (set at 2–4 cm H_2O) to the bag valve outlet. Only an uncuffed endotracheal tube should be used on a neonate.

  Endotracheal (ET) intubation directs suctioning and ventilation directly to the trachea. The decision to intubate may also hinge on the expertise and capabilities of the available providers. Intubation is a skill that must be learned and practiced. The less experienced provider should defer to a more experienced provider if intubation is necessary.

> **The Oxygen Debate**
> Research has raised concerns about potential damage to infants from 100% oxygen used in resuscitation. It has also raised concerns about damage from oxygen deprivation during and after asphyxia. It appears that human infants may benefit from resuscitation with room air instead of oxygen, but at this time the AHA continues to recommend supplementary oxygen for both positive-pressure ventilation and free-flow for central cyanosis. Alternative practices include initiating resuscitation with less than 100% oxygen and titrating upwards as needed, or starting with room air, then adding supplementary oxygen if no improvement within 90 seconds after birth.

The following steps are required for successful intubation of the neonate:

- ► Preoxygnate the baby with a bag and mask. The NRP guidelines use birth weight and gestational age to determine the proper sized ET tube. Use a straight Miller blade.
- ► Place the baby aligned on his back with his neck slightly extended in the sniffing position. Limit intubation attempts to less than 20 seconds. Administer free flow oxygen while you intubate.
- ► Hold the laryngoscope in your left hand between the thumb and the first two or three fingers so the blade hangs down like an L shape. Insert the blade over the right side of the tongue, moving the tongue to the left and advance until the blade reaches the vallecula, just beyond the base of the tongue.
- ► Lift the laryngoscope to allow visualization of the vocal cords *without* levering off the upper gums.
- ► When you see the cords, slip the endotracheal tube through them with the right hand until the heavy black line on the tip of the tube reaches the cords. A stylet is useful to stiffen and curve the tube for easier insertion.
- ► The infant should improve markedly. If the heart rate is still below 60, reevaluate the effectiveness of CPR and make sure the endotracheal tube is still in the trachea.

A rapid increase in heart rate, misting of moisture in the tube, chest rise, and detection of exhaled carbon dioxide confirm successful placement of the endotracheal tube except in some cases of cardiac arrest. The most accurate way of confirming placement is to actually see the tube pass the vocal cords while intubating. If you are sure the tube is correctly placed, secure it with tape or a commercial stabilization device. Unrecognized, accidental placement of an endotracheal tube in the esophagus will kill the baby. "When in doubt, pull it out."

Laryngeal mask airways (LMAs) fit over the laryngeal inlet and can be used to ventilate near-term and full-term neonates. Research suggests that the LMA and endotracheal tube are equally effective at securing the airway of the newborn, but at this point the endotracheal tube is still the gold standard for airway management.

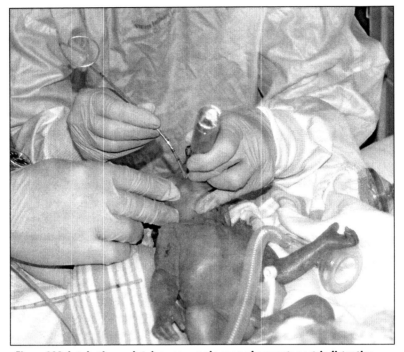

Figure 109. Intubation maintains a secure airway and prevents gastric distention.

▶ *Reassess after 30 seconds.*
  ▶ **7. Consider epinephrine, volume expansion, or both** if adequate ventilation with 100% oxygen and chest compressions fail to raise the heart rate above 60 bpm. (Drugs are rarely required to resuscitate a newborn. Most bradycardia results from inadequate oxygenation and resolves with ventilation.)
    ▶ Administer epinephrine via the endotracheal tube with a 1-ml saline flush, and ventilate. Epinephrine increases the rate and strength of cardiac contractions and raises the blood pressure through vasoconstriction. Newborns should receive 0.1–0.3 ml/kg of a 1:10,000 (0.01–0.03 mg/kg) concentration of epinephrine hydrochloride. Follow with several deep ventilations to move the drug into the lungs. Epinephrine may be repeated every 3–5 min.

- *Reassess after 30 seconds.*
- **8. Establish venous access** through a peripheral vein, intraosseus cannulation, or umbilical vein cannulation if the baby has failed to respond adequately to resuscitation by this time. Absorption appears to be more reliable when epinephrine is given IV.

  If local protocols permit access through the umbilical vein, trim the cord to one inch above the abdomen and identify the three vessels. Normally the opening of the umbilical vein is large and obvious, and the two umbilical arteries are smaller. Some babies have only one umbilical artery. Do not attempt cannulation if you cannot clearly identify the vein. Do not allow this procedure to delay transport.
    - Prepare a sterile field and a #5 French umbilical catheter (or 20-gauge IV catheter) with the needle removed.
    - Flush a 3-way stopcock and connect to normal saline extension set.
    - Insert the catheter into vein until tip is just below the abdominal skin and you can observe free flow of blood.
    - Attach 10 cc syringe partially filled with normal saline and aspirate gently to confirm lack of resistance. If blood does not reflux into syringe, withdraw the catheter slightly and aspirate again.
    - Inject a small amount of saline and check for resistance.
    - Secure with umbilical tape.
- **9. Consider other causes** for depression if the baby still has not responded to resuscitation efforts. In the case of placental abruption, placenta previa, or cord accident, the baby may be in hypovolemic shock as evidenced by pale skin, poor perfusion, or weak pulse.
    - **Hypovolemia**—Administer a fluid bolus of 10 ml per kg of lactated Ringer's or normal saline given slow IV push. This volume is sometimes repeated once. Rapid infusions of large volumes may cause a brain hemorrhage, especially in premature infants.
    - **Narcotic intoxication**—Naloxone administration may be indicated if the mother of a depressed infant might have taken a narcotic within 4 hr of delivery and is not addicted to narcotics. A baby exposed to narcotics may maintain a normal heart rate, but shows poor tone, color, and breathing effort. Do not administer to infants of long-term narcotics users. Naloxone can cause seizures in the neonate if the mother has used narcotics regularly in the weeks before delivery. The dose for neonates is 0.1 mg/kg IV, IM, ET, or SC. It may be repeated every 2 or 3 min as needed to a maximum of 10 mg.

The infant who has required resuscitation is at risk for further decompensation after vital signs have returned to normal. Once a baby has been successfully resuscitated, transport to a facility capable of managing an acutely ill neonate. Frequently reassess vital signs, color, and tone en route. Ensure adequate warmth and a clear airway.

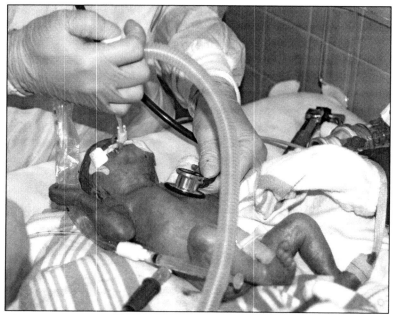

Figure 110. Confirming placement of the endotracheal tube. A rapid increase in heart rate, misting of moisture in the tube, chest rise, equal lung sounds, and detection of exhaled carbon dioxide confirms successful placement of the endotracheal tube.

Respiratory distress in a newborn can develop rapidly and unexpectedly, even in the infant that was vigorous at birth. A grunting "uh. . .uh. . . uh. . ." quality to exhalations suggests that the baby is having respiratory difficulty. Retractions are a sinking in of the flesh between the ribs and above and below the sternum on inspiration and a seesawing motion between the chest and the belly with respirations. Nasal flaring also indicates difficulty breathing. The child with respiratory distress needs rapid transport to the hospital. Supply blowby oxygen as needed and stand ready to use positive-pressure ventilation if needed.

Resuscitating the Preterm Infant

If a preterm infant is delivered at home, anticipate resuscitation and transport. When ventilating the preterm infant, begin with an initial inflation pressure of 20–25 cm H_2O, increasing pressure as necessary for adequate ventilation. The immature lungs of a premature baby are resistant to ventilation, and are easily damaged by overinflation. These babies are also prone to brain hemorrhage, hypothermia, infection, and hypovolemia.

Preterm infants weighing less than 1,500 g develop hypothermia much more rapidly than a full term infant. Warming methods suitable for the term infant might be adequate, including drying and swaddling, warming pads, increased room temperature, and skin-to-skin "kangaroo care" with a blanket covering mother and child. Additional warming techniques are recommended to reduce heat loss, such as covering the infant in food-grade, heat-resistant plastic wrap and placing him under radiant heat if available. Resuscitation measures, including endotracheal intubation, chest compression, and insertion of lines, should be performed while maintaining this warmth. Monitor the baby's temperature closely—premature babies straddle a fine line between under- and overheating, and hyperthermia can worsen cerebral injury.

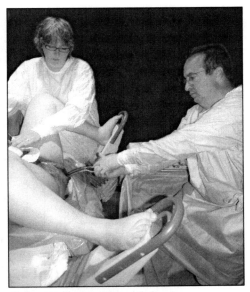

Figure 111. Forceps delivery. Deliveries instrumented with forceps or vacuum are more likely to involve a depressed infant in need of resuscitation.

Meconium
Usually priority 2 or 3, but sometimes priority 1

Meconium staining occurs in about 8–25% of all births after 34 weeks' gestation, and about 10% of these develop meconium aspiration syndrome (MAS), which carries a 4–19 % mortality rate (Clark & Clark, 2008). Babies born with moderate to thick meconium in the fluid are seven times more likely to have neonatal seizures (Wiswell & Fuloria, 2000).

The fetus ordinarily does not move his bowels until after birth. Sometimes, however, a hypoxic event can cause the anal sphincter to relax and expel meconium into the amniotic fluid. A healthy post-term baby may pass meconium *in utero* as his intestines mature and start to function. Breech babies often pass meconium as their abdomens are squeezed through the maternal pelvis. Although meconium itself is sterile, it reduces the antibacterial activity of the amniotic fluid and thereby increases the risk of perinatal bacterial infection. Meconium is irritating to fetal skin and increases the likelihood of erythema toxicum. Opaque particles visible in amniotic fluid on ultrasound can indicate the presence of either vernix or meconium in the waters—but the provider cannot distinguish which until the membranes are ruptured.

When meconium enters the amniotic fluid, the fetus may inhale it and develop lower airway obstructions. A distressed fetus may gasp *in utero*, drawing meconium deeper into the lungs. If meconium is inhaled into the lower airway, meconium aspiration syndrome (MAS) may result. Aspiration interferes with oxygenation not only by obstructing the airway, but by causing surfactant dysfunction, chemical pneumonia, and pulmonary hypertension (Clark & Clark, 2008). Although meconium is sterile, meconium aspiration increases the risk of pulmonary infection. Few babies with meconium-stained fluid will develop MAS, but the ones that do may suffer severe respiratory distress. Complete bronchial obstruction may lead to atelectasis; partial blockage leads to air trapping that can progress to tension pneumothorax.

 Atelectasis—alveolar collapse resulting from insufficient ventilation. It can also represent incomplete expansion of the lungs in the neonate.

Meconium aspiration syndrome appears to correlate with fetal hypoxia. If meconium is thick or particulate, the out-of-hospital midwife should transfer care of the client unless birth is imminent (Vedam, et al., 2007).

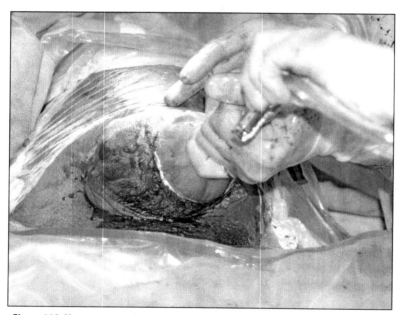

Figure 112. Vacuum extraction in a cesarean delivery. Vacuum extraction can be used to facilitate both vaginal and cesarean deliveries. Though generally safe in experienced hands, the vacuum can cause trauma to the neonate.

Providers were once trained to suction meconium from the infant's airway after the head delivers, but before the shoulders. This technique has not been shown to reduce the incidence of meconium aspiration and may cause fetal bradycardia, so routine intrapartum suctioning is no longer recommended. Amnioinfusion to dilute thick meconium similarly has made no difference in outcomes.

Deliver the infant to the maternal abdomen or the bed and briefly observe his activity. If the baby is vigorous—defined as having a heart rate over 100, spontaneous crying or breathing, and flexed or flailing extremities—proceed with routine care. Apgar score for a vigorous baby will be 8 or greater. If the infant is not vigorous, cut the cord and move him *with minimal stimulation* to a surface where resuscitation can be readily performed. Take care not to chill the infant.

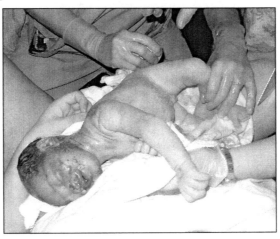

Figure 113. Depressed infant with meconium. If the infant is not vigorous, move him with minimal stimulation to a surface where resuscitation can be readily performed.

Quickly intubate the infant and perform suctioning through the endotracheal tube itself, using a meconium suction adapter. Occlude the suction control port on the aspirator and gradually withdraw the tube. Do not apply suction for more than 3–5 seconds. If no meconium is removed, do not re-suction, but ventilate the infant. If suctioning yields meconium and the heart rate is not significantly bradycardic, reintubate and repeat until little or no meconium is extracted or the heart rate begins to drop. Ventilate and stimulate the infant as usual.

Caution! Endotracheal suctioning can trigger a vagal response that can drop the infant's heart rate to dangerously low levels. If the infant becomes significantly bradycardic, the responder may need to stop suctioning and provide positive-pressure ventilations, even though ventilations could drive the meconium deeper into the respiratory tract.

RESPIRATORY DISTRESS IN THE NEONATE

Meconium Aspiration Syndrome (MAS)
Priority 1

Meconium aspiration syndrome (MAS) can develop when meconium is aspirated into the lower airways. Approximately 10% of all infants with moderate to thick meconium stained amniotic fluid will develop MAS ("2005 American Heart Association Guidelines," 2006). Meconium can create a partial obstruction that allows air to flow into the lungs on inspiration but blocks exhalation, causing hyperinflation of the lungs distal to the blockage. The baby develops air hunger and gasps, potentially bringing more meconium into the lungs as it struggles to breathe. Hyperinflation, hypoxemia, and acidemia cause increased pulmonary vascular resistance, which shunts blood through the ductus arteriosus and away from the lungs. Hypoxemia worsens as blood moves through the fetal

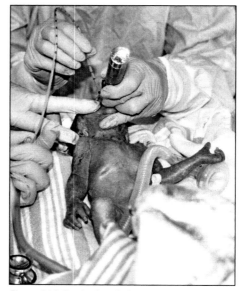

Figure 114. Suctioning. A clear airway is essential, but too-vigorous suctioning can cause bradycardia.

circulation circuit rather than the neonatal system. Hyperinflation of the lungs predisposes the baby to pneumothorax. Babies with MAS, especially if post-

term, frequently develop persistent pulmonary hypertension of the newborn.

Babies with MAS are often hypoxic and depressed at birth, showing floppy "rag doll" tone, retractions, grunting, tachypnea or apnea, cyanosis or pallor, and nasal flaring similar to infants with respiratory distress syndrome. A barrel chest may develop from hyperinflation of the lungs. Increased work of breathing leads to hypoglycemia, hypothermia, respiratory and metabolic acidosis, and electrolyte imbalance. This may progress rapidly to respiratory failure.

Babies with MAS are admitted to the NICU for ventilatory support, IV fluids, chest percussion, and postural drainage. Some

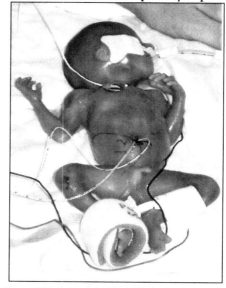

Figure 115. Cusp of viability. This boy was born at about 22 weeks' gestation. His parents wanted "everything" done for him. He was born kicking and even tried to cry, but was too immature to survive. Despite the best technology had to offer, he died in the NICU after 18 hours.

babies must receive specialized treatments, such as extracorporeal membrane oxygenation (ECMO), available only in certain regional hospitals, if they are to survive.

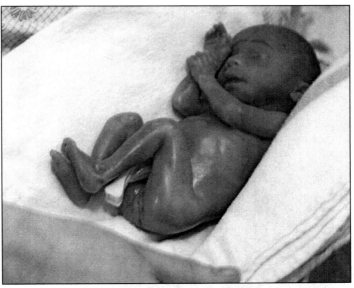

Figure 116. This girl was also born at about 22 weeks' gestation. After the neonatologist explained options to the parents, they decided to keep her comfortable until she died. She survived about 5 minutes.

Infant Resuscitation? Remember "RESUS":
REMOVE meconium.
EVALUATE while warming, drying, stimulating and suctioning.
SUPPORT breathing, oxygenation, and circulation as necessary.
UNDERTAKE ALS if BLS is ineffective.
SEEK underlying causation (hypoglycemia, hypovolemia.).

Transient Tachypnea of the Newborn
Priority 1

Transient tachypnea of the newborn usually affects infants that are full term and of average weight. The infant is born vigorous and then develops progressive respiratory distress. Auscultation of the lungs reveals crackles from excessive fluid, which may result from a failure to empty the lungs of fluid during birth or from aspiration of amniotic fluid. Dyspnea gradually worsens, until by

6 hours of life the infant may have respirations of 100–140 breaths per minute. Out-of-hospital treatment is the same as with any condition that compromises respiration.

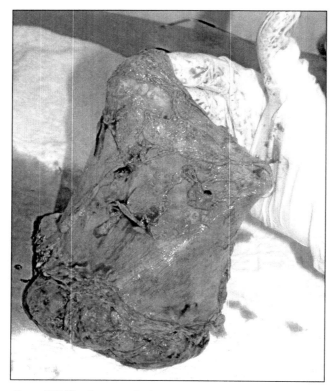

Figure 117. The placenta tells the story. Examination of the placenta from the baby in figure 116 shows evidence of longstanding infection and acute abruption.

When To Withhold Resuscitation

Resuscitation is withheld when gestation, birth weight, or congenital anomalies will bring almost certain death or extremely high morbidity if the baby survives. Examples include gestational age <23 weeks or birth weight <400 g, anencephaly, and chromosomal anomalies incompatible with life. Resuscitation is nearly always initiated in conditions with a reasonable chance for survival and acceptable morbidity, including gestational age ≥25 weeks, most congenital malformations, and Down syndrome. If the individual situation involves questionable prognosis, uncertain survival, and high likelihood of significant morbidity (for example, a 23-week infant), many protocols allow the parents' wishes to influence the choice to resuscitate. Infants who have neither a heart beat nor respiratory effort after 10 min of resuscitation generally do not survive, or survive with grave neurodevelopmental disability. Many protocols support cessation of resuscitation if the infant still shows no signs of life after 10 min of continuous and adequate efforts.

BIBLIOGRAPHY

2005 American Heart Association (AHA) guidelines for cardiopulmonary resuscitation (CPR) and emergency cardiovascular care (ECC) of pediatric and neonatal patients: Neonatal resuscitation guidelines (Electronic version). (2006). *Pediatrics, 117* (5), e1029–e1038. Retrieved March 24, 2008, from http:// pediatrics.aappublications.org/ cgi/content/full/117/5/e1029

Acker, D. (2007). Clinical pearls in application of electronic fetal heart rate monitoring. In B.D. Rose (Ed.), *UpToDate*. Wellesley, MA: UpToDate.

Ailsworth, K., Anderson, J., Atwood, L.A., Bailey, R.E., & Canavan, T. (2006). *ALSO: Advanced life support in obstetrics* (4th ed.). Leawood, KS: American Academy of Family Practice Physicians.

American College of Obstetricians and Gynecologists. (2003, January 31). *Obstetrician-gynecologists and pediatricians say most newborn brain injuries do not occur during childbirth.* Retrieved December 4, 2004, from http://www.acog.org/from_home/publications/press_releases/nr01-31-03-1.cfm

Braner, D., Denson, S. & Ibsen, L. (Eds.). (2007). *Textbook of neonatal resuscitation.* Dallas, TX: American Heart Association.

Chen, H., & Laufer-Cahana, A. (2007). *Ellis-van Creveld Syndrome* (eMedicine, topic 660). Retrieved May 19, 2008, from http://www.emedicine.com/ped/ topic660.htm

Clark, M.B., & Clark, D.A. (2008, December 2). *Meconium Aspiration Syndrome.* Retrieved December 13, 2009, from http://emedicine.medscape.com/article/974110

Fernandes, C.J. (2008). Neonatal resuscitation in the delivery room. In B.D. Rose (Ed.), *UpToDate*. Wellesley, MA: UpToDate.

Fullerton, J., Navarro, A., & Young, S. (2007). Outcomes of planned home births: An integrative review. *Journal of Midwifery and Women's Health 52 (4)* 323–333.

Garcia-Prats, J.A. (2007). Clinical features and diagnosis of meconium aspiration syndrome. In B.D. Rose (Ed.), *UpToDate*. Wellesley, MA: UpToDate.

Gillen-Goldstein, J., & Young, B. (2007). Overview of fetal heart rate assessment. In B.D. Rose (Ed.), *UpToDate*. Wellesley, MA: UpToDate.

Gomella, T.L., Cunningham, M.D., Eyal, F.G., & Zenk, K.E. (2004). *Neonatology: Management, procedures, on-call problems, diseases and drugs* (5th ed.). New York : Lange Medical Books/McGraw-Hill.

Gruenberg, Bonnie U. (2005). *Essentials of prehospital maternity care.* Upper Saddle River, NJ: Prentice Hall.

Kenner, C., & Lott, J.W. (2003). *Comprehensive neonatal nursing: A physiologic perspective* (3rd ed.). Philadelphia: W.B. Saunders.

Kliman, H. (2007). Intrauterine fetal death. In B.D. Rose (Ed.), *UpToDate*. Wellesley, MA: UpToDate.

Liston, R., Sawchuck, D., & Young, D. (2007). Fetal health surveillance: Antepartum and intrapartum consensus guideline (SOGC Clinical Practice Guideline 197, electronic version). Journal of Obstetrics and Gynaecology Canada, 29(9, Suppl. 4), S3–S56. Retrieved May 17, 2008, from http://www.sogc.org/guidelines/documents/ gui197CPG0709.pdf

Moore, K., & Persaud, T. (1998). *Before we are born: Essentials of embryology and birth defects* (5th ed.). Philadelphia: W.B. Saunders.

Riley, L.E. (2007). Varicella-zoster virus infection in pregnancy. In B.D. Rose (Ed.), *UpToDate*. Wellesley, MA: UpToDate.

Sielski, L.A. (2007). Initial routine management of the newborn. In B.D. Rose (Ed.), *UpToDate*. Wellesley, MA: UpToDate.

Sorem, K., & Druzin, M.L. (2004). Electronic fetal monitoring: The difficulty of linking patterns with outcomes (Electronic version). *OBG Management, 16* (2), 31–38. Retrieved March 24, 2008, from http://www.obgmanagement.com/ article_pages.asp?AID=3270&UID

Vedam, S., Goff, M., & Nolan-Marnin, V. (2007). Closing the theory–practice gap: Intrapartum midwifery management of planned homebirths. *Journal of Midwifery and Women's Health, 52*(3), 291–300.

Wiswell, T.E., & Fuloria., M. (2000). Managing meconium aspiration. *Contemporary Ob/Gyn, 45*(7), 113–125.

Epilog: The Past and the Future

In many countries, including the United States, home birth is widely perceived as unsophisticated and dangerous. The uninformed public often assumes that a midwife is an untrained, possibly unclean, self-trained individual serving misguided women who avoid hospitals. The roots of this misconception extend deep into the past and can be changed only by bringing the reality of the modern out-of-hospital midwife into the light of day.

Midwives, traditionally women, have shepherded mother and child through the passage of birth from time immemorial. When things went wrong, women frequently called upon men to assist. They knew no more than the midwives, usually much less, but could provide "forceful and determined effort" to end labor (ACOG, 2001).

From the 5th to the 13th centuries, the Church often obstructed the advance of medical and scientific knowledge in the West. Midwives and other women healers were routinely accused of witchcraft because their methods involved active inquiry and experimentation, rather than prayer and passive reliance on God (Ehrenreich & English, 1973). The Church was frequently the highest authority of the time, and it taught that observations of natural phenomena are not to be trusted because the Devil leads people astray through the senses.

Midwives nonetheless plied their craft despite the risks: if labor was easy, and mother and child survived, they might be accused of sorcery; if not, they might face the Church *and* the grieving family. If it became clear that a baby was unlikely to deliver spontaneously, a barber-surgeon was often summoned to hack the fetus apart and remove it piecemeal in a desperate attempt to save the mother.

Concepts learned from the Islamic world sparked the development of medical schools in medieval universities, but the Church maintained rigid control over the practice of medicine, ensuring that it did not conflict with dogma and requiring physicians to co-manage with priests. Patients who refused confession were not treated (Ehrenreich & English, 1973). Without experimentation and dissection, knowledge of anatomy and physiology was primitive. Without even the rudiments of evidence-based medicine, the medieval physician relied on superstition and religious advice, attempting to cure through bloodletting and astrology while so-called witches—women healers—developed a working knowledge of anatomy and herbal pharmacology.

By the 12th century, medicine was developing an organized structure and becoming institutionalized. As medicine became a profession, laws began to regulate who could enter it. Male physicians, legitimized by the male-dominated Church and State, tended to treat female healers as ignorant or evil and became the experts who judged whether a patient's symptoms were caused by witchcraft. The Church decreed that a woman who dared to heal without formal study is a witch—but women were banned from study (Ehrenreich & English, 1973). Doctors developed their own body of mostly unscientific knowledge, cloaked in Latin and incomprehensible even to the educated layman, and took control of their own educational institutions, the regulation of clinicians, and the supervision of paramedical fields (Rooks, 1997; Roush, 1979).

While the medical profession invented itself, conditions remained appalling. Until the 20th century, the only effective contraception was breast-feeding, which generally spaced babies less than two years apart—or foregoing intercourse entirely. Slightly more than half of all children lived beyond their fifth birthday. In her 40-odd-year lifespan, a woman needed to bear seven or eight babies just to maintain a stable population (Harer, 2001). Always in demand, midwives continued to attend births without benefit of the growing body of obstetrical knowledge. Calling upon increasingly educated practitioners to assist when labor took a life-threatening turn exposed them to greater official scrutiny.

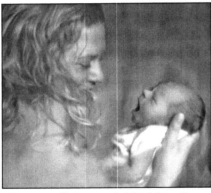

Figure 118. "As long as she's healthy...." *Since prehistoric times, women have prioritized safe delivery and healthy babies.*

In 1560, a Parisian statute included provisions for licensing and registering midwives (Roush, 1979). Instruction was through apprenticeship with the most experienced midwives in the community, and a certificate of good conduct and character was a prerequisite for licensure. Aspiring midwives also learned anatomy and were examined by a board. Upon registration, a midwife was supervised by doctors, and she was required to call a surgeon in case of malpresentation. Priests eventually required midwives to perform intrauterine baptism for fetuses not expected to survive, via nonsterile syringe, a procedure that contributed to mortal infections in the hapless mother (Rooks, 1997). Early English regulations were likewise less concerned with clinical competence than with insuring that the midwife was of sound character. Midwives were forbidden to perform abortions, expected not to use witchcraft, and often required to uncover the paternity of a child (DeVries, 1996; Lay, 2000).

Medicine and midwifery were separate specialties for most of history. Doctors did not concern themselves with normal deliveries, and midwives sought the help of doctors only when faced with complications. The boundary began to blur in the 17th century. In 1671, Jane Sharp wrote *The Midwives Book*, the first midwifery manual by a midwife (Litoff, 1982). Sharp taught accurate anatomy when the subject was considered indecent even for doctors and declared that most births would succeed if assisted only by herbs and a midwife's hands. Doctors had already begun crossing the customary line. Peter Chamberlen (died 1631) developed the obstetric forceps, a device that could have saved thousands of women from the horrors of prolonged obstructed labor. Instead, the Chamberlen family chose to profit by keeping the device secret nearly 100 years (Litoff, 1982), then selling it to the Medical-Pharmaceutical College of Amsterdam (DiLeo, 1996).

Once forceps became generally available, surgeons could extract a fetus whole, shorten labors, and sometimes save mother's and baby's life. They charged high fees for this service and began to compete with midwives, changing childbirth attendance from a neighborly service to a profitable career. Forceps were kept from midwives by legally classifying them as surgical instruments—it was illegal for midwives to practice surgery (Ehrenreich & English, 1973). British physician William Smellie promoted forceps use and encouraged male physicians to attend women in childbirth. Soon it became commonplace for births to be attended by physicians. Midwives bristled at the intrusion onto turf that had been historically theirs (Litoff, 1982).

Midwives attended births in most of colonial America for about 250 years (Stern, 1972). Like physicians, surgeons, and apothecaries, they were mostly self-taught or apprenticeship-trained, and they practiced without educational standards or regulation (Rooks, 1997). Where there were no trained midwives, untrained midwives met the need. Midwives offered lower fees and did not compromise a woman's modesty. Decorum was an important issue, and many opponents of the male accoucheur found a man attending a woman in childbirth offensive (Litoff, 1982).

In the South, most plantations had their own midwives, who attended both black slaves and white mistresses in childbirth. Whereas in Europe midwifery was often associated with sin and low social class, African midwives were honored members of the community (McGregor, 1998). When Africans of different tribes and languages were thrown together in the common culture of slavery, midwives retained their high status.

Childbirth was especially difficult for a slave. She was often bought as a "breeder" and expected to bear as many healthy children as possible. Often her master would impose his sexual desires upon her, and it was his right to dispose of her children as he saw fit. Her body often suffered from inadequate nutrition and depletion by too many pregnancies in rapid succession (McGregor, 1998).

Like many of its practitioners, we all tend to think of modern allopathic medicine as an awakening produced by uniformly humanitarian impulses and producing increasingly beneficial results. Medicine evolved, however, in the social, ethical, and legal contexts of the time, encompassing some values that are incomprehensible to us today. Doctors in the Americas in the 1800s were more enlightened than their 12th-century precursors, but they were immersed in a culture that embraced white superiority and the subjugation and eradication of other races. New procedures were often perfected on slaves or the poor, usually without anesthesia, before being offered to paying white clients (McGregor, 1998). Dr. Marion Simms, celebrated for developing a procedure to repair vaginal fistulas, performed unanesthetized, nonsterile surgeries on his three slave women for 4 years, up to 30 operations per woman, before he found one that worked. When tubal ligation and vasectomy became safe and easy, eugenics became an influential medical and political movement.

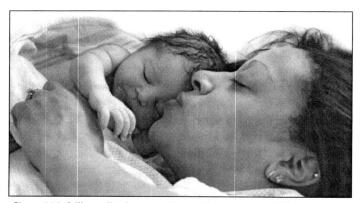

Figure 119. Still at a disadvantage. During the slavery era, African American women were often malnourished, mistreated, and expected to produce as many children as their constitutions would allow. Today, there is still a racial disparity; the African American infant mortality rate is twice that of white infants, and African American women are three to four times more likely than white women to die of pregnancy complications.

By the 1930s, 30 states had laws imposing sterilization upon convicted criminals and those deemed mentally ill or defective, though these laws were frequently challenged, and only California and Virginia applied them regularly. Physicians had standards, however, and many opposed women midwives as unsafe (Gould, 2002).

In 1765 William Shippen, Jr., an American doctor who had studied in England under Smellie, broke with precedent by offering a course in midwifery, including "theory and demonstration." He offered to teach female pupils privately and assist with any of their patients when necessary (Litoff, 1982; Stern, 1972). Few women were literate or wealthy enough for such a program, though, and women generally were discouraged from seeking education. Shippen soon limited his course to men, and for the next century, as midwifery education advanced in Europe, the United States offered no formal educational options for prospective women midwives (Rooks, 1997).

Men, on the other hand, were not accepted as birth attendants in many circles until the educational disparity between doctors and midwives became a chasm. By the end of the 1700s, the United States had four medical schools, none of which accepted female students. Midwives had few means of learning about discoveries in anatomy and physiology or the use of obstetrical instruments. The number of physicians increased, and by the 1800s, affluent women began to rely upon them to attend their labors (Litoff, 1982).

Formal training through the early 1800s gave physicians little advantage over midwives. Modern medical science was in its infancy. Medical schools offered several months to two years of classroom didactics with no access to patients and did not require a high school diploma for entry. Physicians were taught to oppose regular bathing and treat most afflictions with "heroic" methods, such as bloodletting, colonic purges (which could involve mercury compounds), and opium (Ehrenreich & English, 1973). The herbs and dietary changes employed by midwives and lay-healers were often less injurious to the patient. Even so, physicians offered on the reassurance of a diploma and instruments that could haul a child from the womb if Nature did not deliver. Thus, they gained the support of the upper class, to which they usually belonged, and their political power increased.

The safety and competence of midwives varied as enormously as the safety and competence of physicians (Baldwin, 1999). Although European immigrant midwives were often well-educated, domestic midwives were usually trained by apprenticeship, and their clientele generally consisted of the poor and the isolated, chiefly blacks and rural whites.

By 1830, 13 states had passed laws granting physicians the exclusive right to heal (Ehrenreich & English, 1973). A large segment of the public rebelled and founded the Popular Health Movement of the 1830s and 1840s, a social upheaval of early feminists and the working class that empowered people, especially women, to take charge of their own health and asserted that wellness-promoting self-care was more valuable than the harsh ministrations of doctors. This movement spawned new varieties of alternative medicine, which gained nearly as much credibility as the allopathic mainstream—sometimes more. It became unclear which practitioners were the "real" physicians, and by the 1840s, most states had repealed their licensing laws (Ehrenreich & English, 1973). New medical schools admitted women, asserting that they were at least as qualified as men. Gradually, the Popular Health Movement lost popularity and clout as division and contention set in.

Allopathic medicine revived, and in 1848 practitioners founded the American Medical Association. County and state medical societies returned to prominence. In the years that followed, physicians attacked lay-practitioners, sectarian doctors, and women practitioners of every kind (Ehrenreich & English, 1973).

The same year, American midwives finally received a chance for education, at the Boston Female Medical College, established by Samuel Gregory over furious opposition by the Boston Medical Society. Gregory felt strongly that men should not attend women in childbirth and set out to give female providers a 3-month course in midwifery (Litoff, 1982). Detractors said that female midwives and female physicians alike were emotionally, physically, and intellectually inferior and incapable of being birth attendants. Further, they asserted that the uterus and nervous system were linked, and women who pursued serious study would render themselves infertile (Litoff, 1982). By the end of the 19th century most midwives who pursued formal study were educated inadequately, through "diploma mills" run by physicians for profit (Baldwin, 1999; Litoff, 1982).

Obstetrics, however, was also taught haphazardly or not at all in medical schools, which still graduated doctors without scientific education. Modern gynecology did not develop until the principles of anesthesia, antisepsis, and hemostasis were recognized (ACOG, 2001). Residencies in obstetrics and gynecology did not appear until around 1900.

In the late 1800s physicians in France and Germany began to develop a true scientific basis for medicine. In 1883, Johns Hopkins University opened to teach this new kind of medicine, emphasizing research and clinical training and associating the medical school with a full university (Ehrenreich & English, 1973). Millionaires of the Gilded Age established foundations that poured money into institutions that followed the Johns Hopkins model. Smaller, poorer medical schools, mostly sectarian schools open to blacks and women, were denied such generosity, and many folded. Allopathic physicians gained power and used it to exclude other practitioners, monopolizing prescriptive authority and taking control of hospital admitting privileges (Rooks, 1990).

Early in the 20th century, midwives, generally apprenticed-trained lay-midwives, delivered 50% of American babies (Litoff, 1982; Stone, 2000). Obstetricians saw them as competitors and agitated for even the poorest women to deliver in hospitals, not only to increase revenue, but also to obtain teaching subjects for medical students (Dawley, 2000). Indigenous midwives often did little more than provide labor support, catch the baby, deliver the placenta, and perform household chores for the family for a few days after the birth. Even so, a study by a Johns Hopkins professor in 1912 showed that most American doctors were less competent than midwives (Ehrenreich & English, 1973). Physicians' patients became septic significantly more often, and physicians were more likely to employ surgical interventions that endangered mother and child. In Newark, NJ, in 1921, traditional midwives had a maternal mortality rate of 22 per 10,000 births while physicians' patients died at a rate of 87 per 10,000 (Dawley, 2000).

But doctors had more political power and were better organized, so states began to outlaw midwifery. For poor and working-class women, this prohibition often cut off obstetrical care completely. A study of infant-mortality rates in Washington showed that infant deaths increased immediately after midwifery was banned (Ehrenreich & English, 1973).

One reason for the success of American allopathic medicine is its early and well-accepted professional organization. The Boston Obstetrical Society was founded in 1861, and within 5 years New York and Philadelphia obstetricians had their own organizations. The American Gynecological Society was established in 1876 and the American Association of Obstetricians, Gynecologists and Abdominal Surgeons in 1888 (ACOG, 2001). Other organizations sprang up and maintained exclusivity by keeping memberships small.

In 1912, the U.S. Children's Bureau was created to examine and monitor all issues that affected the health of children. Its investigations revealed an alarmingly high infant-mortality rate: only 2 of 15 industrialized countries studied had higher rates of death than the United States. Death rates for women in childbirth were also shocking. Childbirth caused more deaths among young women than any disease except tuberculosis (Litoff, 1982). Midwives bore the brunt of blame for these outcomes and were popularly portrayed as illiterate, filthy, and unskilled (Stone, 2000). Indeed, some carried rusty scissors, used old rags as dressings, and kept stiffened catheters for performing abortions, but the interventions of the unskilled, heavy-handed doctors of the time were as dangerous to the women as the actions of untrained midwives (Rooks, 1997).

Nurse-run "midwifery clubs" tried to educate traditional midwives in such essentials as hand-washing and what to carry in the birth bag. Instructors sought to improve retention by setting key concepts to rhyme and music. American midwives were trained to wash their hands to the tune of "Mary Had a Little Lamb." In Europe, midwives learned anatomy and physiology, chemistry, biology, and clinical skills in 2- and 3-year programs and emerged as competent professionals (Dawley, 2000).

Physician-attended hospital births with nitrous oxide and twilight sleep became fashionable among the well-off. Economic prosperity in the 1920s produced a growing middle class of women expected to be wives and mothers, not to seek careers. They often could not find midwives of like social status and were reluctant to seek lower-class women for midwifery services (Rooks, 1997). Further, after 1920 the birth rate declined precipitously. Birth became a special event, and couples sought the best available care for each experience, which was commonly identified with hospitals and physician-attended delivery (Litoff, 1986).

Medical societies and public-health agencies convened to debate solutions to "the midwife problem." Midwifery rose to the attention of the public through articles in popular magazines, and states evaluated and revised laws and regulations pertaining to midwives. The anti-midwife campaign, designed to block midwifery practice and orchestrated primarily by physicians, reached its peak between 1910 and 1935 and resulted in the virtual elimination of lay-midwives in America (Baldwin, 1999; Stone, 2000). Many obstetricians saw midwives as obstacles to the expansion of obstetrics and believed that they could never garner the respect, credibility, and income that they deserved as long as untrained women could deliver babies. Most asserted that childbirth was inherently dangerous and only a skilled doctor in a modern hospital could save mother and child when things went awry (Litoff, 1982).

Doctors, moreover, could legally offer respite from the pain of childbirth. Dr. Joseph DeLee and other prominent obstetricians asserted that childbirth was no longer a natural function and was so pathological that very few women escape damage (Baldwin, 1999). They recommended total control of parturition as safer than unassisted labor. For modern, scientific delivery, obstetricians were taught to sedate women with scopolamine at the onset of labor to erase all memory of the event, give ether during the second stage of labor, allow the cervix to dilate, cut a large episiotomy, extract the infant with forceps, remove the placenta, give ergot to contract the uterus after delivery, and then repair the perineum (Rooks, 1997). The mother had little part in the proceedings.

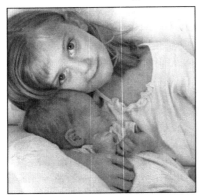

Figure 120. Healthy children. Good prenatal and childhood care confers a lifelong health advantage.

Public-health officials often disagreed with this approach, however, and maintained that if midwives were properly trained and regulated, maternal and infant mortality would decrease substantially. In Europe, well-educated midwives were responsible for a large percentage of deliveries, and infant mortality was far below American rates. American communities that provided high-quality midwifery education, such as in New York City and parts of New Jersey, also had excellent outcomes.

In 1921, the Sheppard-Towner Maternity and Infant Protection Act provided federal money to states for planning maternal-child health services. By 1929, 29 states provided instruction or educational supervision for midwives, but opposition from the AMA allowed the act to expire in that year (Rooks, 1997). Virtually every program that educated midwives improved maternal mortality rates, and whenever midwifery practice declined, maternal mortality and infant morbidity increased—yet most physician organizations continued to oppose midwifery (Rooks, 1997). In 1929, there were 5,300 doctors specializing in obstetrics and gynecology nationwide, though more than 90% of all childbirth was conducted by the general practitioner (ACOG, 2001).

In the early 19th century, nursing was a job, not a profession. Nurses were untrained women, often of ill repute, frequently dirty and sometimes devious, who tended the sick. Women such as Florence Nightingale and Dorothea Dix gave nursing a new focus and a respectable image, and in America nursing schools opened soon after the Civil War. The medical profession was receptive to nurses who were obedient, eager to serve, properly feminine, and no threat to physicians' authority. As the 20th century dawned and modern medicine took hold, nurses proved their value by taking over the menial tasks of patient care (Ehrenreich & English, 1973).

As childbirth moved into hospitals, nursing schools added obstetrics to their core curricula, often preparing nurses to assume the duties of obstetricians and attend women throughout labor until the time of delivery was near. Nursing, not medicine, created the concept of prenatal care; as early as 1888, nurses visited women's homes to monitor fetal growth, assess for edema, and provide information about pregnancy (Dawley, 2000).

One solution to the so-called midwife problem was the introduction of the nurse-midwife, a birth attendant well trained as a nurse and tightly under the physician's control. The medical profession was more comfortable with compliant nurses who had studied midwifery than with lay-midwives, but many still objected to working with midwives of any kind.

Some physicians worked to establish the specialty, however (Scoggin, 1997). Nurse-midwifery held the promise of eliminating competition, for it would provide another alternative to lay-midwifery. It was expected that nurse-midwives' extensive education would help them realize their limitations and not practice independently and that they would treat the poor patients that some physicians were not eager to attend. Their actions would be fully under the control of physicians, who could take over management of cases that deviated from normal.

Mary Breckinridge, on the other hand, showed how well nurse-midwives could function in isolation when she created a system of nurse-midwife-staffed community nursing centers to meet the health care needs of the rural poor in Kentucky. When she researched the living conditions of Leslie County residents in 1923, she found a scattered population of mountaineers. Large families of 10 or more frequently shared one or two rooms without the benefit of running water or outhouses. Breckinridge established the Frontier Nursing Service to serve 1,000 square miles of virtually inaccessible mountains where 15,000 people had no access to a licensed resident physician (Breckinridge, 1952).

Indigenous mountain midwives learned by helping their neighbors in childbirth because nobody else was available (Dammann, 1982). Malnutrition, anemia, dysentery, tuberculosis, measles, and hookworm were common. Typhoid was rampant because of unsanitary waste-disposal. Breckinridge's first nursing center officially opened in Hyden, KY, in September, 1925. Because there was only one nurse-midwifery school in America, FNS either hired British nurse-midwives or sent American nurses to England for schooling. Eventually six decentralized clinics allowed nurses to reach more patients in a day and respond to emergencies in a timelier manner.

The most remote areas could be reached only on horseback, so her nurses rode out in all weather to contend with whatever emergency presented. After analyzing the statistics of the first 1,000 births, the Metropolitan Life Insurance Company suggested that if the country at large were to benefit from the type of service rendered by the Frontier Nursing Service, every year 10,000 mothers' lives would be saved, 30,000 more children would survive the first month of life, and there would be 30,000 fewer stillbirths (Dammann, 1982).

When World War II broke out, most of the British nurse-midwives returned to England. Breckinridge had long dreamed of establishing a nurse-midwifery school in the United States. Having lost 75% of her staff, she realized that it was now a necessity (Tom, 1982). The Frontier Graduate School of Midwifery opened November 1, 1939, to train nurse-midwives to practice in rural areas, and it has been in continuous operation since. Its curriculum followed that of the Central Midwives Board of England and Scotland.

The only domestic predecessor of the Frontier School had opened just 7 years earlier at the Maternity Center Association (MCA) in New York City. MCA founded the Lobenstine Midwifery School in 1931 to prepare nurse midwives to assume responsibility under the guidance of a competent physician (Stone, 2000).

As nurse-midwifery schools opened in universities around the county (seven between 1930 and 1950), nurse-midwives gained professional respect, and their scope of practice shifted from a subordinate role to a collaborative one. The landscape of American obstetrics was changing, though, and by the end of the 1950s the vast majority of births occurred in hospitals. Legislation passed during the anti-midwife campaign had restricted nurse-midwives' ability to practice, and this development severely limited them further because initially they were not welcome in hospitals. In fact, for three decades Mary Breckinridge's small hospital in Kentucky was the only hospital where midwives attended births (Stone, 2000).

Nurse-midwives made inroads into hospital practice during the post-war Baby Boom, when physicians could not cover the explosion of births. Gradually hospitals allowed nurse-midwives to expand their scope of practice to include anesthesia and analgesia, IV solutions, and episiotomy repair. By the mid-1960s, nurse-midwives were managing the contraceptive needs of patients, including IUD insertion (Stone, 2000).

The creation of Medicaid in 1965 had a tremendous impact on the development of nurse-midwifery. Medicaid pays a minimal set figure for medical services to the poor, and obstetricians generally were not interested in providing care for such low reimbursement. Special programs, largely staffed by midwives, sprang up to treat Medicaid-dependent women. In 1970, Title X funding became available for family planning, and nurse-midwives were frequently in charge of providing services.

A study conducted by ACOG in the 1960s showed that a majority of obstetricians still opposed nurse-midwifery. By 1970, childbirth occurred most often in the hospital, accompanied by pain-killing medications and technological innovations like fetal monitoring. Suddenly, social pressures for more-natural deliveries reached critical mass. Grantly Dick-Read's groundbreaking book *Childbirth without Fear: The Principles and Practices of Natural Childbirth* was published in the United States in 1944, and with it began the stirrings of the natural-childbirth movement. Robert Bradley's *Husband-Coached Childbirth* and Ferdinand Lamaze's techniques of psychoprophylaxis furthered American interest in working with natural processes rather than anesthetizing them out of existence (Rooks, 1997). In 1956, La Leche League formed in Chicago to encourage women to feed babies the healthful milk from their own breasts, a notion that had long been out of fashion. Just as large numbers of potential clients turned their attention to the concept of nurse-midwifery, the profession attracted criticism for becoming too medicalized and adopting the techniques of the physician (Rooks, 1997).

Nurse-midwives tended to view themselves as family-centered advocates for childbearing couples, and many were taken aback when Suzanne Arms said in her book *Immaculate Deception* (1975) that nurse-midwives had lost their patient-centered philosophy to the interventionism prevailing in hospitals. Couples sought alternatives to nurse-midwifery, and the often-illegal lay-midwife prospered. Out-of-hospital birth centers, first established in the 1940s and 1950s for poor families in rural areas, began to flourish elsewhere as a safe alternative to home delivery. By 1999, there were 160 freestanding birth centers nationwide.

Today in the United States, the practice of any individual CNM might fall anywhere on the continuum from noninterventionist to technology-reliant. Many deliver at home and in birth centers. The CNM is legal in all 50 states, and all states grant CNMs prescriptive authority. Only 4% of CNMs attend planned home births (Vedam, et al., 2007). ACNM also recognizes Certified Midwives (CMs), non-nurses with training similar to that of CNMs who pass the same examination as the CNM. Few states recognize this new designation.

Certified professional midwives (CPMs) are independent obstetrical practitioners educated in midwifery through self-study, apprenticeship, or direct-entry schooling and certified by the North American Registry of Midwives (NARM). Direct-entry midwifery education is evolving toward greater professional credibility through certification, licensure, and training programs that confer college degrees. CPMs are regulated on a state-by-state basis and deliver at home or in freestanding birth centers. Lay midwives or traditional midwives vary in experience, training, and competence. They are illegal in at least 10 states and unregulated in many others.

Midwifery and obstetrical medicine are complementary professions with overlapping but distinct purposes and knowledge. Philosophy remains a chief difference between midwives and doctors today. Whereas the midwife is trained to focus on holistically enhancing wellness and working optimally with natural processes, the doctor is generally taught to look for and treat pathology. Obstetrician training places emphasis on the things that can go wrong with a pregnancy and teaches doctors to be ever vigilant for them (Baldwin, 1999). Consequently, many obstetricians take control of the birthing process and manipulate it when it deviates from the expected course—a practice beneficial in high-risk pregnancies but often detrimental to low-risk women.

Midwives consider pregnancy a critical, vulnerable, but normal part of a woman's life (Rooks, 1999). They believe that a labor treated as normal tends to stay normal, and every intervention in the normal process is likely to engender more interventions. A midwife is more likely to employ gentle, natural ways of correcting a potential problem in the early stages. Research shows that midwifery practice reduces the incidence of low birth weight and infant and neonatal mortality, decreases cesarean birth rates, lowers rates for assisted vaginal births and epidural anesthesia, raises breastfeeding rates, and results in very high client satisfaction (Rosenblatt, et al., 1997; Payne & King, 2001).

The expertise and equipment available in the hospital do not increase safety in childbirth for low-risk women. The safety advantage of a hospital birth is the availability of technological interventions that can be used if complications should develop—decreasing the rate of complications for the high-risk mother and her infant. The safety advantage of home birth is noninterventionist watchful waiting and respecting the natural process of birthing—decreasing the risk of complications for the low-risk mother and her infant

Low-risk women have much to gain from birthing outside the hospital. As resources are strained by an aging population and insufficient numbers of health care providers, lower-acuity problems are best managed outside of the hospital. Women are usually more comfortable in their own homes surrounded by family. Hospitals harbor virulent strains of antibiotic-resistant drugs. If an influenza pandemic occurred, it would clearly be safer for healthy, immunologically vulnerable mothers to stay out of overtaxed hospitals and away from contagion.

Every state has its own laws on out-of-hospital births and who may attend. Research supports the safety of out-of-hospital birth for low-risk women. Growing evidence demonstrating the safety of home birth is likely to change the legal framework over time, state by state, eventually creating a home-birth-friendly climate in America.

The provision of obstetrical care is influenced by economics, politics, research, client preferences, malpractice issues, credentialing policies in hospitals and within states, and the health professional career decisions of students (Rosenblatt, et al., 1997). Midwifery care should be considered mainstream health care and not an alternative (Baldwin, 1999). Despite the growing popularity of midwifery, the American public has

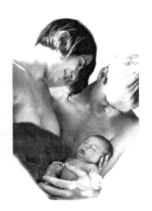

Figure 121. Family-centered practice. The holistic focus of the midwife's practice emphasizes wellness, education, communication, empowerment, and seeing each woman in the context of her life activities, relationships, and value system.

little idea of what the midwife does and the advantages that midwifery care provides (Payne & King, 2001). Public education is needed to show the lay public that for low risk women, midwives can be as safe as physicians and out-of-hospital births can be safer than the hospital.

In an ideal future, we might see more collaboration between obstetricians and midwives, giving women the benefits of both specialties. In a true collaborative practice, midwife and physician work together, share ideas, and develop strategies of care that work for the individual woman. There will be growth in out-of-hospital birthing options. Midwifery care will become the model of low-risk women's health care while physician remains the model for more complicated cases. Collaborative practice not only allows midwife and physician to capture a far greater share of the market together than could have been captured independently, but it also provides the greatest benefit to the consumer (Stapleton, 1998; Payne & King, 2001).

Clearly there is potential for significant increase in the out-of-hospital birthrate in America. An obstetrical crisis impacts not one person, but many. Women seek obstetrical providers who are experienced and educated. Home births are safe only if the provider is well trained in recognizing and managing emergencies.

The growth of the midwifery profession is in the hands of physicians, legislators, managed-care organizations, the public at large, and the midwives themselves. America's women stand to benefit through safety, cost reduction, and satisfaction.

BIBLIOGRAPHY

American College of Nurse Midwives. (2002). *About the American College of Nurse-Midwives*. Retrieved December 7, 2002, from http://www.midwife.org/about

American College of Nurse Midwives & American College of Obstetricians and Gynecologists. (2002). *Joint statement of practice relations between obstetrician-gynecologists and certified nurse-midwives/certified midwives*. Retrieved December 7, 2002, from http://www.midwife.org/prof/ display. cfm?id=274

American College of Obstetricians and Gynecologists. (2001). *History of the American College of Obstetricians and Gynecologists*. Washington, DC: Author.

American College of Obstetricians and Gynecologists. (2002a). *The American College of Obstetricians and Gynecologists: Celebrating 50 years of improving women's health*. Retrieved December 6, 2002, from http://www.acog.org/ from_home/acoghistory.cfm

American College of Obstetricians and Gynecologists. (2002b). *The American College of Obstetricians and Gynecologists*. Retrieved December 6, 2002, from http://www.acog.org/from_home/acoginfo.cfm

Arms, S. (1975). *Immaculate deception: A new look at women and childbirth*. New York: Houghton Mifflin.

Avery, M.D., & Burst, H.V. (2000). The evolution of the core competencies for basic midwifery practice. *Journal of Midwifery and Women's Health, 45* (6), 532–536.

Baldwin, K.A. (1999) The midwifery solution to contemporary problems in obstetrics. *Journal of Nurse-Midwifery 44* (1), 75–79.

Baldwin, L.M., Raine, T., Jenkins, L.D, Hart, L.G., & Rosenblatt, R. (1994). Do providers adhere to ACOG standards? The case of prenatal care. *Obstetrics and Gynecology, 84* (4), 549–556.

Bell, K.E., & Mills, J.I. (1989). Certified nurse midwife effectiveness in the health maintenance organization obstetric team. *Obstetrics and Gynecology, 74*(1), 112–116.

Breckinridge, M. (1952). *Wide neighborhoods*. Lexington: University Press of Kentucky.

Burst, H.V. (1980). The American College of Nurse Midwives: A professional organization. *Journal of Nurse-Midwifery, 25*(1), 4–6.

Dammann, N. (1982). *A social history of the Frontier Nursing Service*. Sun City, AZ: Social Change Press.

Dawley, K. (2000). The campaign to eliminate the midwife. *American Journal of Nursing, 100* (10), 50–56.

DeVries, R. (1996). *Making midwives legal: Childbirth, medicine and the law* (2nd ed.). Columbus: Ohio State University Press.

Dick-Read, G. (1944). *Childbirth without fear: The principles and practices of natural childbirth*. New York: Harper.

DiLeo, G.M. (1996). *The Dirty Secret of the Doctors Chamberlen*. Retrieved December 7, 2002, from http://www.babyzone.com/dileo/forceps.asp

Ehrenreich, B., & English, D. (1973). *Witches, midwives and healers : A history of women healers*. Old Westbury, NY: The Feminist Press.

Gould, S.J. (2002). Carrie Buck's daughter: A popular, quasi-scientific idea can be a powerful tool for injustice. *Natural History, 111*(6), 12–17.

Harer, W.B., Jr. (2001). A look back at women's health and ACOG, a look forward to the challenges of the future. *Obstetrics and Gynecology, 97* (1), 1–4.

Lay, M.M. (2000). *The rhetoric of midwifery: Gender, knowledge, and power*. New Brunswick, NJ: Rutgers University Press.

Litoff, J. (1986). *The American midwife debate: A sourcebook on its modern origins*. Westport, CT: Greenwood Press.

Litoff, J.B. (1982). The midwife throughout history. *Journal of Nurse-Midwifery, 27*(6), 3–11.

McGregor, D.K. (1998). *From midwives to medicine: The birth of American gynecology*. New Brunswick, NJ: Rutgers University Press.

Payne, P.A., & King, V.J. (2001). What can midwives teach family physicians? *Clinics in Family Practice, 3*(2), 349–364.

Rooks, J.P. (1990). Nurse-midwifery: The window is wide open. *American Journal of Nursing, 90*(12), 30–36.

Rooks, J.P. (1997). *Midwifery and childbirth in America*. Philadelphia: Temple University Press.

Rooks, J.P. (1999). The midwifery model of care. *Journal of Nurse-Midwifery, 44*(4), 370–374.

Rosenblatt, R.A., Dobie, S.A., Hart, L.G., Schneeweiss, R., Gould, D., Raine, T.R., et al. (1997). Interspecialty differences in the obstetric care of low-risk women. *American Journal of Public Health*, 87(3), 344–351.

Roush, R.E. (1979). The development of midwifery—male and female, yesterday and today. *Journal of Nurse-Midwifery 24* (3), 27–37.

Scoggin, J. (1997). The historical relationship of nurse-midwifery with medicine. *Journal of Nurse-Midwifery 42* (1), 49–52.

Stern, C. (1972). Midwives, male midwives, and nurse-midwives. *Obstetrics and Gynecology 39*, 308–311.

Stone, S.E. (2000). The evolving scope of nurse midwifery practice in the United States. *Journal of Midwifery and Women's Health 45* (6), 522–531.

Sullivan, N.H. (2000). CNMs /CMs as primary care providers, scope of practice issues. *Journal Of Midwifery and Women's Health, 45* (6), 450–456.

Tom, S.A. (1982). The evolution of nurse-midwifery, 1900–1960. *Journal of Nurse-Midwifery, 27* (4), 4–13.

Vedam, S., Goff, M., & Nolan-Marnin, V. (2007). Closing the theory–practice gap: Intrapartum midwifery management of planned homebirths. *Journal of Midwifery and Women's Health, 52*(3), 291–300.

Index

breathing 41–45, 262–265, 267–268
  difficulty in 125

breech presentation
  complete 226
  undiagnosed—OOH management 235
  delivering 234
  footling 225, 226, 228, 234
  frank 226

brow presentation 219-;220

C

carbon monoxide poisoning 139

carboxyhemoglobin 140, 141

cardiac arrest 177–180

cerclage 189

cervical incompetence 189

changes in consciousness
  Glasgow Coma Scale 136
  states of consciousness 137
  symptoms 135

chlamydia 120, 187, 192

cholecystitis 120–121

cholelithiasis 120–121

chorioamnionitis 118–120, 173, 192–195

clavicular fracture
  use in resolving shoulder dystocia 246

coagulopathy 96, 104

coma
  Glasgow Coma Scale 136

compensated shock (pre-shock, "warm shock") 170

complete breech presentation 226

complete placenta previa 78

compound presentation 220–221

conditions requiring immediate transport 28

controlled cord traction 98

cord prolapse 236–238

costovertebral angle 115, 174

critical thinking

  in diagnosis 19
  in obstetrical emergencies 17

culdocentesis 66, 70

cyanosis, 45, 265–267

cyst, ovarian 117

D

DAMIT (mnemonic) 101

danger signs in pregnancy 48

decelerations 258–260

decision-making conflicts 27
  accountability 29
  communication in an emergency 30
  second birth attendant 29

deflexion 218–119

diabetes 57, 138, 239, 263
  gestational 205
  clinical clues 170

difficulty breathing 113

dilation and curettage 59, 176

disseminated intravascular coagulation 82, 96, 104, 109, 175

dizygotic twins 204

documentation for shoulder dystocia 247

dyspnea125–132, 140, 177, 279

E

early decelerations 258

eclampsia, 141-144, 157–160

ectopic pregnancy, 53–56, 64–66, 68–70, 72–75

edema, 130
  pulmonary 129, 130, 152, 172, 173, 188

embolism 127, 173, 180
  amniotic fluid 109, 172
  pulmonary 125–128

end-organ dysfunction 171

endometritis 119, 174, 192

endotracheal suctioning 277

W

Z

About the Author

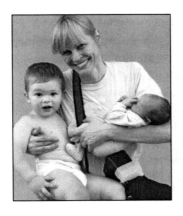

Bonnie U. Gruenberg with friends Aiden and Conor Fenton. These boys were the product of high-risk pregnancies involving Rh isoimmunization, prematurity, occiput posterior presentation, severe postpartum hemorrhage, retained placental fragments, and neonatal pulmonary hemorrhage. Despite their precarious beginnings, both are healthy and thriving.

Bonnie Urquhart Gruenberg is a certified nurse-midwife and women's health nurse practitioner with a master's degree from the University of Pennsylvania. She has held a Connecticut paramedic license since 1991 and has served as an EMT, as an urban paramedic, and as a maternity nurse in two tertiary-care hospitals. Her midwifery training included extensive experience with a busy home-birth practice in Lancaster County, PA, the heart of Amish country. She works as a CNM at a bustling practice in central Pennsylvania, managing the care of ethnically diverse, often high-risk pregnant women.

Bonnie has been published on a wide range of topics in professional journals and elsewhere. Her most recent book, *Essentials of Prehospital Maternity Care* (Prentice Hall, 2005), is the only substantial work for EMS personnel that is dedicated to the management of obstetrical emergencies. In 2002, Eclipse Press published *Hoofprints in the Sand: Wild Horses of the Atlantic Coast*, a hardcover book featuring her text and photographs. She also is a prizewinning artist and photographer who specializes in horses and infants.

She lives in Duncannon, PA, with her husband, Alex. She has two grown sons, Keith and Mark Bryan Scianna, and an amazing Connemara gelding named Fancy, also known as The Pone.

Essentials of Prehospital Maternity Care

Prentice Hall, 2006

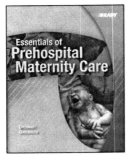

More than half the people encountered by emergency medical services are female, yet formal training for first responders often omits key obstetric and gynecologic issues. *Essentials of Prehospital Maternity Care* is not only the first major-length work for EMTs and paramedics devoted to obstetrical and gynecological emergencies. It also combines generally accepted practices of EMS with the holistic, patient-centered principles of midwifery. The text is rich with current information and results of the latest research. Although this book is designed for classroom instruction, the relaxed style, clear descriptions, and artful illustrations rivet the attention of independent students at any level of expertise.

Paperback • 464 pages • 9.1 x 7 x 1 in
ISBN-10: 0131199900 • ISBN-13: 978-0131199903 • $28.00

Available from the publisher, at bookstores, and online.

Hoofprints in the Sand
Wild Horses of the Atlantic Coast
Eclipse Press, 2002

The herds of feral horses inhabiting the barrier islands of Maryland, Virginia, North Carolina, and Georgia are in crisis. Despite a harsh environment and pressures exerted by encroaching humanity, these horses have clung to their scattered ranges for hundreds 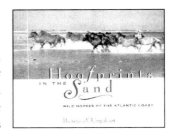 of years. Now they must compete with native species for dwindling resources and with vacationers and developers for shrinking space. Their geographic range and genetic diversity have declined. They are caught up in controversy, passion, and misunderstanding—are they ancient or modern, wildlife or pests, treasure or trouble? *Hoofprints in the Sand: Wild Horses of the Atlantic Coast* combines thoughtful text and solid information with arresting images by the author. This book explores not only the history and genetics of these horses, but also what these horses signify and what they tell us about ourselves. The result is a vivid portrait of threatened animals and the changing islands that are their home.

Hardcover • 224 pp. • 10.9 x 8.3 x 0.7 in
ISBN-10: 1581500742 • ISBN-13: 978-1581500745 • $24.95

Out of print, but still available at bookstores and online.

The BEST Deal

from Birth Muse Press

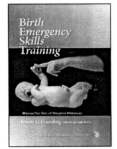

Birth Emergency Skills Training

The last word on managing obstetrical emergencies for out-of-hospital midwives. With 121 illustrations; 33 tables; abundant references; and a wealth of mnemonics, reminders, tips, and points to consider.

Paperback • 310 pages • 10 x 7 x 0.7 in
ISBN 10: 0-9790020-0-1 • ISBN 13: 978-0-9790020-0-7
$36.00

the BOOK

— **Buy the *BEST* book and CD, get *The Midwife's Journal* FREE!** —

BEST CD-ROM

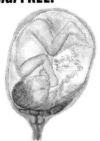

The full text of the book—plus COLOR illustrations— in two widely supported e-book formats: untagged PDF (for viewing and printing with desktop or notebook computers) and Microsoft Reader (for viewing on computers or hand-held devices). **EXTRA CONTENT:** many informative PowerPoint presentations used in the BEST course.

Compatible with recent versions of Windows and Mac OS
ISBN 10: 0-9790020-1-X • ISBN 13: 978-0-9790020-1-4 • **$55.00**

the CD

The Midwife's Journal: Birth Log and Memory Book

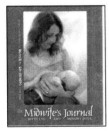

Contains provisions for recording 100 vaginal births and 20 cesareans, a section for addresses and telephone numbers, a variety of useful tables and charts, and plenty of space for notes and anecdotes. Designed to endure years of heavy use.

Hardbound • 96 pages • 11 x 8.5 x 0.7 in
ISBN 10: 0-9790020-0-1 • ISBN 13: 978-0-9790020-2-1 • **$18.99**

NEW!

Order online at **www.birthmusepress.com** or detach (or photocopy) this form.

Name _____

Address _____

Phone _____ E-mail _____

_____ *BEST* books @ $36.00 .... $ _____

_____ *BEST* CDs @ $55.00 .... $ _____

_____ *Midwife's Journals* @ $18.99 .... $ _____

Shipping in continental USA: $5.00 for first book, $2.50 per book thereafter. E-mail **info@birthmusepress.com** for other rates. ⇨

Shipping .... $ _____

PA residents, please add 6% sales tax. ... $ _____

Total *(check or money order only)* .... $ _____

Birth Muse Press
17 Pinetree Drive
Duncannon, PA 17020

☐ Free *Midwife's Journal*
(with purchase of *BEST* book and CD)

Created with Adobe® InDesign®
using **Minion Pro**, **Myriad Pro**, and
various dingbat fonts.

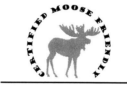

*No moose were harmed
during production of
this book.*

Birth Muse Press
Duncannon, PA
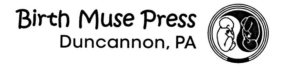

CPSIA information can be obtained at www.ICGtesting.com
Printed in the USA
BVOW01s0219020215

385970BV00005B/86/P